AFTER-DINNER MINTS, SOFT DRINKS, COFFEE . . . HEALING HERBS? YOU BET.

DRAMAMINE SUBSTITUTE—The most effective antinausea herb is a snap to take. Find out how to use this common ingredient in cookies and soft drinks for motion sickness (and it lasts 57% longer than Dramamine). Page 271.

TAGAMET RIVAL—Mainstream medicine has recently proven that an herbal remedy can be as effective for intestinal ulcers as America's leading prescription drug. And it's not the least bit exotic or expensive—in fact, it was once a common penny candy. Page 342.

WEIGHT-LOSS MIRACLE—The oldest herbal remedy known is a mainstay in bronchial decongestants, but it's also one of the best ways to increase basal metabolic rate and burn up those calories! Page 230.

CLUSTER HEADACHE RELIEF—Rubbed inside the nostril and outside the nose, this common kitchen spice reduces pain for 75% of sufferers. And it works for other pain, too—muscle and joint aches, shingles, and diabetic foot pain. Page 437.

ANTIPERSPIRANT—The French call this herb "toute bonne" and Germans have put it in a commercial antiperspirant. Now you can smell sweeter—and sweat 50% less—without resorting to harsh aluminum salts. Page 467.

AND DON'T MISS HOW CHOCOLATE CAN BE
GOOD FOR YOU! (Page 176)

" . . . successfully bridges the practical with the scientific. The book is well organized, readable, and, most impor- tant, presents information accurately and ____ibly."
—Sheldon Saul He____ ____ ____ ____ ____ r of
Medicine, Universit____ ____ ____ ____ e Doctor's
Vitamin and Miner____ ____

The Bantam Library of *Prevention* Magazine Health Books

The Doctors Book of Home Remedies

The Doctors Book of Home Remedies II

The Doctors Book of Home Remedies for Children

High-Speed Healing

The *Prevention* Pain-Relief System

Women's Encyclopedia of Health & Emotional Healing

And ask your bookseller about these other Bantam Health and Nutrition Books

The Bantam Medical Dictionary

The Best Treatment

The Herb Book

Modern Prevention

The Pill Book

The Pill Book Guide to Children's Medications

The Pill Book Guide to Everything You Need to Know About Prozac

The Pill Book Guide to Safe Drug Use

Symptoms

The Vitamin Book

The
HEALING
HERBS

THE ULTIMATE GUIDE
to the Curative Power
of Nature's Medicines

by Michael Castleman

Medical Reviewer: Sheldon Saul Hendler, M.D., Ph.D.
Biochemist, Researcher, and Assistant Clinical
Professor at the University of California San Diego

BANTAM BOOKS
New York   Toronto   London   Sydney   Auckland

*This edition contains the complete text
of the original hardcover edition.*
NOT ONE WORD HAS BEEN OMITTED.

THE HEALING HERBS
*A Bantam Book/published by arrangement
with Rodale Press*

PUBLISHING HISTORY
*Rodale Press edition published 1991
Bantam edition/August 1995*

ISBN 0-553-56988-0

Published simultaneously in the United States and Canada

Bantam Books are published by Bantam Books, a division of Bantam
Doubleday Dell Publishing Group, Inc. Its trademark, consisting of the
words "Bantam Books" and the portrayal of a rooster, is Registered in
U.S. Patent and Trademark Office and in other countries. Marca
Registrada. Bantam Books, 1540 Broadway, New York, New York
10036.

PRINTED IN THE UNITED STATES OF AMERICA
OPM 0 9

NOTICE

The Healing Herbs is meant to increase your knowledge of the latest developments in the use of plants for medicinal purposes. Because everyone is different, a physician must diagnose conditions and supervise the use of healing herbs to treat individual health problems. Herbs and other natural remedies are not substitutes for professional medical care. We urge you to seek out the best medical resources available to help you make informed decisions.

To Melissa Joan Rubin
January 22, 1966–October 4, 1987

Balm—*Melissa officinalis*

Melissa causeth the mind and heart to become merry . . . and driveth away all troublesome cares and thoughts. . . .
Culpeper's Herbal, 1652

CONTENTS

ACKNOWLEDGMENTS

At home: Anne Simons, M.D., Jeffrey and Maya Castleman.

At Rodale Press: Alice Feinstein, Debora Tkac, William Gottlieb, and Sharon Faelten.

At John Brockman and Associates: Katinka Matson and John Brockman.

And: Paul Bergner, editor, *Medical Herbalism*; Mark Blumenthal, executive director, American Botanical Council, and editor, *HerbalGram*; Wade Boyle, N.D., historian, author; Maureen Buehrle, executive director, International Herb Growers and Marketers Association; Lyle E. Craker, Ph.D., editor, *Herb, Spice, and Medicinal Plant Digest*; Ara der Marderosian, Ph.D., pharmacognosist, author; James A. Duke, Ph.D., herbalist, author, U.S. Department of Agriculture Research Service; Eclectic Medical Publications; Peter Finkle, research director, Yerba Prima; Steven Foster, herbalist, author; H. Winter Griffith, M.D., author; Sheldon Saul Hendler, M.D., Ph.D., author; Christopher Hobbs, herbalist, author; *Lawrence Review of Natural Products*; Albert Y. Leung, Ph.D., pharmacognosist, author; Lawrence Liberti, M.S., pharmacognosist, author; Lloyd Library; Robert McCaleb, president, Herb Research Foundation; Daniel Mowrey, Ph.D., herbalist, author; Michael Murray, N.D., herbalist, author; Paula Oliver, herb grower, author; Jeanne Rose, herbalist, author; Lynda Sadler, research director, Traditional Medicinals; Linda Sparrowe, editor, *The Herb Quarterly*; Varro E. Tyler, Ph.D., pharmacognosist, author; Susun Weed, herbalist, author; Michael Weiner, Ph.D., herbalist, author; Rudolph Fritz Weiss, M.D., herbal physician, author.

Ancient Remedies and Modern Medicine

T *he Healing Herbs* provides the information you need to use the earth's wonderful bounty of medicinal plants confidently, effectively, and above all, safely. It examines 100 herbs used in traditional healing, traces their history, folklore, and medicinal use, and summarizes the latest scientific research on their many benefits (and in some cases, their potential hazards).

The World Health Organization estimates that healing herbs are the primary medicines for two-thirds of the world's population—some four billion people. Herb critics concede herbal healing's leading role in Third World health care but say it's obsolete in today's high-technology, laboratory-based American medicine. That's hardly the case. Even in the United States, 25 percent of all prescriptions still contain active ingredients derived from plants, and the average physician writes eight herb-based prescriptions every day. Not only that, even the most vociferous herb critics use healing herbs all the time—usually without realizing it.

Coffee, Coke, and Clorets

When was the last time *you* used a healing herb? You may not realize it, but you use herbs that have medicinal properties all the time. We all do. Perhaps you started your day with a cup of coffee or tea. Coffee is not only America's favorite morning stimulant, but scientists have shown it's also an effective bronchial decongestant. Tea is less stimulating than coffee, but it has also been found to be an effective decongestant. And it's a good source of flouride, so it would help in preventing tooth decay.

Do you enjoy soft drinks? Most of today's carbonated beverages were originally herbal medicines. Thousands of years ago, the ancient Chinese drank ginger tea for indigestion, a use supported by modern science. During Elizabethan times, the English developed their own ginger-based stomach-soother, ginger beer, which evolved into today's ginger ale.

Coca-Cola began as an attempt to develop an herbal headache remedy. Coke was invented in the 1880s by an Atlanta pharmacist who stocked the tropical kola nut because 19th-century physicians prescribed it to treat respiratory ailments. Not too long ago, an article in the *Journal of the American Medical Association* suggested giving cola drinks to children with asthma as preventive medication.

The last time you dined out, did your plate come with a sprig of parsley? Parsley garnishes are another echo of herbal healing. People used to munch this herb to freshen their breath after meals. Parsley is high in the breath-sweetening plant pigment chlorophyll—the *Clor* in Clorets breath mints and one of the active ingredients in Certs.

And speaking of restaurants, perhaps your last check arrived with an after-dinner mint. These candies harken back to ancient times, when people sipped mint tea after feasts to settle their stomachs, another traditional medicinal use supported by modern science.

The Source of Today's Drugs

America's medicine cabinets are filled with drugs. Did you know the very word *drug* links us to herbal healing? It comes from the early German *droge*, meaning to dry, as in drying herbs, the first step in processing herbs into medicines. But the link goes beyond word origins. Many drugs in home medicine cabinets have herbal roots.

Aspirin was originally created from two healing herbs, white willow bark and meadowsweet. In fact, meadowsweet's old scientific name, *Spirea*, gave us the *spirin* in aspirin.

For the congestion of colds, flu, or hay fever, millions of Americans reach for Sudafed. Its active ingredient, pseudoephedrine, was developed from the world's oldest healing herb, *ma huang*, which Chinese physicians have prescribed for 5,000 years to treat chest congestion.

Thousands of years ago, people noticed that several aromatic herbs helped treat tooth pain. We now know tooth decay and gum disease are caused by oral bacteria, and science has shown that the herbs traditionally used to treat dental ailments kill these germs. One antibacterial herb is peppermint, which is why peppermint oil (menthol) is an ingredient in many toothpastes. An active component of thyme—thymol—is an ingredient in Listerine.

Constipation is one of America's most common health complaints, and most laxatives are herbal products. Metamucil is almost entirely psyllium seed. Cascara sagrada is the active ingredient in Stimulax, Comfolax, and Cas Evac. And Movicol owes its laxative action to buckthorn.

If there are children in your home, chances are there's a cherry-flavored cough syrup in your medicine cabinet. The cherry flavor is no accident. The American Indians treated coughs with wild cherry bark, and we're still using it today.

A Blind Spot in Medical Training

British and European physicians often prescribe herbal medicines along with—or instead of—pharmaceuticals. Some American physicians support herbal healing, but most remain skeptical. Some are downright hostile. Why?

The answer has to do with a major blind spot in American medical training. Medical schools ignore the history of healing, so most physicians have no idea that until this century, most medicines were herbal. And pharmacology professors rarely mention that a large percentage of U.S. prescription medications are still derived from plants.

From time to time, a leading medical journal reports an herb's effectiveness. For example, a recent report in the *Journal of the National Cancer Institute* suggests that garlic prevents stomach cancer. But most herb studies are published in obscure journals (many in German), publications the typical physician never sees. As a result, most American doctors are unfamiliar with the vast scientific literature demonstrating herbs' safety and effectiveness for an enormous number of ills.

The sad fact is, the typical American physician's only real exposure to herbal healing involves the small but steady stream of medical journal articles reporting harm from the irresponsible use of healing herbs. The number of people harmed by herbs is only a tiny fraction of the number harmed by pharmaceuticals and accepted medical procedures. Nonetheless, the majority of what physicians know about herbs is decidedly negative, so it's no wonder they feel skeptical of herbal healing.

Fortunately, this situation is changing as herb studies make their way into more prestigious journals. Headache specialists now recommend feverfew to prevent migraines because several well-publicized studies have shown its effectiveness. Many physicians now suggest ginger to prevent motion sickness and the nausea associated with cancer chemotherapy because a study published in the respected British medical journal *Lancet* shows that it prevents nausea better than a standard treatment, Dramamine. Many cardiologists now recommend a diet high in garlic, based on studies showing it to be remarkably effective in reducing cholesterol and other risk factors for heart disease.

Surgeons routinely spur the healing of surgical incisions with preparations containing a chemical (allantoin) extracted from comfrey. And some gastroenterologists now recommend a slightly modified form of licorice for ulcers, based on studies showing it to be about as effective as the standard treatment, Tagamet. Healing herbs even play a role in cancer chemotherapy. Two substances, vincristine and vinblastine, extracted from the Madagascar periwinkle are now used to treat childhood leukemia and Hodgkin's disease.

Scientists are taking a new look at a whole gamut of ancient healing remedies. And in the process, they are taking the guesswork and the hocus-pocus out of using Nature's medicines. It is now easier—and safer—than ever to take advantage of the healing power of herbs.

How to Use This Book

On the other hand, some people become so enamored of herbal healing that they reject mainstream medicine entirely. This is a serious mistake. Herbal healing can make an important contribution to human well-being, but it also has its limits. Responsible herbalists should consult physicians and use pharmaceuticals appropriately. In general, if a minor ailment does not respond to herbal self-treatment within two weeks, consult a physician.

For some conditions, all you need is an herbal remedy: aloe for minor burns, dill for infant colic, or clove oil for fast, temporary toothache relief.

Of course, many conditions require professional care—for example, high blood pressure, diabetes, heart disease, and congestive heart failure. But healing herbs can still play an important role in your overall treatment plan as complements to standard therapies and in consultation with your physician.

Before you start using healing herbs:

- Read chapter 2 to gain a basic understanding of herbal safety issues. All the herbs discussed in *The Healing Herbs* can be used safely *if* they are used responsibly. However, when used improperly, some may cause harm.
- Before using any herb discussed in chapter 5, pay special attention to the sections titled "Rx and "The Safety Factor."
- Before you ingest any healing herb, read chapters 3 and 4 to make sure you understand how to obtain and prepare it. For example, an infusion is not tea.
- If you'd like to use herbs for any condition requiring professional treatment, take *The Healing Herbs* with you the next time you consult your physician. The references list near the end of the book outlines the scientific sources for the information on each herb.

PART ONE

There is nothing in the most advanced contemporary medicine whose embryo cannot be found in the medicine of the past.

Maximilien E. P. Littré

Chapter 1

From Magic to Medicine: 5,000 Years of Herbal Healing

The healing properties of plants have not changed. What was a healing herb a thousand years ago is still a healing herb. Physicians of the ancient world were expected to know their herbs. Plants gave healing powers to those who studied them, worked with them, and respected them. In many lands and in many times, healers spent a good part of their lives in field and forest gathering green medicines. They remembered what they learned, and they passed it on.

Today we benefit from the accumulated herbal wisdom of the ages.

Our special vantage point enables us to peer back through history, harvesting for our own benefit only those herbs that have stood the test of time. But even the herbal uses that didn't pan out are fascinating. While the story of the healing herbs has its comic episodes, it's also a dramatic story of human sacrifice, complete with medical heroes—men and women whose work deserves to be recognized.

Before jumping into our story, however, we need to answer one question. What *is* a healing herb? The word *herb* comes from the Latin for grass. Technically, herbs are plants that wither each autumn, plants other than shrubs or trees. But many shrubs and trees are used in herbal healing, such as barberry, bay laurel, and slippery elm, for example. To an herbalist, "healing herbs" include *every* plant with medicinal value.

8

Animal Attractions

The plants that we know as healing herbs existed long before the first human appeared on earth. No one knows how long it took for humans to discover the curative power of plants, but prehistoric sites in Iraq show the Neanderthals used yarrow, marsh mallow, and other healing herbs some 60,000 years ago.

Prehistoric humans no doubt noticed that when animals appeared ill, they would often eat plants they ordinarily ignored. Our ancestors sampled these plants, and in many cases noticed curious effects: wakefulness, sleepiness, laxative action, increased urination, etc. The herbs that caused these effects were incorporated into prehistoric shamanism, and later into medicine.

Observing animal behavior continues to point humanity to healing herbs today. Recently, naturalists at Tanzania's Gombe National Park noticed sick chimpanzees swallowing leaves from a bush called Aspilia. Subsequently, scientists discovered that Aspilia leaves contain a powerful antibiotic (thiarubrine-A).

Aromatic Magic

Early humans were also attracted to healing herbs' aromas. They rubbed strong-smelling herbs on their bodies to repel insects and hide their human scent from animals they feared or hunted. They also adorned themselves with sweet-smelling herbs to please their mates.

But foul odors, not fragrant ones, were key to the development of herbal healing. Early humans used such plants as rosemary, thyme, dill, and virtually all of today's culinary spices to mask the stench of rotting meats. Today we use culinary herbs and spices only as flavor enhancers. But to our prehistoric ancestors, flavor was incidental to food preservation.

Prehistoric humanity had no refrigeration, and meats spoiled quickly. Spoilage destroyed precious food reserves, and early humans learned through painful experience that eating rotten meats causes illness and sometimes death. No doubt, some prehistoric hunter or homemaker accidentally lay some rotting meat on a bed of wild mint, sage, basil, or other aromatic herb, hoping its fragrance would mask the meat's malodorousness. It did, and amazingly, the meat didn't spoil as quickly.

Herbal School of Hard Knocks

Our ancestors also discovered many healing herbs simply by trial and error. They learned the hard way that some plants heal while others harm. They had little control over their world or their bodies. Their average life expectancy was barely 30 years. Because life was so full of threatening, often fatal, surprises, *anything* that made life more predictable acquired an aura of magic and healing.

Major herbal effects, such as vomiting or hallucinations, made big impressions, but prehistoric humans also recognized many herbs' more subtle healing benefits. We'll never know what possessed some ancient Chinese peasant to brew a tea from the small, ungainly stalks of *ma huang* (ephedra). But 5,000 years ago, someone did and stumbled upon the world's oldest medicine, a decongestant. (Pseudoephedrine, a laboratory analog of ephedra, is still widely used in cold formulas today.) Similarly, we'll never know how many roots the ancient Indians dug up before they discovered ginger more than 4,000 years ago. Or why the American Indians had a hunch that black cohosh might induce labor. But all over the world, ancient peoples dug, dried, chewed, pounded, rubbed, and brewed the plants around them, and through trial and error, they discovered the vast majority of healing herbs we still use today.

Isolated Cultures, Similar Herbs

Herbal trial and error becomes even more remarkable when we consider that cultures separated by thousands of miles arrived at similar uses for many healing herbs, apparently independently.

Herbal healing includes four major traditions: Chinese, Ayurvedic (in India), European (including Egyptian), and American Indian. Until the 15th century, Old World cultures were isolated from the Americas. Nonetheless, Old and New World herbalists used many herbs similarly.

Angelica and licorice. Asians, Europeans, and Native Americans all used these herbs to treat respiratory ailments.

Hop and the mints. All the ancient herbal traditions used these herbs as stomach soothers.

Blackberry and raspberry. These two popular herbs have been used around the world to treat diarrhea.

Uva ursi. Asians, Europeans, and Native Americans all discovered this herb's diuretic properties.

White willow. All the herbal traditions used this herb to treat pain and inflammations.

During the 19th century, chemists used this "herbal convergence" to point them to the plants that provided extracts for the first pharmaceuticals. According to a report published in the journal *Science*, of the 121 prescription drugs derived from higher plants, about 74 percent came to drug companies' attention because of their use in traditional herbal healing.

Homage to the "Wise Women"

Most medical histories chronicle great discoveries by great men, from Hippocrates, the father of medicine, to Alexander Fleming, who discovered penicillin. Their contributions should not be underestimated, but from ancient times down to the present day, a relatively small number of male physicians have made the great discoveries and ministered to the kings and princes, while an enormous number of women herbalists have taken care of everyone else.

Women healers have gone by many names: midwives, wise women, green women, witches, old wives, and nurses.

Most physicians have never taken women's folk healing very seriously, and scientists often dismiss folk wisdom as "old wives' tales."

But the fact is, medically untrained women still provide most of the world's primary care. Even in the United States, most people view physicians as the health-care choice of last resort. The medical profession promotes the idea that family doctors are our "primary providers," but studies show that before people call health professionals, *about* 90 *percent* consult a friend or family member, and those "health advisers" are overwhelmingly women.

Not only that, women have always been the primary consumers of health care. Today women account for an estimated two-thirds of all physician visits and three-quarters of all prescriptions. It's no coincidence many herbs were used historically to calm the womb, trigger menstruation, induce abortion, promote or dry up mothers' milk, and treat infant colic and infectious diarrhea (still a leading cause of infant death in the Third World). These were the daily concerns women patients brought to their women healers.

Sometimes medically unschooled women herbalists introduced university-trained physicians to powerful medicines. For example, a woman folk healer introduced a British physician to foxglove for congestive heart failure. Foxglove contains the heart drug digitalis. But by and large, physicians looked down on folk healers as ignorant practitioners of inferior medicine, much the way most doctors view herbal healing today. The fact is, women herbalists have played a key—and largely undocumented—role in medical history. Just as herbs are the forgotten sources of many medicines we use today, the "wise women" represent the forgotten healers whose thousands of years of collective experience taught us how to use them.

Judging by the number of herbs used primarily to treat women, these unsung healers apparently helped create all four of the great herbal traditions. Nevertheless few women are ever mentioned by name in the written history of herbs.

Shen Nung and *The Classic of Herbs*

The origins of Chinese herbalism are lost in the mists of time, but legend has it that around 3400 B.C., mythological emperor/sage Shen Nung invented agriculture and discovered that many plants have medicinal value. He tested herbs on himself, recorded their effects, and died after consuming too much of one that was poisonous.

Chinese herbalists credit Shen Nung as author of China's first great herbal, the *Pen Tsao Ching* (*The Classic of Herbs*), which listed 237 herbal prescriptions using dozens of herbs, including ephedra, rhubarb, and opium poppy. Succeeding emperors ordered new herbals, each more elaborate than the last. In 1590, Li Shih-Chen published his landmark 52-volume *Pen Tsao Kang Mu* (*The Catalogue of Medicinal Herbs*), listing 1,094 medicinal plants and an astounding 11,000 herbal formulas.

Starting in the mid-19th century, European colonialists introduced Western medicine into China and dismissed traditional Chinese herbalism and acupuncture as nonsense. The Chinese felt the same way about the "foreign devils'" medicine, and the two systems seemed irreconcilable.

Shortly after the establishment of the People's Republic in 1949, the Chinese government decided China's huge medically underserved population could benefit from the integration of Western and Chinese medicine. It hasn't been easy to combine these two systems, but 40 years into the process, considerable progress has been made. In China today, Western-trained physicians practice alongside traditional herbalists and acupuncturists. Chinese and Western physicians examine the same patients, confer with each other, and often coordinate their recommendations.

A turning point in American acceptance of Chinese medicine occurred in 1972, when President Nixon first visited China. Network news broadcast astonishing footage of a woman having abdominal surgery while fully conscious, her only anesthesia a few acupuncture needles in her earlobes and feet. Soon afterward, a *New York Times* columnist who'd accompanied Nixon used acupuncture successfully to control his pain after an appendectomy. His first-person account in the nation's most influential newspaper helped open the United States to acupuncture and Chinese herbalism.

Jivaka and the Vedas

India's herbal tradition is almost as old as China's. It, too, has its legendary heroes. Around the time of the Hebrew Exodus from Egypt in approximately 1200 B.C., a poor young Indian named Jivaka wanted to study medicine. As the story goes, he approached the great Punarvasu Atreya, founder of India's first medical school. Jivaka had no money, so he offered to become Atreya's servant in exchange for medical training. After seven years, he asked the great professor when his studies would be completed. Instead of answering, Atreya challenged him to search the countryside and collect all the plants he considered medically useless. Jivaka did not return for many days. When he finally appeared, he was sullen and empty-handed. He told his mentor he was unable to find a single plant without healing power. Professor Atreya replied, "Go! You now have the knowledge to be a physician."

Ancient Indians called their medicine *ayurveda*, from two Sanskrit words, *ayur*, "life," and *veda*, "knowledge." Ayurvedic medicine developed from the Vedas, India's four books of classic wisdom. The oldest, the 4,500-year-old Rig Veda, contains astonishingly detailed descriptions of eye surgery, limb amputation, and formulas for medicines using 67 healing herbs, including ginger, cinnamon, and senna.

One herb Ayurvedic healers introduced was *Rauwolfia serpentina*. This plant is the source of resperine, still used in Western medicine to manage high blood pressure.

After A.D. 600, Ayurvedic healing influenced Arab medicine, which combined Greco-Roman, Middle Eastern, and Asian therapies. Arab physicians in turn introduced some Ayurvedic practices into Europe.

During the 19th century, the British introduced Western medicine into India; however, an estimated 70 percent of Indians and Pakistanis still rely on Ayurvedic physicians and the healing herbs they prescribe.

The "Stinking Ones" of the Nile

Although a hint of Chinese and Indian herbal tradition reached Europe by way of the Arabs, Western herbalism owes far more to another ancient land—Egypt. In 1874 in the Valley of the Tombs near Luxor, the German Egyptologist Georg Ebers discovered the world's oldest surviving medical text, a 65-foot papyrus dating from around 1500 B.C. The *Ebers Papyrus* summarized more than 1,000 years of ancient Egyptian medicine and listed 876 herbal formulas made from more than 500 plants, including about one-third of the herbs in today's Western pharmacopoeia.

Some Ebers formulas strike the modern reader as bizarre—for example, a shampoo made from a dog's paw, decayed palm leaves, and a donkey hoof, all boiled in oil, then rubbed on the head. But others sound surprisingly contemporary—for example, the recommendation to bandage moldy bread over wounds to prevent infection. Modern antibiotics are derived from molds.

But the Egyptians' affection for fragrant herbs paled next to their obsession with two herbs many ancients considered foul-smelling, garlic and onion. The Egyptians believed garlic and onion strengthened the body and prevented disease (a view supported by modern science). They ate so much that the Greek historian Herodotus called them "the stinking ones." (Six cloves of garlic were found in the tomb of King Tut.)

By about 500 B.C., Egyptian herbalists were considered the finest in the Mediterranean, and the rulers from Rome to Babylon recruited them as court physicians. Aspiring physicians, including many from Rome and among them Galen, went to Egypt to study with the medical masters of the Nile. Thus, Egyptian herbal healing began to influence Western medicine.

European Herbal Healers (and Assassins)

The first truly medical botanist was Pedanius Dioscorides. Born in Turkey in A.D. 40, Dioscorides was Greek, but he served as a physician with the Roman legions of Emperor Nero. In A.D. 78, he published De Materia Medica (On Medicines), Europe's first real herbal. It discussed 600 plants, 90 of which are still used today.

De Materia Medica remained a standard medical reference for 1,500 years. And after the invention of printing in the 1450s, De Materia Medica was one of the first books published.

Roman herbalists were as likely to be killers as healers. The imperial court of the Roman Empire bubbled with intrigue as hostile factions plotted murder to gain political power. Among assassination methods—knifing, "accidents," and poisoning—the herbal approach was most popular. Death occurred some time after the deed, allowing for escape or alibi. And in an age before autopsy, when apparently healthy people often sickened and died suddenly, wily poisoners might escape unsuspected. As a result, rulers throughout the Roman Empire were obsessed with the identification of herbal poisons and the development of antidotes.

When Rome fell, the barbarians seized not only Rome's lands and wealth but also its vast stores of herbs and spices. During one attack, the barbarians demanded horses, money—and 3,000 pounds of black pepper.

Monasteries and Liqueurs

After the fall of Rome, European medicine was dominated by the Catholic Church, which officially viewed illness as punishment from God and treatable only by prayer and penance. Unofficially, however, Catholic monks preserved Greco-Roman herbalism by copying the ancient texts.

Among the monastic orders, the Benedictines were the most avid herbalists. They were the first Europeans to adopt the Arab practice of transferring herbs' healing powers to alcohol. They flavored wine with digestion-promoting herbs and created the forerunners of today's liqueurs, one of which still bears the order's name.

Charlemagne, emperor of the Holy Roman Empire, was so impressed by the Benedictines' herb gardens, he ordered all the monasteries in his vast realm to plant "physic gardens" to ensure an adequate supply of healing herbs. Charlemagne called herbs "friends of the physician and cook."

The most notable Benedictine herbalist was Hildegard of Bingen (1098–1179), abbess of the Rupertsburg Convent in the German Rhineland. A nun from age 15, Hildegard claimed visions of God commanded her to treat the sick and compile her herbal formulas. Her book, *Hildegard's Medicine*, combined mystical Catholicism and early German folk medicine with her own extensive experience using herbs.

Hildegard was unique. She wrote an original medical work at a time when the few Europeans who were literate, mostly monks, contented themselves with copying the Greeks and Romans. And she was the only medieval woman who left any account of "wise woman" healing practices. Some of Hildegard's advice sounds silly. For poor vision, she advocated rubbing the eyes with a topaz soaked in wine. But many of her recommendations were quite sensible. She advocated a balanced diet and tooth brushing with aloe and myrrh, both of which have antibacterial, decay-preventive properties.

Around the time the Benedictines invented liqueur, Germanic Angles and Saxons were settling England. They brought European herbalism with them and learned how the native Celts and their priests, the Druids, used healing herbs. Around A.D. 950, a nobleman named Bald persuaded England's King Alfred to commission the first British herbal. The book combined Anglo-Saxon and Celtic herbalism with Greco-Roman and Arab practices. Called the *Leech Book of Bald*, it discusses 500 plants, including vervain and mistletoe, both sacred to the Druids.

Wise Women: From Healers to Witches

Hildegard of Bingen was lucky she lived in the 11th century. If she'd practiced herbalism from 1300 to 1650, she probably would have been burned as a witch.

It's not clear what caused Europe's 350 years of witch-hunts. Feminists link them to the rise of secular medicine as a male-dominated profession. Others blame the witch-hunts on bubonic plague, the Black Death, which swept Europe in waves and killed half its population.

Whatever the cause, after 1300 the image of the folk herbalist changed from wise woman to witch. The witch-hunts started in Germany and eventually reached all of Europe. Accusations of "sexual intercourse with the Devil" were typically accompanied by testimony that the alleged witch practiced herbal medicine and made healing mixtures, cosmetics, love potions, aphrodisiacs, abortion-inducing preparations, and poisons.

Accusations of poisoning were particularly damning. It's quite possible that some women herbalists continued the Roman tradition of herbal assassination. But this was the era before the discovery of the "dose-response relationship,"—the idea that the greater the dose, the greater the effect. Many so-called witches' plants, poisonous in large amounts, cause no harm in therapeutic or cosmetic amounts.

The witch-hunts failed to eradicate women's herbalism, but they succeeded in driving it underground. More than a century after the last witch-hunts, the "old woman" who helped popularize foxglove—source of the heart drug digitalis—said it was a "secret family recipe." Her forebears had good reason to keep it secret.

Nicholas Culpeper: England's Herbal Robin Hood

With the invention of printing in the 1450s, herbals proliferated, especially in England.

Nicholas Culpeper was by far England's most influential

herbalist. His *Complete Herbal and English Physician*, first published in 1652, has been in print ever since in more than 100 editions, a record surpassed only by the Bible and the works of Shakespeare.

But Culpeper was—and still is—loathed as well as loved. His herbalist contemporary, William Coles, denounced him as "a man very ignorant in simples [herbal medicines]." And today, scientists scoff at Culpeper's devotion to astrology.

Egotistical and brash, Culpeper came of age during the English Civil War, which pitted King Charles I and the aristocracy against Oliver Cromwell and the Puritan Parliament. The Puritans won, abolished the monarchy, and executed Charles. Culpeper came from an aristocratic family, but he was a Puritan and fought for Cromwell. He took a musket ball in the chest, which left him in poor health the rest of his life and influenced his decision to study medicine.

As an aristocrat, Culpeper attended Cambridge, where he fell in love and planned to elope. But his fiancé was killed when lightning struck her carriage on her way to their secret rendezvous. Beside himself with grief, Culpeper left Cambridge and became an apothecary's apprentice, a major social step down for anyone who had attended Cambridge.

Culpeper was an anomaly. Cambridge trained, he could read Greek and Latin as well as the physicians, and he resented the snobbery of former classmates who looked down on apothecaries. Furthermore, as a Puritan, he was outraged that the monarchist College of Physicians ignored the medical needs of the largely Puritan lower classes. Culpeper's solution was to become England's medical Robin Hood.

In 1649, Culpeper translated the College of Physicians' Latin manual, the *Pharmacopoeia Londinensis*, into English, calling it *The London Dispensatory and Physical Directory*. It gave apothecaries and others illiterate in Latin their first look at the thousands of formulas that constituted the state of the art in 17th-century English medicine. Culpeper's audacity earned him the physicians' undying hatred. But apothecaries, midwives, and the common people lionized Culpeper for giving them access to professional medical information.

To make herbal medicine even more accessible, Culpeper

published his *Herbal* in 1652. It was revolutionary because it gave equal weight to the official herbalism of the ancient masters and the folk wisdom of England's "country people."

Contemporary critics usually dismiss Culpeper because of his devotion to astrology. Culpeper's real problem was that he rarely met an herb he didn't consider a panacea. He touted dozens of herbs "to heal all inward and outward hurts." He called about a third of the herbs in his *Herbal* sure cures for "the bites and stings of venomous creatures." And he promoted scores of herbs to "bring down women's courses" (promote menstruation).

Perhaps Culpeper can be forgiven his exaggerations. In the 1650s, very little was known about the body, and statements that seem gross misrepresentations today may not be all that farfetched. Physicians call most medical problems self-limiting, that is, if you wait long enough, they go away by themselves. Take almost any herb for "inward or outward hurts," and most do clear up—with or without all the herbs Culpeper recommended.

Unfortunately, Culpeper's promotion of any herb for every ill has haunted herbalism ever since. Several of today's best-selling herbals still tout Culpeper's exaggerations as Truth, with a capital T, providing easy targets for attacks from herb skeptics. Nicholas Culpeper was a seminal figure in botanical medicine, but his *Herbal* should be viewed as history, not as a reference for contemporary herbal healing.

Sickly Colonists, Robust Indians

The fourth great herbal tradition grew up on the distant shores of the New World. Europeans considered America's Indians "ignorant savages"—except when it came to health and healing. Explorers and colonists were all too familiar with the plagues, pestilence, and suffering back home. They marveled at the Indians' good health, physical stamina, and fine teeth. Not surprisingly, colonists became eager students of Indian herbal medicine.

Puritan Boston minister/physician Cotton Mather wrote that

Indian healers produced "many cures that are truly stupendous." And when John Wesley, founder of Methodism, visited America in the 1730s, he wrote the Indians had "exceedingly few" diseases, and their medicines were "quick and generally infallible." Later, even ardent Indian haters in the U.S. Army marveled at the effectiveness of Indian wound treatments. And many early American physicians touted their apprenticeship to Indian herbalists.

Of course, Indian healers also had their critics, mostly among the university-trained physicians. Philadelphia doctor Benjamin Rush, a signer of the Declaration of Independence, declared, "We have no discoveries in the materia medica . . . from the Indians. It would be a reproach to our schools of physic if modern physicians were not more successful than Indians."

How wrong Rush was. The Indians introduced white settlers to many valuable healing herbs: black and blue cohosh, black haw, boneset, cascara sagrada, echinacea, chaparral, goldenseal, lobelia, Oregon grape, sarsaparilla, slippery elm, wild cherry, and witch hazel.

Of course, American colonists grew both culinary and medicinal herbs in their "kitchen gardens." Thomas Jefferson was a typical herb grower. His 1,000-square-foot garden at Monticello contained 26 herbs.

Thomson's Botanic Medicine

Early America's leading herbalist was Samuel Thomson (1760–1843). Born in Alstead, New Hampshire, he studied with a midwife and Indian healers. Around 1800, his daughter became seriously ill. Unsure of his skills, Thomson called a physician, who pronounced her incurable. Then Thomson cured her with herbs and hot baths inspired by Indian sweat lodges. Soon after, he declared himself a "doctor."

Thomson detested the "regular" physicians of his day, who relied on bleeding, violent laxatives, and mercury. These treatments were called heroic medicine, but the only heroes were the patients. Consider the case of George Washington. One day in 1799, the elderly but otherwise healthy father of our country developed a sore throat with a fever and chills. Chances are he had strep throat or some other minor infection, which probably would have cleared up with rest, hot liquids, and herbal antibiotics such as garlic and onion. Instead, Washington's heroic physicians bled him of 4 pints of blood, leaving him anemic and weak, then gave him laxatives and mercury. He was dead within 24 hours.

Samuel Thomson developed a medical system based on herbs and hot baths, inspired by European herbalism and mineral baths and by Indian herbalism and sweat lodges. His favorite herb was lobelia or Indian tobacco, which in large amounts causes vomiting.

In 1809 Thomson was arrested for murder for allegedly administering a fatal dose of lobelia. He was acquitted due to lack of evidence that lobelia is poisonous. After Thomson's acquittal, New Hampshire's regular physicians still considered him a menace. They persuaded the New Hampshire legislature to forbid him by name from practicing medicine in the state. Thomson went national.

In 1839, at the height of his popularity, Thomson claimed three million adherents. This was probably an exaggeration, but there's no doubt Thomsonian herbalism was enormously popular. Thomson boasted that half of Ohio practiced his herbal healing. His critics said only one-third.

After Thomson's death in 1843, his medical system fell from fashion. Some practitioners, the naturopaths, continued the Thomsonian herb/bath tradition. One was Dr. John Kellogg of Battle Creek, Michigan, who invented the nation's first health food, the cornflake, and founded Kellogg's cereal company. But Thomsonian medicine was largely replaced by homeopathy and eclectic herbalism.

The Eclectics: America's Scientific Herbalists

Despite the "regular" physicians' reliance on bleeding, violent laxatives, and mercury, most 19th-century medicines were herbal. In 1820, two-thirds of the treatments in the U.S.

Pharmacopoeia were botanical. In 1880, the figure was almost three-quarters.

In the 1820s, a group of antiheroic practitioners—Thomsonians, Indian-trained herbalists, and disillusioned "regulars"—created the Reformed Medical Society to promote nonheroic, largely herbal healing. In 1830, the Society met in New York to found a Reformed medical school.

The Reformers were mostly easterners, but the East's cities were strongholds for what they called regular medicine. The Reformers decided to locate their school on the free-thinking western frontier, then located at the Mississippi River. Thomsonian medicine was popular in Ohio, so the Reformers established their school near Columbus. They adopted the term *eclectic* to describe their herb-based approach, which combined European, Asian, Indian, and slave herbalism.

In 1845 the Eclectics moved their Eclectic Medical Institute to Cincinnati. It was the nation's first medical school to admit women, many of whom were Thomsonian herbalists interested in more training. But in 1877, the Eclectics "yielded to the prejudices of the profession," according to Eclectic historian Henry Felter, and barred women.

The Eclectics were scientific herbalists. They experimented with herbs, analyzed them chemically, extracted their active constituents, published their findings in scientific journals, and were prominent in the early pharmaceutical industry.

The years 1880 to 1900 marked the heyday of Eclectic medicine. Its practitioners numbered about 8,000. But Eclectic popularity declined in the 20th century. The institute graduated its last class in 1939.

The Eclectic legacy lives on today in the herbal medicine programs at the nation's two naturopathic medical schools, the National College of Naturopathic Medicine in Portland, Oregon, and John Bastyr College in Seattle, Washington.

Hoxsey's Herbal Cancer Treatment

The period from 1920 through the 1960s might be called the Lost Decades of herbal healing. Medical schools ignored herbs.

Pharmaceutical drugs replaced herbal tinctures in the nation's pharmacies. Even many culinary herbs fell from popularity. But herbal healing didn't die. It simply reverted to what it had been for most of its history, folk medicine practiced by women and some men who grew and gathered their own herbs and prescribed them as the classic herbals recommended.

A few diehards continued to promote herbal healing. Dr. Benedict Lust, the father of modern naturopathy, came to the United States from Germany in 1895, opened the nation's first health food store, and established sanitariums in New Jersey and Florida based on healing baths and herbal medicines. His nephew, John Lust, wrote *The Herb Book*.

Jethro Kloss, a sanitarium manager and health food pioneer, published *Back to Eden* in 1939. Subtitled *A Story of the Health and Restoration to Be Found in Herb, Root, and Bark*, the book has been in print ever since.

But the most flamboyant and controversial herbalist of the mid-20th century was Harry Hoxsey, who loudly proclaimed that his herbal formula cured cancer. A former Appalachian coal miner, Hoxsey graduated from high school with a correspondence diploma and had no formal medical training. He attributed his Hoxsey Cancer Formula to his great-grandfather who had witnessed a cancer-stricken horse recover after eating various herbs. Hoxsey started prescribing the family formula in the 1930s, and by the 1950s, his Dallas clinic was the world's largest privately owned cancer center with branches in 17 states.

Hoxsey's claims outraged Texas medical authorities, and a Dallas prosecutor arrested him for fraud more than 100 times in the 1930s. The Hoxsey formula didn't work for everyone, but the prosecutor could not find any patients who felt defrauded, and Hoxsey presented hundreds who swore his formula had cured their cancers.

The Food and Drug Administration (FDA) eventually closed Hoxsey's clinics for violating federal drug-labeling regulations. His herbal ingredients were not approved as cancer treatments.

Ironically, Hoxsey died of prostate cancer. He took his formula, but it didn't work for him.

The Hoxsey formula is still available today at the Bio-Medical

Center in Tijuana, Mexico. Recent studies show that nine of its ten herbal ingredients have antitumor action: barberry, buckthorn, burdock, cascara sagrada, red clover, licorice, poke, prickly ash, and bloodroot.

The FDA Versus Healing Herbs

Patent medicines laced with alcohol, cocaine, and even heroin raised cries for national drug legislation, but *The Jungle*, Upton Sinclair's exposé of the meat-packing industry, finally convinced Congress to prohibit the adulteration or mislabeling of foods and drugs.

Congress established the FDA in 1928, but it had little authority. Then in 1937, a new antibiotic, Elixir of Sulfanilamide, killed 107 people because its liquid base was toxic. The following year, Congress passed the Food, Drug, and Cosmetic Act, which led to the first U.S. drug regulations. (Homeopathic medicines were specifically exempted because of lobbying by a homeopath who was a congressman at the time.)

In the late 1950s, a supposedly safe European sleep aid, Thalidomide, caused serious limb malformations in 8,000 children of women who took it while pregnant. The scandal led to more stringent FDA regulations that require drugs to be proven safe and effective before release. Unfortunately, the FDA ignored the vast majority of healing herbs, leaving them in regulatory limbo, and in effect prohibiting medicinal claims for them unless they survived the FDA approval process.

This process requires manufacturers of new drugs—or packagers of age-old herbs not "grandfathered in"—to file New Drug Applications (NDAs), which must include elaborate studies persuasively demonstrating the product's safety and effectiveness in strict laboratory and clinical trials. Such trials are extremely costly—an estimated $50 to $100 million per product.

Only the nation's pharmaceutical companies have the financial resources to run the FDA gauntlet. But there's a catch. Drug companies are not inclined to spend millions to prove the safety and effectiveness of a medicine anyone can go out and grow. They want exclusive rights to the drugs they invest in, which means they want to invest in unique chemicals they can patent.

Healing herbs cannot be patented. So drug company researchers isolate healing herbs' active constituents, tinker with them to make them chemically unique, and patent drugs developed from these "new" chemicals. As a result, few physicians and consumers have any idea that the chemicals in many of the pills and capsules they use have herbal roots.

Under current FDA regulations, the prohibition against unapproved medicinal claims includes *a ban on warnings about possible side effects*. In other words, it's illegal for herb packagers to list possible problems, even though such warnings are clearly in the public interest. As a result, most healing herbs are sold not as medicines but as food supplements, which do not require preapproval testing but which also allow no healing claims or warnings about potential risks. Ironically, by forbidding appropriate warnings, the FDA is violating its major mission: to protect the public health.

Other countries treat healing herbs differently. In Germany, medicinal herbs must be proven safe, but they need not pass the elaborate and costly effectiveness tests required for new pharmaceuticals. Except in cases where herbs' traditional healing uses have been proven false, the German government accepts traditional claims, requiring only cautionary labeling about potential side effects. As a result, hundreds of herbal products line German pharmacy shelves today, and mainstream German physicians are as likely to prescribe valerian-based sleep aids as pharmaceutical sleeping pills.

Canada may take similar steps. The Canadian government's Expert Advisory Committee on Herbs and Botanical Preparations has recommended a new class of drugs, "Folklore Medicines," which would be exempt from expensive effectiveness tests as long as they were shown to be pure, safe, and accurately labeled with warnings where appropriate.

U.S. herbalists, led by the American Botanical Council (ABC) of Austin, Texas, hope to persuade the FDA to create a Folklore Medicine drug category here. But as this book goes to press, ABC Executive Director Mark Blumenthal says the FDA has given no indication it intends to treat age-old herbs differently from new pharmaceuticals.

The Herb Renaissance

Starting in the late 1960s, many Americans began changing their attitudes about health and healing. They decided to invest their energy in preventing illness, rather than treating it after the fact. One step in that direction was a retreat from salt as the nation's main seasoning, because of research linking it to high blood pressure, heart disease, and stroke. Many Americans retired their saltshakers and rediscovered culinary herbs and spices. Here are just a few examples of the results.

Selected U.S. Herb Importation (tons)

Herb	1959	1986
Fennel	500,000	5,000,000
Oregano	467,000	12,000,000
Red pepper	5,000,000	14,000,000

Most herbs show similar enormous increases. Domestic production has also soared—everything from large-scale herb farming to the millions of Americans who grow a few herbs in their gardens or in pots on their kitchen windowsills.

Today, herbal products line the shelves in health food stores and supermarkets. Authorities estimate that retail sales of healing herbs, kitchen spices, herb books, herbal beverage teas, and herbal cosmetics and personal care products top $3 billion a year.

The herbal healing boom involves the convergence of many trends.

Increased interest in self-care. Mainstream medicine has produced miracles, but it has also grown expensive and impersonal. To save time, money, and limit their dependence on doctors, many Americans have turned to prevention and self-care. Healing herbs fit neatly into lifestyles focused on sound nutrition, fitness, and stress management.

Increased interest in alternative healing arts. Homeopathy, naturopathy, Chinese, and Ayurvedic medicine have become more popular in recent years. These healing arts use herbal medicines.

Reaction against high technology. The very wizardry of high technology creates a yearning for more down-to-earth approaches to human problems. When there's a choice, many Americans prefer healing herbs to the pharmaceuticals often derived from them.

Increased environmental consciousness. Pollution, industrial development, and the destruction of tropical rain forests are causing record numbers of plant extinctions. As a result, scientists are scrambling to preserve our plant heritage and screen new herbs as potential medicines. Several years ago, the Drug Research and Development Branch of the National Cancer Institute (NCI) launched an ambitious project to test plants for anti-cancer activity. NCI scientists have investigated 70,000 extracts from 7,500 species and have found 750 with antitumor effects. But much work remains. Of the estimated 250,000 plant species on earth, scientists estimate only about 15 percent have been screened for medicinal uses.

Increased global consciousness. A 1974 World Health Organization report concluded that adequate worldwide health care could not be achieved unless Third World nations were encouraged to nurture traditional herbal healing.

Looking Toward the Future

The herbal renaissance has had a profound effect on U.S. drug researchers, resulting in a surge in healing herb research. The most exciting possibilities involve herbal treatments for human immunodeficiency virus (HIV), which causes AIDS. In the fall of 1986, Dr. Hin-wing Yeung, a professor of herbal medicine at the Chinese University of Hong Kong, wandered unannounced into the AIDS research facility at San Francisco General Hospital. He'd read of U.S. researchers' inability to develop HIV drugs that were safe and effective. The safe drugs didn't work, and the effective drugs were too toxic. Yeung asked AIDS researcher Dr.

Michael McGrath if he'd ever treated HIV-infected cells with trichosanthin, a protein in Chinese cucumber root. Dr. McGrath had never heard of the plant.

Yeung gave him a vial containing some of the herb extract, and when McGrath added it to a test tube of HIV-infected cells, he couldn't believe his eyes. The trichosanthin seemed to kill only the cells infected with the AIDS virus. Uninfected cells remained alive and well.

Since then, trichosanthin, or Compound Q, has been tested in AIDS patients. It's no miracle cure, but preliminary results suggest the herbal extract has benefit.

Another promising anti-AIDS herb is St.-John's-wort, a European plant used in healing for centuries. In 1988, a report published in the *Proceedings of the National Academy of Science* showed a chemical in the plant, hypericin, inhibits the growth of a virus that causes one form of leukemia. That virus is a retrovirus. So is HIV. The researchers speculated hypericin might help treat AIDS.

Physicians treating AIDS patients began prescribing St.-John's-wort, and in November 1989, AIDS *Treatment News* published a survey of 112 patients' experiences with hypericin. Like trichosanthin, it's no cure, but most respondents reported intriguing benefits: improved immune function, reduced fever, reduced swelling of lymph nodes, and improvements in appetite, energy, and mood.

AIDS researchers have since launched clinical trials of both trichosanthin and St.-John's-wort. Perhaps these herbs will play a role in curing the late 20th century's most baffling disease. But even if they don't, it's clear that the world's oldest medicines, the herbs humanity has used for more than 5,000 years, will continue to play a key role in health and healing as the 20th century becomes the 21st.

Chapter 2

Tempest in a Teapot: Are Healing Herbs Safe?

Any discussion of herb safety opens the door to an Alice-in-Wonderland world where some passionate advocates insist herbs are "completely safe," while some equally passionate critics condemn them as "poison."

"Are herbs safe to use?" asks Donald Law, Ph.D., in *The Concise Herbal Encyclopedia*. "The answer is yes. No plant that could have any possible unpleasant effects is ever recommended by any botanic physician nowadays. We have not centuries, but millenia of experience behind us. We know thoroughly the effects of the medicines we use. . . . Do not let complicated medical works worry you to death."

On the other hand, in *The New Honest Herbal*, Varro Tyler, Ph.D., writes: "Partisans in the [herb] revival are more evangelistic than critical. . . . Practically all [herbals] recommend large numbers of herbs . . . based on hearsay, folklore, and tradition; in fact, the only criterion which seems to be rigorously avoided is scientific evidence. Some are so indiscriminate, they appear to recommend everything for anything . . . Particularly insidious is the myth . . . that there is something almost magical about herbs which prevents them from inflicting harm. Think how completely false this argument is! Even those unfamiliar with the execution of Socrates by poison hemlock more than 2,000 years ago are probably not inclined to collect and eat wild mushrooms indiscriminately."

Most U.S. medical journal articles on herbs focus on their dangers. Coltsfoot and comfrey allegedly cause cancer and liver damage. Chamomile has been accused of triggering potentially fatal allergic reactions. Licorice allegedly causes a serious hormonal disorder. And ginseng has been linked to "corticosteroid poisoning." Herb advocates dismiss such charges as absurd. The more paranoid hint darkly at an anti-herb conspiracy among the medical journals, all financed mostly by pharmaceutical advertising.

The fact is, healing herbs are neither "completely safe" nor "poison." They are like other medicines. Take too little, and nothing much happens. Take the right amount of the proper herb, and you enjoy healing benefits. Take too much for too long, and you run into trouble.

Is Noomba Safe?

Not long ago, anthropologists discovered a remote tribe in New Guinea, the Sipsep, who greeted them with noomba, a bitter but tasty drink they claimed the gods had given their ancestors to keep them strong and healthy. The anthropologists tried noomba—and immediately felt more alert, energetic, and productive. They could run faster and hike farther without fatigue. One who had asthma claimed she breathed easier after drinking the herbal brew. Noomba caused only two problems: insomnia if the anthropologists drank it before bed, and a headache for a day after they stopped drinking it on a trip to the coast.

Despite these annoyances, the anthropologists grew to love noomba and took a great deal home with them. It was an immediate hit with their university colleagues. At a cocktail party, some medical researchers asked if they could study the herb. The anthropologists readily agreed.

It didn't take long for the researchers to report disturbing findings:

- Noomba was classically addictive. Over time, users developed a tolerance; that is, they required more and more noomba to obtain the same increase in alertness and productivity. The headache the anthropologists had reported was actually just one symptom of physical withdrawal from the addiction. Other withdrawal symptoms included constipation, sleepiness, and a craving for other stimulants.

- Noomba's stimulating effect caused not only insomnia but also anxiety, irritability, anemia, diarrhea, heartburn, stomach upset, muscle tension, and, in a few cases, outbursts of uncontrolled rage.
- Even more disturbing, a five-cup-a-day noomba habit (which many of the anthropologists had) raised cholesterol and blood pressure, and *doubled* their risk of heart attack.
- Some studies suggested noomba impaired fertility. And in experiments involving pregnant animals, the herb caused birth defects.
- Finally, some animal studies linked noomba to several cancers.

What do *you* think? Is noomba safe? Would you drink it? How would you feel if your children became noomba addicts? Are increased alertness, stamina, and productivity worth physical dependence, insomnia, heartburn, diarrhea, infertility, cancer, heart disease, and birth defects?

The truth is, noomba was not discovered recently in New Guinea. It arrived in Europe about 500 years ago from Arabia. Noomba is actually coffee, and all the effects mentioned above apply to America's favorite herbal beverage.

Is coffee safe? That depends. Most Americans enjoy the stimulation of a cup or two each morning. But most "java junkies" know that large amounts of its powerful stimulant, caffeine (also found in tea, colas, chocolate, and maté), can cause problems.

Coffee is probably the most dangerous herb discussed in this book. It's the only one that's addictive, and in large amounts, it causes more problems than most others. Yet it's one of the world's most popular herbs, and most people consider it safe in moderate amounts.

A Double Standard

When asked if animal tests of drug and chemical safety could be applied to humans, one scientific wit replied, "If they confirm my opinions, I believe them. If not, I don't."

"Herbs have been victimized by a scientific double standard," says Mark Blumenthal, executive director of the American Botanical Council in Austin, Texas, which promotes healing-herb research. "When animal studies show therapeutic value, many scientists say you can't apply the results to humans. But when even a single mouse suffers harm from any dose of a medicinal herb, these same scientists are up in arms, saying no one should use the herb."

Life is inherently risky. Nothing is absolutely safe. "Safety" is a judgment call, a risk/benefit appraisal. Is chicken safe? Every year several Americans choke to death on chicken bones, and according to recent estimates, many thousands develop food poisoning because chicken may be contaminated with salmonella bacteria. Yet most people wouldn't hesitate to call chicken safe. Are automobiles safe? Almost 50,000 Americans die each year in car wrecks, yet just about everyone believes the automobile's benefits outweigh its risks.

Herb critics often use emotionally loaded terms like "hazardous" and "poison" to describe healing herbs. If they are, in fact, poisonous, it might be instructive to consult the nation's Poison Control Centers about their experience with them. In 1985 the American Association of Poison Control Centers (AAPCC) reported an estimated 170,000 plant and mushroom poisonings in the United States, which led to six deaths, four from death-cap (*Amanita*) mushrooms, one from poison hemlock, and one from water hemlock. Healing herbs caused no deaths. Among nonfatal plant ingestions, 86 percent involved children under age six who became sick eating houseplants, particularly *Dieffenbachia* or dumb-cane, so named because ingestion causes burning in the mouth, which can interfere with speech.

That same year, the AAPCC reported 227 nonsuicide

deaths from prescription and over-the-counter (OTC) pharmaceuticals: 90 from antidepressants, 87 from pain relievers, 62 from sedatives, 21 from blood pressure medications, 11 from asthma drugs, and 6 from amphetamines.

Figures for drug fatalities (227) and herb fatalities (0) cannot be compared directly because so many more people use pharmaceuticals. But they suggest that healing herbs are not a major public health hazard.

Pharmaceuticals appear even more hazardous in a 1989 Department of Health and Human Services (HHS) report, which estimates 243,000 elderly Americans are hospitalized each year for adverse reactions to pharmaceuticals, while another 163,000 other older adults experience "serious mental impairment caused or aggravated by drugs." The study deplores "widespread mismedication," calling it "the nation's other drug problem." HHS investigators criticized drug makers for testing new products primarily on young adults and largely ignoring their effects on the elderly. They chided physicians for neglecting to adjust dosages downward for the elderly, who are more sensitive to drugs than younger people. And they faulted the elderly for sharing their medicines too freely.

This report was news for one day, then it was basically forgotten. But reports of harm from healing herbs seem to live forever. Ginseng was linked to an "abuse syndrome" and "corticosteroid poisoning" in a 1979 study published in the *Journal of the American Medical Association*. The study was terribly flawed, and even herb critics have repudiated it. Yet, 11 years later, a *New York Times* article called ginseng hazardous.

Because healing herbs have been criticized so far out of proportion to their actual risks, some herb advocates automatically dismiss new reports of harm as nothing more than proof of the continuing medical prejudice against Nature's healers. This is a serious mistake. Any pharmacologically active substance capable of doing good when used properly, can also do harm when used improperly. That's why each herb discussed in *The Healing Herbs* includes a comprehensive list of its potential risks—not because any are dangerous in recommended amounts, but because herbalists need to respect *everything* herbs do and use them in ways that maximize their benefits and minimize their risks.

The Problem of Dose Control

Many Americans believe herbs are safer than pharmaceuticals because they are "natural." Herb critics counter that pharmaceuticals are safer because users know precisely how much they're ingesting, while herb users can only guess at dosages with raw plant material.

Herb critics have a point. Herb potency depends on plant genetics, growing conditions, maturity at harvest, time in storage, the possibility of adulteration, and preparation method. A cup of instant coffee contains about 65 milligrams of caffeine. A cup of cappuccino has more than 300.

On the other hand, one need look no farther than the suicide statistics to know that precise pharmaceutical dose control does not guarantee drugs will be *used* safely. In addition, different people often have very different reactions to the same dose of many drugs.

How do *you* react to drugs? For headache, the adult aspirin dose is two tablets every 4 hours. But through experience, some people learn that one tablet provides sufficient relief, while others must take three.

In general, healing herbs cause fewer side effects than pharmaceuticals. Pharmaceuticals tend to be highly concentrated, and pills and capsules have little taste, factors that make it easier to take an overdose. In herbs, active constituents are typically less concentrated and most taste bitter, which helps discourage overdose. Nonetheless, anyone who uses healing herbs must strive for good dose control.

The doses recommended in this book represent a consensus of the opinions found in both traditional herbals and scientific references. In the few cases where sources disagreed significantly, *The Healing Herbs* recommends the smaller amount, in the belief that it's best to err on the side of caution.

Dose recommendations typically involve a range of ½ to 1 teaspoon of dried herb per cup of water. Start at the low end

if you're over 65, have a chronic illness, are taking other medications, are generally sensitive to drugs, or are using herbs to
treat a child. Feel free to start with stronger preparations if
you're an otherwise healthy adult under 65 and not particularly
sensitive to drugs. Then pay attention to your reactions and
adjust your herb amounts accordingly.

Do Herbs Cause Cancer?

No doubt about it: Many healing herbs contain chemicals
that cause cancer in laboratory animals. But that does *not* necessarily mean they are hazardous. Since the mid-1980s,
scientists have come to a new understanding of cancer-
causation (carcinogenesis) that has important implications
for anyone interested in healing herbs.

Chemicals that cause cancer (carcinogens) used to be considered time bombs. The theory was that if you ingested even
a minute amount of any carcinogen, you were at significant
risk for cancer. As a result, identifying and avoiding carcinogens became a national passion.

Bruce Ames, Ph.D., chairman of the Biochemistry
Department of the University of California at Berkeley, has
long been one of the nation's leading carcinogen detectives.
Dr. Ames knew the vast majority of carcinogens also cause
genetic mutations in bacteria. In 1975, he developed a test
that allowed reasonably reliable carcinogen testing to be
done quickly and inexpensively.

Dr. Ames himself was most suspicious of industrial chemicals, and sure enough, many turned out to be carcinogenic.
Most had been introduced since the 1950s. It takes 20 to 30 years
for carcinogens to cause cancer, so many authorities predicted a major surge in U.S. cancer rates by the late 1970s,
particularly among people born after 1950 who had been exposed to all the new man-made carcinogens that came into existence since their births.

But the predicted chemical cancer surge didn't occur. To be
sure, some cancer rates increased: lung (from smoking),
melanoma (from sun exposure), and breast (for reasons not

entirely clear). Workers in some industries (chemical, steel, asbestos, agriculture, and nuclear) who were exposed to staggering amounts of chemical carcinogens suffered higher cancer rates. And children exposed to high levels of carcinogens from living near toxic waste sites also showed high cancer rates. But the predicted across-the-board increases did not materialize. For most Americans, cancer has remained what it has always been—a degenerative disease that typically develops in older adults. Of course, it's prudent to avoid known carcinogens (cigarette smoke, asbestos, pesticides, excessive sun, etc.), but the "time bomb" theory simply did not explain observed reality.

Dr. Ames also tested some food plants. In the early 1980s, he stunned the world with the news that natural carcinogens account for 5 *to* 10 *percent* of the dry weight of virtually all food plants. Dr. Ames theorized plants had evolved their toxic chemicals as protection against insects and disease-causing microorganisms. In a landmark 1987 report published in the journal *Science*, he wrote that wheat, corn, and peanut butter contain the powerful carcinogen aflatoxin. Celery is packed with carcinogenic psoralens. Mushrooms contain carcinogenic hydrazines. And anything toasted, grilled, barbecued, or broiled contains carcinogenic by-products of burning. Dr. Ames estimated the average person consumes 10,000 *times* more natural carcinogens (by weight) than man-made carcinogenic chemicals.

Then why doesn't everyone develop cancer? Because, researchers discovered, most food plants also contain chemicals that *prevent* cancer.

These discoveries have led to a new perspective on cancer. We ingest carcinogens in everything we eat, so it's not possible to insulate ourselves from them. Fortunately, the harmful effects of these cancer-causing substances are usually offset by natural cancer-preventive substances, such as vitamins C and E, and beta-carotene, a form of vitamin A.

According to the new understanding of carcinogenesis, people who eat a diet high in carcinogens should experience higher cancer rates than those whose diet is rich in anti-cancer substances. Population studies bear this out. Fats tilt the balance toward cancer, while fiber tilts it away. Red meats, fast foods, and junk foods are high in fat and low in fiber. Whole grains and fresh fruits and vegetables are high in fiber and low in fat. People who eat a high-fat, low-fiber diet suffer considerably more cancer than those who eat primarily whole grains and fresh fruits and vegetables. The research is so compelling, the American Cancer Society recommends a low-fat, high-fiber diet to prevent many cancers.

Like all food plants, healing herbs also contain both pro- and anti-cancer substances. Some herb critics, who focus only on herbal carcinogens, have charged that several healing herbs "cause cancer." Carcinogenic chemicals isolated from their herbal sources and administered to laboratory animals have indeed caused cancer. But the actions of herbal carcinogens are typically offset by the plants' anti-cancer substances, particularly in people who eat a cancer-preventive, low-fat, high-fiber diet.

For the sake of comprehensiveness, *The Healing Herbs* mentions herb constituents shown to be carcinogenic or toxic in any way. However, it also lists herbs' anti-cancer substances, which help protect herb users against harm. Those with personal or strong family histories of cancer might decide, in consultation with their physician, not to use particular herbs because of their carcinogen content. But unless an herb carries a specific warning, otherwise healthy adults need not fear cancer from ingesting recommended amounts for recommended periods.

Safety Guidelines

Each herb discussed in this book includes specific safety recommendations, but here are some general guidelines.

Don't take herb identity for granted. Most herbs are identified accurately. But adulteration is still possible, particularly among such costly herbs as saffron, ginseng, goldenseal, and echinacea. Learn what healing herbs smell, feel, and taste like. When in doubt, do not ingest the herb.

Use only recommended amounts for recommended pe-

riods. When herbs have caused harm, the vast majority of cases have involved people who consumed huge amounts for long periods.

If you're over 65 or sensitive to other drugs, start with low-strength preparations. Many elderly people develop increased sensitivity to drugs.

Be extra cautious if you have a chronic disease. Healing herbs may interact with other drugs you might be taking. Check with your physician and pharmacist about possible problems.

Pay attention to any symptoms of toxicity. If you develop stomach upset, nausea, diarrhea, and/or headache within an hour or two of taking any healing herb, stop taking it and see if your symptoms subside. When in doubt, call your local Poison Control Center (listed in the white pages under "Poison"), or your physician or pharmacist. If you experience a severe reaction, call your doctor immediately.

Be extra careful when using herb oils. Aromatic herbs' "essential" or "volatile" oils are highly concentrated, and amounts that seem small may cause serious harm. As little as a teaspoon of pennyroyal oil can cause death. Many herb oils are available commercially. If you use any, take only a drop or two at a time.

With few exceptions, pregnant and nursing women should not use medicinal amounts of healing herbs. Herbs that cause no problems for adults may harm the unborn and newborns. Pregnant women should use herbs medicinally only with the consent and supervision of their obstetrician.

With few exceptions, medicinal amounts of healing herbs should not be given to children under age 2. If you give herbal medicines to infants, be sure to use very dilute preparations. Also, get the okay from your pediatrician.

Chapter 3

Storing and Preparing Healing Herbs

When you're used to snapping open a plastic bottle and popping one of those convenient capsules into your mouth, the prospect of dealing with dried plant material can be a little daunting.

Don't let it intimidate you. If you use prepackaged commercial products, preparing and using the healing herbs need be no more complicated than making a cup of tea. Simply follow directions on the package label.

On the other hand, you may *enjoy* growing and preparing your own herbs. Here's what you need to know to use the healing herbs if you grow or gather your own.

Directions for Drying

Healing herb formulas almost always begin with dried plant material, so fresh herbs—either wild or garden-grown—should be dried before they're stored or used.

Traditionally, most herbs were simply tied in bunches and hung in a warm, dry, shady spot until they crumbled easily. Roots were washed, split, and spread in a single layer on a clean surface. Traditional drying methods are still used today. In fact, some herb shops sell herbs in dried bunches.

But traditional drying has two disadvantages. It often requires more room than foragers or gardeners have, and it takes time—a few days to a few weeks for many leaves, stems, and flowers, and sometimes many months for barks or roots. To preserve the aromatic volatile oils in many herbs, the faster the drying time, the better. That's why most commercial herb producers use special equipment for drying herbs. The same process can be done at home by placing herbs on a cookie sheet or piece of clean window screen in a 95°F oven. Oven drying is convenient and inexpensive, but it has two drawbacks. In places where many herbs are harvested in the heat of the summer, the last thing people want to do is turn their oven on. And many ovens don't heat evenly, so some plant material might char while the rest remains too moist.

Another approach is to purchase a small produce dryer, a tabletop appliance with built-in removable trays that uses a hot-air fan to dry not only herbs but other garden produce as well. One good model is the Equi-Flow Dehydrator, which costs around $230 and can be ordered from The Gardener's Supply Catalog, 128 Intervale Road, Burlington, VT 05401.

Power for Powdering

Once dry, most herbs are powdered, reducing them to the form most convenient to use. Traditional herbalists used a mortar and pestle, a method that still works well for those who process only small amounts of herbs.

A more modern approach is to use a small coffee grinder (carefully cleaned to remove all traces of coffee). For gardeners who produce large amounts of herbs, larger grinders are available.

Setup for Storing

This may come as a shock to those who store their kitchen spices in clear glass jars, but light is one of the two biggest destroyers of herb flavor and medicinal potency. The other is oxygen.

To best preserve herbs' medicinal constituents, store them in opaque glass or ceramic containers. Fill containers full to limit the amount of oxygen they contain. As you use your herbs, add cotton wadding to the containers to limit the amount of oxygen inside them.

When stored carefully, aromatic herbs (such as sage, rosemary, and thyme) can remain potent for more than a year, and nonaromatic herbs (such as alfalfa and chaparral) considerably longer.

Moisture is another herb killer. If your herbs get wet, redry them quickly to prevent the growth of mold.

Insects also take their toll. Drying kills many pests, but watch for signs of infestation. When not using your herbs, keep the containers closed tight.

Procedures for Preparing

Healing herbs are typically used as infusions, decoctions, compresses, tinctures, ointments, and capsules. They may also be added to baths.

How to Make an Infusion

Infusions are extracts made from herbs with medicinal constituents in their flowers, leaves, and stems. Infusions are *not* teas. Some herbalists use the terms interchangeably, but the two are quite different. Infusions are prepared like teas, but they are steeped longer so they become considerably stronger.

The standard traditional infusion recipe calls for $1/2$ to 1 ounce of dried herb steeped in a pint of boiling water for 10 to 20 minutes. Infusions do not have a long shelf life. They should be made as needed, so many of today's herbalists recommend $1/2$ to 1 rounded teaspoon per cup of boiling water steeped for the same amount of time. Of course, after 20 minutes, infusions are no longer hot. They may be drunk at room temperature or reheated. A handy way to reheat them is to use a microwave oven with a temperature probe.

You can use fresh herbs instead of dried to make an infusion by simply doubling the amount of herb.

Making infusions can be as therapeutic as drinking them. While your infusion is steeping, inhale the warm, steamy vapors. They can act as a nasal decongestant and may help relieve the discomfort of colds, flu, cough, bronchitis, and allergies. As you inhale the vapors, close your eyes and visualize your immune system attacking your illness and making you well. Studies show that such meditative visualizations stimulate the immune system to fight many diseases more effectively.

The main problem with herbal infusions is their taste. Most healing herbs taste quite bitter. This is Nature's way of discouraging overdose, but if you can't get your medicine down, it can't do any good. To make infusions more palatable, add sugar, honey, or lemon, or mix them with herbal beverage blends. If you still can't stomach an infusion, try a different preparation.

How to Make a Decoction
Similar to infusions, decoctions are extracts made from roots and barks. Compared with flowers, leaves, and stems, the active chemicals in roots and barks are more difficult to extract, so instead of steeping, you gently simmer the dried herb material in boiling water for 10 to 20 minutes.

How to Make a Tincture
Tinctures are extracts made with alcohol rather than water. They are highly concentrated, so they're more portable than infusions or decoctions—or even the herbs themselves. They also remain potent longer.

To make tinctures, commercial herb marketers typically use pure grain alcohol, which is 198 proof. But home tincture makers can use 100 proof vodka or brandy. Vodka is less expensive. The standard tincture recipe calls for 1 ounce of crushed dried herb steeped in 5 ounces of distilled spirits for six weeks. Here are some tips for tincture-making:

- Seal tincture containers tightly.
- Despite sealing, some containers may ooze. Don't store developing tinctures on valuable furniture.
- Label tinctures with the herb used and the date you put them up so you'll know when six weeks have passed.

- Shake the mixture every few days to encourage alcohol uptake of the herb's medicinal constituents.
- Keep tinctures out of direct sunlight.
- Most herbalists recommend using brown glass containers to minimize light damage.
- Some tinctures change color as they develop. Don't be surprised.
- As tinctures develop, the liquid level often goes down slightly. Top it off with more distilled spirits.
- After six weeks, many herbalists recommend straining out the plant material. This is fine, but it's not necessary.
- Store tinctures in a cool place.
- Keep tinctures out of the reach of children. They are quite potent, and a small amount might trigger a harmful reaction.

Those who do not drink alcohol can make tinctures using warm (but not boiled) vinegar. Herbalists recommend wine or apple cider vinegar, not the white variety. The directions are the same.

Using Capsules

Powdered herbs can also be packed inside standard gelatin capsules. Capsules are a convenient way to carry healing herbs while you travel or to take herbs that taste unpleasant. Many herb supply catalogs offer capsules and capsule-packing devices. (You'll find a list on page 49.)

Capsules come in different sizes. The "00" size is standard.

If you make capsules, measure how much powdered herb fits into the capsules you're using so you won't exceed the dosage recommended in this book. Capsules can also be opened up and the contents used to make infusions, decoctions, or compresses.

Store capsules away from light and out of the reach of children.

External Preparations

You can make your own herbal ointment by adding 1/2 to 1 teaspoon of tincture per ounce of commercial skin lotion.

For external use, particularly for cuts, burns, and other skin problems, dip a clean cloth in a cool infusion or decoction and drape it over the affected area for 20 minutes. Repeat as needed.

To make baths more relaxing, fill a cloth bag with a few handfuls of aromatic herbs and run your bathwater over it. For additional aroma, leave the herb bag in the water as you bathe.

Chapter 4

How to Obtain Healing Herbs

There are three ways to obtain healing herbs: gather them, grow them, or buy them.

Gathering Your Own

If you enjoy long walks in meadows and forests, gathering herbs can be great fun. Of course, not all healing herbs grow in the United States, but many do. To go "herbing," you'll need a good field guide. The best is *A Field Guide to Medicinal Plants: Eastern and Central North America*, written by noted herbalists Steven Foster and James A. Duke, Ph.D. This book discusses more than 500 healing herbs and includes 500 pen-and-ink drawings and 200 color plates. Any bookstore can order it for you.

Some herbs, such as dandelion, are easy to recognize and safe to pick. In fact, with dandelion, your neighbors will probably thank you for pulling it out of their lawns. But other herbs, particularly ginseng, are more difficult to find.

Some healing herbs have thorns: blackberry, raspberry, nettle, and rose. Wear gloves, long pants, and long sleeves to gather these favorites.

Other herbs, such as angelica root and cascara sagrada bark, are safe to ingest when dried but hazardous when fresh.

A few herbs' medicinal parts are safe, but their other parts cause problems. Blue cohosh's medicinal root is safe when used properly, but its berries are poisonous. Rhubarb's medicinal root can be used safely, but its leaf blades are poisonous.

Finally, a few poisonous plants resemble healing herbs. Three poisonous species of hemlock look like parsley, and some herb gatherers have died because they mistook poison hemlock—also known as "fool's parsley"—for the familiar garnish.

If you stalk the wild healers, dress appropriately, read up on the herbs in chapter 5 to see if they're safe or problematic, use a good field guide, and most important, when in doubt about any plant's identity, don't ingest it.

Growing Your Own

Chapter 5 contains directions for cultivating the healing herbs that grow in the United States, but to get started, you'll still need seeds, cuttings, or root divisions.

Cuttings can be difficult to obtain. You have to know an herb gardener. But cuttings are rarely necessary.

Most nurseries carry quite a few culinary herb seeds. Standard seed catalogs usually contain dozens of herbs as well. Most nurseries also carry herb seedlings. If you don't see the herbs you want, ask if your nursery can obtain them for you.

But for the committed herb gardener, nothing compares with the specialty catalogs published by many of the nation's hundreds of commercial herb growers. Most charge a small fee for the catalog. Some of the best are:

- Companion Plants, 7247 North Coolville Ridge Road, Athens, OH 45701. Has 300 varieties of plants and 100 varieties of seeds.
- The Rosemary House, 120 South Market Street, Mechanicsburg, PA 17055. Carries 100 varieties of plants and 200 varieties of seeds.
- Taylor's Herb Gardens, Inc., 1535 Lone Oak Road, Vista, CA 92084. Stocks 100 varieties of plants.

- Abundant Life Seed Foundation, P.O. Box 772, Port Townsend, WA 98368. Carries 150 varieties of seeds.

This list does not even scratch the surface of herb-gardening resources. Fortunately, several national directories of herb businesses are available (at a cost of about $10), many of which sell plants and seeds as well as dried herbs.

- *The Herb Gardener's Mail-Order Source Book* by Elayne Moos. Woodsong Graphics, P.O. Box 238, New Hope, PA 18938. A marvelous resource with 130 listings.
- *North Wind Farms Directory* by Paula Oliver. Route 2, Box 246, Shevlin, MN 56676. Oliver publishes the herb-grower's trade journal, *Business of Herbs*. Her directory is aimed at commercial herb growers, but it's also quite useful for home herb gardeners. Contains 800 listings. Updated annually.
- The International Herb Growers and Marketers Association (IHGMA), P.O. Box 281, Silver Spring, PA 17575. Membership, which costs around $80 per year, includes a bimonthly newsletter and a membership directory with more than 600 listings. If you'd rather not join the organization, you can subscribe to the newsletter.

You Can Always Buy

Supermarkets now carry many herbal beverage teas, some of which can be brewed into medicinal infusions (see chapter 3). For a better selection, try a health food store. Most carry dozens of bulk herbs, medicinal herb blends, tinctures, oils, and tablets. Popular brands of medicinal herb preparations are produced by HerbPharm, Native Herbs, Nature's Herbs, Nature's Way, Solgar, Traditional Medicinals, Yerba Prima, and Zand, among others.

Bulk herbs, tinctures, oils, and tablets can also be purchased by mail. Many of the gardeners' resources listed above also sell dried herbs and herb preparations. In addition, the following catalogs offer large selections.

- *Nature's Herbs*, 1010 46th Street, Emeryville, CA 94608. Catalog free. 350 herbs and spices.
- *HerbPharm's Whole Herb Catalog*, P.O. Box 116, Williams, OR 97544. Catalog free. 100 herb oils, 20 German extracts, 25 formulas.
- *The Herb and Spice Collection*, P.O. Box 118, Norway, IA 52318. Catalog free. 60 culinary herbs and spice blends, 150 medicinal herbs.
- *Phyto-Pharmica*, P.O. Box 1348, Green Bay, WI 54305. Catalog free. Specializes in hard-to-find herbs, such as deglycyrrhiziniated licorice, but sells only to licensed health professionals: doctors, chiropractors, acupuncturists, nurses, psychologists, etc. Ask a supportive practitioner to obtain the catalog and order for you.

Noteworthy Herb Publications

Another way to find herbs—and learn more about them—is to read the herb press. Recommended publications include:

- *HerbalGram*. The quarterly magazine of the American Botanical Council and the Herb Research Foundation. An excellent, authoritative source of the latest herb research with an emphasis on herbal healing. American Botanical Council, P.O. Box 201660, Austin, TX 78720.
- *Medical Herbalism*. A bimonthly newsletter aimed at herbal medicine practitioners, but an important resource for anyone interested in herbal healing. P.O. Box 33080, Portland, OR 97233.
- *The Herb Quarterly*. A wonderful magazine with a broad scope, including herb gardening, cookery, crafts, history, and medicine. P.O. Box 548, Boiling Springs, PA 17007.
- *The Herb Companion*. A lavishly photographed bimonthly that emphasizes herb gardening and cookery. 201 East Fourth Street, Loveland, CO 80537.

PART TWO

He causeth the grass to grow for the cattle and herbs for the service of humanity.

Psalm 104:14

Chapter 5

100 Healing Herbs

This chapter profiles 100 of the world's estimated 5,000 widely used medicinal plants. Why these 100?

- **They're available.** The selected herbs are generally Western herbs, from the Egyptian, European, and Native American traditions. Several Westernized Asian herbs have been included—cinnamon, ginger, ginseng, rhubarb, tea, etc. But despite their medicinal effectiveness, plants unique to Chinese herbalism have been omitted because they are not widely available in the United States.
- **They're useful.** All the selected herbs have practical applications for everyday medical concerns.
- **They're reasonably safe.** Like other medicines, many of the 100 herbs may cause harm when used improperly. That's why the herb profiles emphasize precautions, dosage limits, and possible hazards. But the selected herbs are reasonably safe when used as recommended.
- **They're familiar.** All the herbs and spices used in cooking today were originally prized mainly for food preservation and healing. Few people appreciate the green pharmacies they already have in their kitchens.
- **They're fascinating.** The Pied Piper was as much an herbalist as a musician (see Valerian). Bayer was originally skeptical of aspirin (see Meadowsweet). A 19th-century battle over abortion popularized a modern remedy for menstrual cramps (see Black Haw). And the cowboys who drank sarsaparilla were less interested in refreshment than in preventing venereal diseases (see Sarsaparilla).

ALFALFA

Hope for the Heart

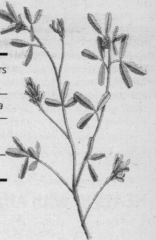

Family: Leguminosae; other members include beans, peas

Genus and species: *Medicago sativa*

Also known as: Chilean clover, buffalo grass, lucerne (in Britain)

Parts used: Leaves

Farmers have long prized the alfalfa plant as animal forage, and in the last 20 years people who graze on salads have come to appreciate this herb's sprouts as well. But it's the alfalfa *leaves* that may contain its real healing power. They may help reduce cholesterol and help prevent heart disease and some strokes.

An Ancient Healer

What's good for your cattle is good for you, too, or so the ancient Chinese thought. Their animals ate alfalfa so enthusiastically, the Chinese began preparing the herb's tender young leaves as a vegetable, and soon traditional Chinese physicians were using it to stimulate appetite and treat digestive problems, particularly ulcers.

Ancient India's traditional Ayurvedic physicians also used

53

alfalfa to treat ulcers. They prescribed it for arthritis pain and fluid retention as well.

Ancient Arabs fed their horses alfalfa, believing it made them swift and strong. They called it *al-fac-facah*, "father of all foods." The Spanish changed the name to *alfalfa*.

Spain introduced alfalfa into the Americas, where it became a popular forage crop, particularly in the Great Plains. Like the ancient Chinese, the pioneers believed that what was good for their cattle was good for them. They used alfalfa to treat arthritis, boils, cancer, scurvy, and urinary and bowel problems. Pioneer women used it to bring on menstruation.

After the Civil War, alfalfa fell out of favor as a healing herb, and it wasn't until the 1970s that it returned to popularity via the salad bowl.

HEALING with Alfalfa

Most of alfalfa's ancient healing uses have long been disproved, but modern scientists may have discovered a potential healing benefit our ancestors never dreamed of: Alfalfa as an agent in the war against heart disease, stroke, and cancer, the nation's top three killers.

Heart Disease and Stroke. Animal studies show that alfalfa leaves help reduce blood cholesterol levels and plaque deposits on artery walls. High cholesterol levels and plaque deposits lead to heart disease and stroke. Alfalfa sprouts produce a similar, but less significant, effect. Animal results don't necessarily apply to people, but one case report in the British medical journal *Lancet* documented a major cholesterol reduction in a man who ate large amounts of alfalfa.

Cancer. One study suggests that alfalfa helps neutralize carcinogens in the intestine. Another, published in the *Journal of the National Cancer Institute*, shows it binds carcinogens in the colon and helps speed their elimination from the body.

Alfalfa seeds also contain two chemicals (stachydrine and homostachydrine) that promote menstruation and can cause miscarriage. Pregnant women should not eat alfalfa seeds (see "The Safety Factor" on page 56).

Bad Breath. Alfalfa is a source of chlorophyll, the active ingredient in most commercial breath fresheners. Sip an alfalfa infusion if you're concerned about bad breath.

Intriguing Possibility. In laboratory studies, alfalfa helps fight disease-causing fungi. It might one day be used to treat fungal infections.

Dead-End File. While contemporary herbalists generally endorse the age-old view that alfalfa treats ulcers, they may have to eat their words. Scientific research has found no support for this traditional use of the herb.

Herbalists also recommend alfalfa for bowel problems and as a diuretic to treat fluid retention. Unfortunately, these traditional uses have not held up under scientific scrutiny, either.

Some supplement manufacturers promote alfalfa tablets as a treatment for asthma and hay fever. But a study published in the *Journal of the American Medical Association* shows these claims have no merit. Alfalfa contains neither bronchodilators for treatment of asthma nor antihistamines, which relieve hay fever.

Despite its traditional use as a menstruation promoter, scientists have found no uterine stimulants in alfalfa leaves.

R$_x$ for Alfalfa

Save the sprouts to dress up your salads; its leaves are the part used in herbal healing. Alfalfa leaf tablets and capsules are available at herb outlets, natural food stores, or wherever supplements are sold—follow package directions.

When using the bulk herb, prepare medicinal infusions from 1 to 2 teaspoons of dried leaves per cup of boiling water. Steep 10 to 20 minutes. Enjoy up to 3 cups a day to take advantage of its cholesterol-reducing potential. The infusion has a haylike aroma and tastes like chamomile, with a slightly bitter aftertaste.

Medicinal infusions of the leaves should not be given to children under age 2. For older children and people over 65, start with low-strength preparations and increase strength if necessary.

The Safety Factor

No one should ever eat alfalfa seeds. They contain relatively high levels of the toxic amino acid canavanine. Over time, large quantities of alfalfa seeds may introduce enough cana-vanine into the body to cause the reversible blood disorder pancytopenia, according to a report in *Lancet*. This condition impairs the platelets, which are necessary for clotting, and the white blood cells, which fight infection.

The canavanine in alfalfa seeds has also been linked to systemic lupus erythematosus, a serious inflammatory dis-ease that can attack many organs, particularly the kidneys. Alfalfa seeds have reactivated the disease in some people who were in remission, according to a report published in the *New England Journal of Medicine*. Another study showed the seeds actually induce lupus in monkeys. Anyone with lupus should stay away from alfalfa seeds.

Alfalfa also contains saponins, chemicals that may destroy red blood cells and—at least theoretically—cause anemia. Because of this, some herb critics warn against ingesting al-falfa (and the many other healing herbs that contain saponins) in any form. Such dire warnings seem unjustified. For otherwise healthy, nonpregnant, nonnursing adults, al-falfa is considered safe in amounts typically recommended. There have been no reports of otherwise healthy people de-veloping anemia from using recommended amounts of heal-ing herbs containing saponins. However, anyone with anemia should use this herb only with his doctor's approval, if at all.

Leaf It Be

Alfalfa leaf is on the Food and Drug Administration's list of herbs generally regarded as safe.

Alfalfa should be used in medicinal amounts only in con-sultation with your physician. If alfalfa causes minor dis-comforts, such as stomach upset or diarrhea, use less or stop using it. Let your doctor know if you experience unpleasant effects or if the symptoms for which the herb is being used do not improve significantly in two weeks.

Sprout Your Own

If you can't find alfalfa leaves in your local store, growing your own is a snap. Alfalfa is a deep-rooting, bushy perennial that grows to 3 feet and resembles tall clover. The leaves are divided into three leaflets. The herb's lavender, pale blue, or yellow flowers bloom from May through October, depending on location.

Alfalfa grows best in loamy soil. It tolerates clay but not sand, which lacks sufficient nutrients. Seeds are usually sown in autumn in rows 18 inches apart. Prepare the soil with manure and rock phosphate. Young plants require regular watering, but once established, they become fairly drought tolerant. Harvest alfalfa as the plant blooms. Cut plants back to within 3 inches of the ground, then hang them to dry.

ALLSPICE

The Caribbean Cure

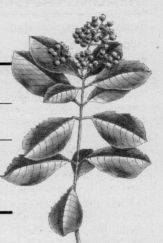

Family: Myrtaceae; other members include myrtle

Genus and species: *Pimenta officinalis, P. dioica*

Also known as: Pimento, pimenta, Jamaican pepper, clove pepper

Parts used: Mature, but unripe, green berries

Many people know the Caribbean as a place to find sunshine, sailboats, and calypso music amidst a warm tropical breeze. But few know the Caribbean as a place to find folk healing at its finest.

Folk healing has been alive in the Caribbean for centuries. Some of its medicinal magic is found in the spice that's native to the islands but known universally to just about any cook—allspice.

Allspice, which combines the flavors of cinnamon, pepper, juniper, and clove, is used as a digestive aid, pain reliever, and anesthetic. Jamaicans drink hot allspice tea for colds, menstrual cramps, and upset stomach. Costa Ricans use it to treat indigestion, flatulence, and diabetes. Cubans consider it a refreshing tonic. And Guatemalans apply crushed allspice berries externally to treat bruises and joint and muscle pains.

HEALING with Allspice

Allspice berries contain an oil that is the source of all its healing powers.

Digestive Aid. Allspice oil is rich in the chemical eugenol, also found in clove and several other healing herbs. Eugenol may promote activity of digestive enzymes.

Pain Reliever. Eugenol has also been found to be an effective pain reliever, lending credence to the Guatemalan practice of applying the crushed berries to painful muscles and joints.

Anesthetic. Dentists use eugenol as a local anesthetic for teeth and gums, and the chemical is an ingredient in the over-the-counter toothache remedies Numzident and Benzodent. Allspice oil may be applied directly to painful teeth and gums as first aid until professional care can be obtained.

R$_x$ for Allspice

When using powdered allspice as a spice, season food to taste.

For toothache, apply the oil directly to the tooth or gum, one drop at a time, using a cotton swab. Take care not to swallow it.

As a digestive aid, prepare an infusion using 1 to 2 teaspoons of allspice powder per cup of boiling water. Steep 10 to 20 minutes and strain. Drink up to 3 cups a day. You'll find that allspice has a warm, pleasant harmony of flavors: cinnamon, pepper, juniper, and cloves.

Medicinal doses should not be given to children under age 2. For older children and people over 65, start with low-strength preparations and increase strength if necessary.

The Safety Factor

Powdered allspice adds a warm, rich flavor to foods, but its highly concentrated oil should never be swallowed. As little as 1 teaspoon can cause nausea, vomiting, and even convulsions.

Although allspice oil is effective when applied externally, this may not always be a good idea. In people with sensitive skin, particularly those with eczema, the oil may cause inflammation.

Allspice is a mild antioxidant. Antioxidants help prevent the cell damage that scientists say eventually causes cancer. On the other hand, in laboratory tests, eugenol weakly promotes tumor growth. This makes allspice one of many healing herbs with both pro- and anti-cancer effects. At this point, scientists aren't sure which way the balance tilts. Until they are, people with any history of cancer should probably not use medicinal doses of allspice.

Allspice is on the Food and Drug Administration's list of herbs generally regarded as safe. For otherwise healthy nonpregnant, nonnursing adults, allspice is considered safe in amounts typically recommended. Allspice should be taken in medicinal amounts only in consultation with your doctor. If allspice causes minor discomforts, such as stomach upset or diarrhea, use less or stop using it. Let your doctor know if you experience any unpleasant effects or if the symptoms for which the herb is being used do not improve significantly in two weeks.

South of the Border

Native to Central America and the Caribbean, and now cultivated in South America, the 40-foot allspice tree has large, leathery, oblong leaves and produces clusters of 1/2-inch berries in July and August. It is not grown in the United States.

ALOE

Soothe Those Wounds

Family: Liliaceae; other members include lily, tulip, garlic

Genus and species: *Aloe vera* and an estimated 500 other *Aloe* species

Also known as: Cape, Barbados, Curaiao, Socotrine, or Zanzibar aloe

Parts used: The jellylike gel found in the leaves, and the bitter, yellow juice (latex) extracted from specialized cells of the leaves' inner skin

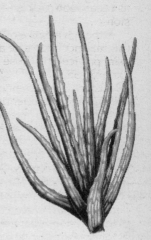

Every kitchen should have a potted aloe on the windowsill. That way, when minor burns, scalds, or cuts occur, it's easy to cut off one of the thick, fleshy leaves and squeeze its clear gel onto the injury. Aloe gel dries into a natural bandage. It may promote wound healing and help prevent infection.

Another part of aloe, the latex (extracted from special cells on its inner leaf skin), is a powerful laxative—so potent, in fact, that many authorities say it should not be taken internally.

A Cause of War

Aloe has been used in healing since the dawn of history. Egyptian medical writings from 1500 B.C. recommend it for infections, skin problems, and as a laxative—uses supported by modern science.

Aloe is one of the few nonnarcotic plants to cause a war. When Alexander the Great conquered Egypt in 332 B.C., he heard of a plant with amazing wound-healing powers on an island off Somalia. Intent on healing his soldiers' wounds— and denying this healer to his enemies—Alexander sent an army to seize the island and the plant, which turned out to be aloe.

The Greek physician Dioscorides recommended aloe externally for wounds, hemorrhoids, ulcers, and hair loss. The Roman naturalist Pliny prescribed it internally as a laxative.

Arab traders carried aloe from Spain to Asia around the 6th century and introduced it to India's traditional Ayurvedic physicians, who used it to treat skin problems, intestinal worms, and menstrual discomforts. Chinese healers used it similarly.

More recently, pioneers used aloe gel to treat wounds, burns, and hemorrhoids. These uses continue to this day.

HEALING with Aloe

Contemporary herbalists use aloe in some of the same ways Dioscorides used it almost 2,000 years ago—externally for burns and wounds.

Wounds, Burns, Scalds, Scrapes, Sunburn. Scientific evidence of aloe's wound-healing power was first documented in 1935 when an American medical journal reported the case of a woman whose x-ray burns were successfully treated with aloe gel scooped straight from leaves cut from the plant. Since then, several studies have supported the herb's ability to spur the healing of first- and second-degree burns and other wounds. One report claims aloe also eases the discomfort of poison ivy rash.

Infection Fighter. Aloe gel may not only spur wound healing, it may also help prevent infection in injured skin. Several studies show aloe effective against many different bacteria that can invade a wound.

Skin Creams. Cleopatra massaged aloe gel into her skin to make it shine. The herb is still widely used in skin-care products. But if you're after beautiful skin, do what the legendary Egyptian beauty did—use the fresh leaf gel, not the "stabilized" (preserved) gel used in commercial shampoos and skin products. Stabilized aloe has none of the fresh herb's skin-healing benefits. If you enjoy the fragrance of aloe shampoos and skin lotions, fine. Just don't expect them to turn you into Cleopatra.

Intriguing Possibilities. Studies show that aloe may kill the fungus (*Candida albicans*) that causes vaginal yeast infections. Its possible effectiveness against the yeast fungus has led some herbalists to recommend using the herb to treat the infection itself. But just because it kills the fungus in laboratory tests doesn't mean it can wipe out the infection in the human body. No scientific studies support this use, and a Food and Drug Administration advisory panel found insufficient evidence to recommend aloe as a yeast treatment.

In laboratory tests, one chemical (aloe-emodin) in aloe has shown promise against leukemia, but National Cancer Institute scientists say experimental preparations are still too toxic to give to leukemia sufferers. Although aloe has been used externally in folk medicine as a treatment for skin cancer, its effectiveness has never been studied scientifically.

A European study suggests aloe gel reduces blood sugar (glucose) levels in experimental animals and humans with diabetes. The gel is not usually taken internally, but if other studies confirm this effect, aloe might one day be used to help manage diabetes.

Rx for Aloe

To help soothe wounds, burns, scalds, and sunburn, and to help avoid infection, select a lower (older) leaf, cut several inches off, slice it lengthwise, apply the gel, and allow it to dry. Make sure you clean the wound properly with soap and water first. As for the injured leaf, it quickly closes its own wound. The rest of it may be used in the future.

To enjoy the cosmetic benefits of aloe, apply gel from the

leaf to freshly washed skin. Discontinue use if it seems to irritate your skin.

The Safety Factor

Aloe gel is safe for external use by anyone who does not develop an allergic reaction. Aloe is best used in consultation with your doctor. Tell your doctor if wounds do not heal significantly within two weeks or appear to be getting worse.

Never a Laxative

Aloe latex contains laxative chemicals (anthraquinones) with such powerful purgative action that they are called cathartics. Other laxative herbs (senna, rhubarb, buckthorn, and cascara sagrada) also contain anthraquinones, but aloe's action is considered the most drastic—and least recommended—because it often causes severe intestinal cramps and diarrhea. Many herbalists discourage its use, but some supplement companies sell aloe laxative tablets. If you use them, never exceed the package dose recommendation and reduce your dose or stop using the product if you develop intestinal cramps.

If you're looking for a natural laxative, your best bet is to seek other herbs with proven, but milder, results, such as psyllium (see page 423) and cascara sagrada (see page 144).

Aloe latex should not be ingested by pregnant women. Its cathartic nature may stimulate uterine contractions and trigger miscarriage. It should not be used by nursing mothers. The latex enters mother's milk and may cause stomach cramps and violent catharsis in infants.

Aloe's cathartic power may also aggravate ulcers, hemorrhoids, diverticulosis, diverticulitis, colitis, or irritable bowel syndrome. Anyone with a gastrointestinal illness should not use aloe latex as a laxative.

In general, aloe latex is not recommended for internal use.

Possible Side Effect

Although aloe gel may help heal injured skin, one case study reported eczema-like welts in a man who had used it for several years—proving that too much of a good thing may cause problems.

Easy to Grow Indoors

Aloe is the perfect houseplant for people with brown thumbs because it requires little water and no other care. Aloe prefers sun, but tolerates shade and doesn't mind poor soil. The only conditions this hardy succulent cannot tolerate are poor drainage and temperatures below about 40°F. Bring potted aloes indoors before the temperature falls lower.

Aloe periodically produces off-shoots, which may be removed and replanted when they are a few inches tall. Simply uproot or unpot the plant, work the soil gently to separate the offshoot, and return the mother plant to its bed or pot.

ANGELICA

An Angel of an Herb

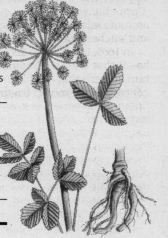

Family: Umbelliferae; other members include carrot, parsley

Genus and species: *Angelica archangelica* (European); *A. atropurpurea* (American); *A. sinensis* (Chinese); and other species

Also known as: Wild celery, masterwort; in China, *dang-gui, dang-qui*

Parts used: Roots, leaves, seeds

Root

Although angelica has been used in magic and medicine for several thousand years, some scientists have dismissed this herb as medically worthless. They may have been too quick to condemn it, however. Recent research reveals several intriguing benefits and even supports a few of the traditional uses for this long-respected herb.

A Mystical Past

European angelica has been viewed as a magical herb for more than 1,000 years. European peasants made angelica leaf necklaces to protect their children from illness and witchcraft. Angelica was reputed to be the only herb witches never used, and its presence in a woman's garden or cupboard was once used as a defense against charges of witchcraft.

During the 16th and 17th centuries, the juice from crushed

angelica roots was combined with other herbs to make "Carmelite water," a medieval drink said to cure headache, promote relaxation and long life, and protect against poisons and witches' spells.

In 1665, Europe was decimated by bubonic plague. Legend has it that a monk dreamed he met an angel who showed him an herb that could cure the scourge. The herb was angelica, and the monk so named it in honor of the angel in his dream. The name stuck, and angelica water was incorporated into the official English plague remedy, "The King's Excellent Plague Recipe," developed by the Royal College of Physicians in London. History provides no clear verdict on the effectiveness of the "Excellent Recipe," but perhaps the old monk's dream was prophetic. Bubonic plague is a bacterial disease, and modern science has discovered that certain substances isolated from angelica have some antibacterial action.

Ancient Healing Tonic

In Asia, where Chinese angelica (*dang-qui*) has been used since the dawn of history, the herb was once considered the tonic for all gynecological problems. Traditional Chinese and Indian Ayurvedic physicians still prescribe it for menstrual problems, arthritis, abdominal pain, and colds and flu.

During the 17th century, angelica became a popular treatment for colds and other respiratory ailments. Its stems are hollow and allow air to pass through them. Under the Doctrine of Signatures—the medieval belief that an herb's physical appearance reveals its healing benefits—hollow-stemmed plants were considered beneficial for respiratory problems.

When European colonists arrived in North America, they found many Indian tribes using American angelica the same way their own healers used the European species—to treat respiratory ailments, particularly tuberculosis.

Eventually the colonists began using large doses to induce abortion.

The 19th-century American Eclectic physicians recommended angelica for heartburn, indigestion, bronchitis, malaria, and typhoid.

HEALING with Angelica

Contrary to legend, angelica does not deliver humanity from epidemic disease. In fact, most of this herb's traditional uses have not stood up to scientific scrutiny. Contemporary herbalists generally recommend angelica mostly for digestive problems and to help clear mucus, uses that may have some validity.

Respiratory Ailments. The Doctrine of Signatures scores one. German researchers have discovered that angelica relaxes the windpipe, suggesting that it may have some value in treating colds, flu, bronchitis, and asthma, after all.

Digestive Aid. The same German investigators found that angelica also relaxes the intestines, lending some credence to its traditional use in treating digestive complaints.

Arthritis. Japanese researchers have reported that the herb has anti-inflammatory effects, meaning there may be something to angelica's traditional Asian use as an arthritis treatment.

Intriguing Possibilities. Preliminary research reports from China suggest angelica increases red blood cell counts. This means the herb may someday prove beneficial in treating anemia. Chinese researchers also report angelica increases the ability of blood to clot. If they're correct, that's good news for people with clotting impairment. It also means that anyone at risk for heart disease should avoid this herb. Increased blood clotting can lead to decreased blood flow to the heart and in some cases might trigger a heart attack.

The Chinese have also found that angelica improves liver function in people suffering from cirrhosis and chronic hepatitis. Their research is preliminary, however. No specific recommendations can be made at this time about using angelica for liver problems.

Rx for Angelica

Angelica reportedly gives relief from colds, flu, and bronchitis. It is sometimes used as a digestive aid or for arthritis relief. There are a variety of ways to prepare this herb, depending on your personal preference.

For an infusion, use 1 teaspoon of powdered seeds or leaves per cup of boiling water. Steep 10 to 20 minutes.

For a decoction, use 1 teaspoon of powdered roots per cup of water. Bring to a boil and simmer 2 minutes. Remove from heat and let stand 15 minutes. Drink up to 2 cups a day. Angelica decoctions taste bitter.

In a tincture, use $1/2$ to 1 teaspoon up to twice a day.

When using commercial extracts, follow package directions.

Angelica should not be given to children under age 2. For older children and people over 65, start with low-strength preparations and increase strength if necessary.

The Safety Factor

Angelica has never been shown to stimulate uterine contractions, but given its traditional use to induce menstruation and abortions, pregnant women should not use medicinal amounts.

Angelica contains chemicals known as psoralens. When exposed to sunlight, people who have ingested psoralens often develop a rash (photosensitivity).

Psoralens also may promote tumor growth, leading the authors of a report in the journal *Science* to advise against taking angelica internally. On the other hand, a recent animal study showed another angelica constituent (alpha-angelica lactone) has an anti-cancer effect. Angelica's role in human cancer, if any, remains unclear. However, people with a history of cancer should probably not use it until this question has been resolved.

Pretty Poison

Fresh angelica roots are poisonous. Drying eliminates the hazard. Herb gardeners should be sure to dry angelica roots thoroughly before using them.

Finally, unless you are a confident field botanist, do not collect angelica in the wild. It's easy to confuse with water hemlock (*Cicuta maculata*), an extremely poisonous plant.

Other Cautions

The Food and Drug Administration includes angelica in its list of herbs generally regarded as safe. For otherwise healthy nonpregnant, nonnursing adults who have no history of cancer, heart attack, or photosensitivity, angelica is considered relatively safe in amounts typically recommended. Angelica should be used in medicinal amounts only in consultation with your doctor. If angelica causes minor discomforts, such as stomach upset or diarrhea, take less or stop using it. Let your doctor know if you experience any unpleasant effects or if the symptoms for which the herb is being used do not improve significantly in two weeks.

Harvest and Have a Feast Day

Angelica often blooms around May 8, the feast day of St. Michael the Archangel, which is the source of this herb's Latin name, *archangelica*.

Angelica grows to 8 feet and resembles celery, hence its common name, wild celery. It's a biennial that dies after producing seeds. It grows from seeds or root divisions. Seed viability is relatively brief, only about six months, but refrigeration extends it up to a year. Germination may take a month. Sow angelica in the fall or spring ½ inch deep in well-prepared beds. Allow plants 2 feet in all directions.

Angelica thrives in rich, moist, well-drained, slightly acidic soil. It prefers partial shade. Leaves may be harvested in the fall of the first year, roots during the spring or fall of the second year.

Angelica is not usually considered a culinary herb, but fresh leaves provide a zesty accent to soups and salads. It has a fragrant aroma and a warm, vaguely sweet taste reminiscent of juniper, followed by a bitter aftertaste. Steamed stems may be eaten with butter, and chopped stems add flavor to roast pork.

ANISE

The Licorice-Flavored Cough Remedy

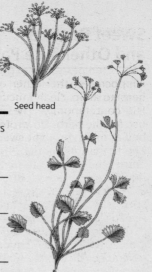

Seed head

Family: Umbelliferae; other members include carrot, parsley; Star anise: Magnoliaceae; other members include magnolia

Genus and species: *Pimpinella anisum;* star anise: *Illicium verum*

Also known as: Aniseed, sweet cumin; star anise: Chinese anise, *illicium*

Parts used: Fruits ("seeds")

Anise sends down a long taproot. But its roots in the history of herbal healing are equally deep.

Since the time of the pharaohs, the aromatic seeds (actually fruits) of this small plant have had many uses. Its alluring fragrance made it one of the world's earliest perfumes—and smelling salts. Ancient Greeks used it to prevent seizures.

Today the herb is best known as a popular spice. And its rich taste of licorice is used to make candy. In fact, most "licorice" candies contain no licorice. They are flavored with anise. Its taste can also be detected in many commercially made cough syrups and lozenges. For some, its flavor is even intoxicating: The Greeks, for example, are known to love their anise-based ouzo, the French their *pastis*. But anise's greatest potential is not found in the candy jar or liquor cabinet. It's found in the medicine chest.

Sweet Dreams
and Other Nice Payoffs

Hippocrates, the father of medicine, recommended the herb to help clear mucus from the respiratory system. His contemporary, Theophrastus had a more romantic use for the herb. He wrote that anise, when kept by one's bed at night, brought sweet dreams with its sweet aroma. The Roman naturalist Pliny recommended chewing fresh anise seed as a breath freshener and digestive aid after big meals.

Ancient Chinese physicians made similar use of the Asian species of this herb, star anise—as a digestive aid, flatulence remedy, and breath freshener.

The Romans cultivated the herb extensively for its fragrance, flavor, and medicinal properties. Anise was one of several spices used to make a cake called *mustaceum*, which was often served as a dessert and digestive aid at Roman feasts. Historians consider *mustaceum* the forerunner of the modern wedding cake.

Early English herbalist John Gerard suggested anise for "hicket" (hiccups). It has also been prescribed as a milk promoter for nursing mothers and as a treatment for water retention, headache, asthma, bronchitis, insomnia, nausea, lice, infant colic, cholera, and even cancer.

America's 19th-century Eclectic physicians recommended anise primarily as a stomach soother for nausea, gas, and infant colic.

In Central America, nursing women still use star anise to promote the flow of milk.

Anise was so important as a cash crop throughout the ancient Mediterranean, it was used as a medium of exchange for payment of taxes. In the Bible, Matthew 23:23 says: "Ye pay tithes of mint, anise, and cumin." Anise was so popular in medieval England as a spice, medicine, and perfume that in 1305 King Edward I placed a special tax on it to raise money to repair London Bridge.

HEALING with Anise

Contemporary herbalists continue to recommend anise as it has been used for more than 2,000 years—for cough, bronchitis, upset stomach, and flatulence. Some also suggest taking it for morning sickness. Still, one popular herb guide flatly states: "None of [anise's purported] medicinal properties has been investigated scientifically." Clearly, someone hasn't been reading the medical journals.

Cough Remedy. Science has supported anise's traditional use as a treatment for coughs, bronchitis, and asthma. According to several studies, the herb contains chemicals (creosol and alpha-pinene) that loosen bronchial secretions and make them easier to cough up.

Digestive Aid. Another chemical (anethole) in anise acts as a digestive aid, which supports its traditional use after meals.

Women's Health. Anise also contains chemicals (dianethole and photoanethole) similar to the female sex hormone estrogen. Scientists suggest their presence probably accounts for the herb's traditional use as a milk promoter in nursing mothers.

Anise has only mild estrogenic activity, but it may help relieve menopausal discomforts.

Men's Health. Female sex hormones similar to estrogen are used to treat some cases of prostate cancer. Of course, by itself anise cannot treat this disease, but men taking hormone therapy for prostate cancer should discuss anise's mild estrogenic action with their physician. Taking the herb in addition to standard medication can't hurt—and it might help.

Intriguing Possibility. One report shows that anise spurs the regeneration of liver cells in laboratory rats, suggesting a possible value in treating hepatitis and cirrhosis. While there are no studies that support using anise to treat liver disease in humans, anise looks promising in this area.

R_x for Anise

For an infusion, gently crush 1 teaspoon of anise seeds per cup of boiling water. Steep for 10 to 20 minutes and strain. Drink up to 3 cups a day.

In a tincture, take $1/2$ to 1 teaspoon up to three times a day.

Diluted anise infusions may be given cautiously to infants to treat colic. For older children and people over 65, begin with low-strength preparations and increase strength if necessary.

The Safety Factor

Many herbalists recommend anise during pregnancy to treat morning sickness. The herb has never been associated with miscarriage or birth defects, but the medical consensus is that pregnant women should steer clear of all drugs, including medical doses of herbs.

Estrogen—and even herbs such as anise that have mild estrogenic activity—may conceivably cause harm. Estrogen is an ingredient in birth control pills, so any woman whose physician advises her not to use the Pill should consult her doctor about anise's estrogenic activity before using medicinal quantities of the herb. Estrogen may contribute to migraine headaches and abnormal blood clotting and promote the development of certain types of breast tumors.

Other Cautions

Anise is on the Food and Drug Administration's list of herbs generally regarded as safe. In medicinal amounts, it is considered safe for otherwise healthy nonpregnant, nonnursing adults. High doses of anise oil—on the order of several teaspoons—may cause nausea and vomiting. Anise should be used in medicinal amounts only in consultation with your doctor. If anise causes minor discomforts, such as stomach upset or diarrhea, use less or stop using it. Let your doctor know if you experience any unpleasant effects or if the symptoms for which the herb is being used do not improve significantly in two weeks.

A Licorice-Scented Garden

Anise is an erect annual that reaches 2 feet. Its smooth stem supports feathery leaves divided into many leaflets, and umbrella-like clusters of tiny white or yellow flowers, which bloom in midsummer and produce small, downy, ribbed fruits in late summer.

Anise grows from seeds planted at a depth of 1/8 inch after danger of frost has passed. Rich, well-drained soil and full sun are best, but the herb tolerates poorer soils. Seeds require a temperature of about 70°F to germinate, typically in one to two weeks.

Anise's long taproot precludes successful transplanting beyond the seedling stage. Thin seedlings to 18-inch spacing. Anise is easy to grow, but it may become spindly or suffer wind damage in unsheltered locations.

Harvest the seeds when they have turned from green to grayish brown by cutting the entire flower head before the seed clusters have broken open. Collect the flowers in a paper bag to prevent seed scatter. Dry seeds on paper or cloth in a sunny location. Store in tightly sealed opaque containers to preserve the volatile oil.

Anise and star anise should not be confused with Japanese anise (*Illicium landeolatum*), which is poisonous.

APPLE

One-a-Day Protection

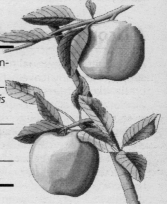

Family: Rosaceae; other members include rose, almond, strawberry

Genus and species: *Malus sylvestris* or *Pyrus malus*

Also known as: No other common names

Parts used: Fruit

An apple a day keeps the doctor away. The old rhyme is truer than ever—particularly if the doctor is a gastroenterologist, cardiologist, or oncologist. Apples may be good for both diarrhea and constipation and may help prevent heart disease, cancer, and some types of stroke—America's top three killers.

Although few contemporary herbalists consider the apple to be an herb, it has a venerable tradition as a healing agent. So much of what the ancient herbalists believed about the healing powers of this delectable fruit has been scientifically supported that it's time to let the apple resume its respected place on the herbal roster.

An Ancient (and Modern) Treatment

The ancient Egyptians, Greeks, and Romans loved apples and developed dozens of varieties, but it was ancient India's traditional Ayurvedic physicians who first prescribed them to relieve diarrhea. Applesauce is still a diarrhea treatment today.

Traditional Chinese physicians have used apple bark for centuries to treat diabetes, another use supported by modern science.

The medieval German abbess/herbalist Hildegard of Bingen prescribed raw apples as a tonic for healthy people and cooked apples as the first treatment for any sickness.

Around the same time in England, people said, "To eat an apple before going to bed/Will make the doctor beg his bread." This evolved into our saying about "an apple a day."

Not everything the English had to say about apples was so apt, however. Seventeenth-century English herbalist Nicholas Culpeper recommended apples "for hot and bilious stomachs . . . inflammations of the breast and lungs . . . [and] asthma." He also suggested boiled apples mixed with milk as a treatment for gunpowder burns.

The Americas had no native apples, but the Pilgrims brought apple seeds with them, and the fruit quickly became, well, as American as apple pie.

Apples, apple bark, and apple cider soon became mainstays of American folk medicine. A century ago, Eclectic physicians recommended raw apples for constipation, baked or stewed apples for minor fevers, apple bark decoction for "intermittent fever" (malaria), and apple cider "as a refreshing drink for patients with fever."

HEALING with Apples

Modern medical science has found that Johnny Appleseed's passion fruit has tremendous value in healing—thanks to its pulp, which is high in pectin, a soluble form of fiber.

Diarrhea. Some studies show that pectin helps relieve diarrhea because intestinal bacteria transform it into a soothing, protective coating for the irritated intestinal lining. In addition, pectin adds bulk to the stool, which helps resolve both diarrhea and constipation.

Some diarrhea is caused by bacterial infection. One study

shows apple pectin is effective against several types of bacteria capable of causing diarrhea. No wonder pectin is the "pectate" in the over-the-counter diarrhea preparation, Kao-pectate.

Constipation. Physicians recommend diets high in fiber to add bulk to the stool. Bulk stimulates normal bowel contractions and relieves constipation.

Heart Disease and Stroke. Pectin may help reduce blood cholesterol, a key risk factor for heart disease and some types of stroke. In the presence of pectin, the cholesterol we eat remains in the intestinal tract until it is eliminated. So eat an apple for dessert when you have meat and dairy products, and enjoy some protection from their cholesterol.

Cancer. The American Cancer Society recommends a high-fiber diet to help prevent several forms of cancer, particularly colon cancer. Pectin binds certain cancer-causing compounds in the colon, speeding their elimination from the body, according to a study published in the *Journal of the National Cancer Institute*.

Diabetes. Physicians also recommend high-fiber diets to control diabetes. Several studies show that apple pectin helps control blood sugar (glucose) levels in diabetics.

Lead Poisoning. European studies suggest apple pectin helps eliminate lead, mercury, and other toxic heavy metals from the body. Cleansing the body of these poisons is yet another reason for people who live in polluted cities to enjoy the proverbial apple a day.

Wound Infection. Although the pectin in apple fruit is this herb's major medicinal component, apple *leaves* contain an antibiotic (phloretin). If you cut yourself out in the orchard, crush some apple leaves and press them onto the wound as first aid until you can wash and bandage it.

Rx for Apples

Eat the whole fresh fruit to enjoy a wide range of healthful benefits. Green apples tend to taste tart, but they usually have more "snap." Red apples are usually sweeter, but may have a mealy texture. Wash apples with soap and water before eating to eliminate any pesticide residues.

The Safety Factor

U.S. Department of Agriculture herb authority (and poet) James A. Duke, Ph.D., sums up apple safety this way:

> An apple a day keeps the doctor away,
> Or at least that's what some people say.
> But one man, we read,
> Ate a cupful of seed,
> And this man died.
> Overdosed. Cyanide.

Strange but true: Apple seeds contain high levels of cyanide, the powerful poison. It takes an estimated 1/2 cup of seeds to kill the average adult, but considerably less to kill children and the elderly. Many parents are familiar with the stomachaches young children develop when they eat apple cores. The small number of seeds in the typical core poses little risk of serious poisoning, but children should be taught not to eat apple seeds.

Eat all the fresh apples you want, just stay away from the seeds. If apples cause minor discomforts, such as diarrhea or constipation, eat less or stop eating them. If diarrhea or constipation does not improve within a week, consult a physician.

Do not attempt to treat diabetes, high cholesterol, or colon disease solely with herbs. In such cases, apples should be used to complement professional medical care.

Grow Your Favorite Variety

Archeologists have found evidence that humans have been enjoying apples since at least 6500 B.C. Prehistoric apples resembled today's crab apples—small, dry, and mealy. But as agriculture developed, apples became one of the world's first hybridized orchard fruits.

Today about 300 apple varieties grow in the 50 states. Special varieties have been developed for just about every set of growing conditions in North America. Consult a nursery for the varieties best suited to your locale.

Full-size apple trees grow to about 40 feet and spread over 1,600 square feet (40 by 40). However, genetic dwarf apple varieties produce delicious, full-size fruit but grow to only 6 to 12 feet and spread over less than 150 square feet (12 by 12).

Plant the rootstock in a sunny location. Water regularly. Prune at planting, then annually. Different apple varieties have different fertilizer requirements and different pest problems. Consult your nursery.

BALM

Honey of a Healer

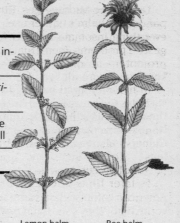

Family: Labiatae; other members include mint

Genus and species: *Melissa officinalis*

Also known as: Lemon balm, bee balm, melissa, sweet balm, cure-all

Parts used: Leaves

Lemon balm   Bee balm

Bees love this fragrant herb, which explains its generic name, *melissa*—Greek for "bee." Balm is also a honey of a healer. It was popular among herbalists for some 2,000 years and is still sweet news for today's herbal enthusiasts.

Be Merry—and Other Ancient Ideas

The ancient Greek physician Dioscorides applied balm leaves to skin wounds and added the herb to wine to treat a variety of illnesses. The Roman naturalist Pliny recommended it to stop bleeding. During the 10th century, Arab doctors recommended balm for nervousness and anxiety. The great 11th-century Arab physician Avicenna wrote, "Balm causeth the mind and heart to become merry."

Medieval Europeans adopted the Arabs' use of balm for nervousness and anxiety. Melissa water, or *Eau de Melisse*, became so popular as a tranquilizer and sedative that Charlemagne ordered the herb grown in all the "physic gardens" in his realm to guarantee an adequate supply.

During the Middle Ages, European herbalists greatly expanded on balm's earlier uses, prescribing it for just about everything: insomnia, arthritis, headache, toothache, sores, digestive problems, menstrual cramps, and as a menstruation promoter—so many ailments, in fact, that balm became known as a cure-all.

In his influential herbal, 17th-century English herbalist Nicholas Culpeper echoed Avicenna, commenting, "It causeth the mind and heart to become merry, and driveth away all troublesome cares and thoughts arising from melancholy. . . ." Culpeper also recommended balm for "faintings and swoonings . . . to help digestion . . . open obstructions of the brain . . . [and] procure women's courses [menstruation]."

In later times, however, the pendulum swung. North American colonists had surprisingly few uses for the bees' favorite herb. They used balm mainly to treat menstrual cramps and to induce sweating, an old treatment for fever. Despite its long history as a tranquilizer, America's 19th-century Eclectic physicians considered balm only as a "moderate stimulant." Nevertheless, today it's still known as a powerful healer.

HEALING with Balm

Contemporary herbalists tout balm's traditional uses: It's still used to induce sweat and menstruation and is recommended to treat headache, flatulence, hypertension, stress, bronchitis, indigestion, asthma, and infant colic. Modern science has not supported all of balm's traditional uses—it has abandoned the 19th-century notion that balm is a stimulant, and Culpeper was off base by saying it "opens obstructions of the brain." But studies show this herb may have even greater healing potential.

Wound Treatment. Score one for Dioscorides. Balm contains chemicals (polyphenols) that may help fight several infection-causing bacteria, among them *Streptococci* and mycobacteria. Balm also contains eugenol, an anesthetic, that may help relieve wound pain.

Herpes and Other Viral Infections. Balm helps fight mumps, herpes, and other viruses. American pharmaceutical companies have ignored balm's possible antiviral action, but Europeans have not. In Germany, where herbal medicine is more mainstream than it is in the United States, balm extract is an active ingredient in Lomaherpan Creme, an ointment used to treat cold sores and genital herpes. Unfortunately, this product is not available in the United States.

A Natural Tranquilizer. Researchers have discovered that balm oil—the source of the plant's pleasant fragrance—may have tranquilizing properties, supporting the herb's traditional use as a relaxant. In Germany, balm is widely used as a tranquilizer and sedative.

Digestive Aid. German researchers have discovered that balm relaxes the smooth muscle tissue of the digestive tract, thus supporting its age-old use as a digestive aid.

Women's Health. Herbs that relax the digestive tract may also calm another smooth muscle, the uterus. This potential effect could help support balm's traditional use in treating menstrual cramps. However, balm has also been historically recommended as a uterine stimulant to promote menstruation. No contemporary research clarifies this confusing situation. For this reason, pregnant women should not use it. Other women might try it to begin menstruation.

Rx for Balm

For a relaxing bath, tie a handful of balm in a cloth and run your bathwater over it. In addition to feeling its tranquil effect, you'll love its lemony aroma.

To help treat wounds, make a hot compress using 2 teaspoons of leaves per cup of water. Boil 10 minutes, strain, and apply with a clean cloth.

For a light, lemony-tasting infusion, which may help soothe the stomach, fight infection, or ease menstrual pain, use 2 teaspoons of leaves per cup of water. Steep 10 to 20 minutes. Drink up to 3 cups a day.

In a tincture, use $1/2$ to $1 1/2$ teaspoons up to three times a day.

When using commercial preparations, follow package directions.

Medicinal infusions or tinctures of balm should not be given to children under age 2. For older children and people over 65, start with low-strength preparations and increase strength if necessary.

To help treat a minor cut, crush some fresh balm leaves and apply them directly to the wound.

The Safety Factor

Two recent studies show that balm interferes with the thyroid-stimulating hormone, thyrotropin. There are no reports of this herb causing thyroid problems, but anyone with a thyroid condition should discuss balm's thyrotropin-inhibiting effect with a physician before using it.

Balm is on the Food and Drug Administration's list of herbs generally regarded as safe. The medical literature contains no reports of toxicity. For otherwise healthy nonpregnant, nonnursing adults who do not have thyroid conditions, balm is considered safe in amounts typically recommended.

Balm should be used in medicinal amounts only in consultation with your doctor. If balm causes minor discomfort, such as stomach upset or diarrhea, take less or stop using it. Let your doctor know if you experience any unpleasant effects or if the symptoms for which the herb is being used do not improve significantly in two weeks.

Sweeten Up Your Garden

Balm is a branching, erect perennial that grows to 2 feet. It has the mint family's characteristic square stems and small, two-lipped, white or yellow flowers, which bloom in bunches throughout the summer. The aboveground parts die back each winter, but the root is perennial.

Balm grows easily from seeds sown in spring or from cuttings or root divisions. Seeds germinate indoors or out and often do best when left uncovered. Simply keep them moist. Germination typically takes three to four weeks.

Balm likes well-drained soil with a pH near neutral. Thin seedlings to 1-foot spacing. The herb prefers partial shade. It wilts in full sun and loses some aroma.

For medicinal use, the leaves should be harvested before the plant flowers. Cut the entire plant a few inches above the ground. Dry it quickly or the leaves may turn black. Balm loses much of its fragrance when dried. After drying, powder the leaves, then store them in tightly sealed opaque containers to preserve the volatile oil.

BARBERRY AND OREGON GRAPE

Powerful Antibiotics—and More

Family: Berberidaceae; other members include May apple, mandrake, blue cohosh

Genus and species: *Berberis vulgaris;* Oregon grape: *B. aquifolium* or *Mahonia aquifolium*

Also known as: Berberry, berberis, jaundice berry

Parts used: Root bark

W ho says herbs can't compete with drugs? In one study, berberine, the active constituent in barberry, proved more potent against bacteria than chloramphenicol, a powerful pharmaceutical antibiotic. But there's a lot more to this herb than mere infection treatment. Barberry, and its close relative, Oregon grape, also may stimulate the immune system, reduce blood pressure, and even shrink some tumors.

Ancient Healer

Barberry has played a prominent role in herbal healing for more than 2,500 years. The ancient Egyptians used it to prevent plagues, a use that was probably effective considering its antibiotic action. India's traditional Ayurvedic healers prescribed it for dysentery, another use confirmed by modern science.

"Jaundice Berry"

During the early Middle Ages, European herbalists were guided by the Doctrine of Signatures, the belief that a plant's physical appearance revealed its therapeutic benefits. Barberry has yellow flowers, and its roots produce a yellow dye. These features were linked to the yellowing of the skin and eyes during jaundice, a symptom of liver disease. As a result, barberry was widely used to treat liver and gallbladder ailments and earned the name "jaundice berry."

In addition to using barberry for liver and gallbladder problems, traditional Russian healers recommended it for inflammations, high blood pressure, and abnormal uterine bleeding.

When the colonists introduced barberry into North America, the Indians recognized it as a relative of the native Oregon grape, a hollylike plant that they considered a powerful healer. Many tribes adopted barberry enthusiastically and used it to treat dysentery, mouth ulcers, sore throat, wound infections, and intestinal complaints.

The 19th-century American Eclectic physicians prescribed barberry as a purgative and treatment for jaundice, dysentery, eye infections, cholera, fevers, and "impurities of the blood," a euphemism for syphilis.

The Hoxsey Formula

Barberry was an ingredient in the popular—but highly controversial—Hoxsey Cancer Formula, an alternative cancer therapy marketed from the 1930s to the 1950s by ex–coal miner Harry Hoxsey (see page 23).

HEALING with Barberry

Most present-day herbalists limit their recommendations to gargling barberry decoction for sore throat and drinking it for diarrhea and constipation. But if they read the medical journals, they'd recommend it for a great deal more.

Antibiotic. The berberine in barberry has remarkable infection-fighting properties. Studies around the world show it kills microorganisms that cause wound infections (*Staphylococci*, *Streptococci*), diarrhea (*Salmonella*, *Shigella*), dysentery (*Endamoeba histolytica*), cholera (*Vibrio cholerae*), giardiasis (*Giardia lamblia*), urinary tract infections (*Escherichia coli*), and vaginal yeast infections (*Candida albicans*).

Immune Stimulant. Berberine may also fight infection by stimulating the immune system. Studies show that it activates the macrophages (literally, "big eaters"), white blood cells that devour harmful microorganisms.

Pinkeye. Barberry's traditional use in treating eye problems is alive and well in Germany, where a berberine preparation, Ophthiole, is used to treat sensitive eyes, inflamed lids, and pinkeye (conjunctivitis). Unfortunately, the product is not available in the United States. A compress made from an herbal infusion may prove helpful, however.

High Blood Pressure. Barberry contains chemicals that may help reduce elevated blood pressure by enlarging blood vessels, thus lending support to the herb's traditional Russian use as a treatment for high blood pressure.

Intriguing Possibilities. Perhaps old Harry Hoxsey was right. One study shows that barberry helps shrink some tumors.

Another shows it has anti-inflammatory activity, suggesting possible value in treating arthritis.

More research needs to be done in both areas before any specific recommendations can be made.

Dead-End File. A few contemporary herbalists continue to recommend barberry as "one of the best remedies for correcting liver function." British researchers have isolated substances in the plant which promote the flow of bile, but barberry is not considered therapeutic for jaundice or other liver problems. So much for "jaundice berry."

R$_x$ for Barberry

For a decoction, use $1/2$ teaspoon of powdered root bark, boiled in a cup of water for 15 to 30 minutes. Drink cool. Drink up to 1 cup a day. The taste is quite bitter. Mask it with honey or an herbal beverage blend.

Barberry should not be given to children under age 2. For older children and people over 65, start with a lower-strength preparation and increase strength if necessary.

To make a compress to treat pinkeye, soak a clean cloth in a barberry infusion.

The Safety Factor

In high doses, barberry can cause nausea, vomiting, convulsions, hazardous drops in blood pressure, and depression of heart rate and breathing. Those with heart disease or chronic respiratory problems should be careful not to take large doses and should take this herb only with the knowledge and approval of their physicians.

Berberine may stimulate the uterus. Thus, pregnant women should not use it.

Barberry is a powerful herb and it should be used cautiously by otherwise healthy nonpregnant, nonnursing adults. Barberry should be used in medicinal amounts only in consultation with your doctor. If barberry causes minor discomforts, such as stomach upset or diarrhea, use less or stop using it. If it causes dizziness or faintness, stop using it. Let your doctor know if you experience any unpleasant effects or if the symptoms for which the herb is being used do not improve significantly in two weeks.

You Can Always Make Jam

Barberry is a perennial shrub that reaches 8 feet. It has smooth gray bark, long spines, and hanging clusters of bright yellow flowers that bloom in spring.

Barberry grows easily in the Northeast and Midwest. Plant seed in the fall in fertile, moist, well-drained soil. Germination occurs the following spring. The shrub can also be propagated from cuttings.

Barberry prefers sun but tolerates shade. Prune and thin the branches in the spring after the shrub flowers. Neglected shrubs become overgrown and unhealthy, but can be rejuvenated by fertilizing and cutting back to within a foot of the ground in late winter. In areas with cold winters, shelter the plant from the wind. Harvest the root bark in spring or fall, and dry.

This herb's edible berries are used to make jams and jellies. The berry juice may substitute for lemon juice.

BASIL

Pesto Versus Parasites

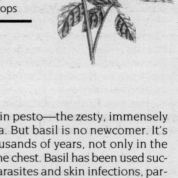

Family: Labiatae; other members include mint

Genus and species: *Ocimum basilicum, O. sanctum*

Also known as: Sweet basil, St. Josephwort

Parts used: Leaves and flower tops

Basil is a key ingredient in pesto—the zesty, immensely popular sauce for pasta. But basil is no newcomer. It's been a favorite for thousands of years, not only in the kitchen but also in the medicine chest. Basil has been used successfully to treat intestinal parasites and skin infections, particularly acne. It may also stimulate the immune system.

Reviled and Revered in Folklore

Considering basil's current popularity, it's amazing what a contradictory reputation it has had down through the ages. To the ancient Greeks and Romans, the herb was a symbol of hostility and insanity. They believed that to grow truly fragrant basil, one had to shout and swear angrily while sowing its seeds. Even today in French "sowing basil" (*semer le basilic*) means "ranting."

Other folk traditions have associated the herb with love. During recent centuries, when an Italian woman placed a potted basil plant on her balcony, it signaled that she was ready to receive her lover. And in northern Europe, lovers exchanged basil sprigs as signs of faithfulness.

In India, basil has long been revered as a sacred herb. The native species is even called *Ocimum sanctum*, "holy basil." It is considered sacred to the gods Vishnu and Krishna and believed to be a protector in life and death. Haitians also believe in basil's protective powers. Shopkeepers in Haiti sprinkle basil water around their stores to ward off evil spirits and bring prosperity.

Is It Bad or Good?

Basil's reputation in healing has been equally contradictory. The ancient Greek physician Dioscorides and the influential Roman doctor Galen both warned against taking basil internally, saying it caused insanity and spontaneous generation of internal worms.

But the Roman naturalist Pliny and Arab physicians 1,000 years later defended it as a great healer, as did the Chinese, who used it to treat stomach, kidney, and blood ailments.

During the 11th century, the German abbess Hildegard of Bingen used basil in a complicated mixture that included "powder from a vulture's beak," to treat cancerous tumors.

By the 17th century, basil was widely used in Europe to treat colds, warts, and intestinal worms. Then the French botanist Tournefort published a tale that tarnished the herb's reputation for years:

> "A certain Gentleman of Sienna, being wonderfully taken and delighted with the Smell of Basil, was wont very frequently to take the Powder of the dry Herb, and snuff it up his Nose; but in short Time, he'd turn'd mad and died; and his Head being opened by Surgeons, there was found a Nest of Scorpions in his Brain."

Used on Everything

As the centuries passed, the scorpion story faded. Basil has never become a major healing herb in North America, but around the world, it has been used as frequently in healing as in cooking. The medicinal plant database at the U.S. Department of Agriculture shows basil has been recommended for just about every conceivable ailment: alcoholism, boredom, childbirth recovery, cholera, colds, constipation, convulsions, cough, cramps, croup, deafness, delirium, depression, diarrhea, dropsy (congestive heart failure), and dysentery—and this list just takes us through the D's!

In the Philippines, basil poultices are applied to ringworm infections, and pregnant women drink basil tea to induce labor. In El Salvador, the herb is placed in the ear to treat deafness. And in Malaya, basil is used to expel intestinal worms and promote menstruation.

If they mention basil at all, American herbalists suggest it as a digestive aid, appetite stimulant, and milk promoter in nursing women.

HEALING with Basil

One best-selling herb guide states: "No modern medical studies have confirmed any of basil's supposed effects." This is hardly the case. Basil's merits have certainly been overblown around the world—putting it in your ear won't cure deafness—but the herb has proven to have definite benefits.

Intestinal Parasites. Basil oil really does kill intestinal parasites, thus confirming its traditional use in Malaya and lending credence to its age-old use as a stomach soother and treatment for a broad range of intestinal ailments.

Acne. Indian researchers have reported that basil kills bacteria when applied to the skin. They have used basil oil successfully to treat acne.

Immune Stimulant. One animal study shows basil stimulates the immune system by increasing production of disease-fighting antibodies by up to 20 percent. This may help explain its supposed effectiveness against bacteria and its traditional uses in treating many infectious illnesses.

R$_x$ for Basil

Scientifically prepared basil oil is more concentrated than even the strongest home infusion or tincture. But if you've become frustrated by the ineffectiveness of other acne remedies, it probably won't hurt to try a strong, fragrant infusion or tincture of basil. Apply with a cotton ball to freshly washed skin.

For an infusion, use 2 to 3 teaspoons of dried leaves per cup of boiling water. Steep 10 to 20 minutes. Drink up to 3 cups a day and enjoy basil's rich, warm aroma and minty, mildly peppery taste.

In a tincture, use ½ to 1 teaspoon up to three times a day.

Use either a tincture or an infusion to take advantage of basil's infection-fighting potential.

Basil should not be given in medicinal quantities to children under age 2. For older children and people over 65, start with low-strength preparations and increase strength if necessary.

The Safety Factor

Basil is one of many healing herbs containing both pro- and anti-cancer substances. On the cancer-prevention side, it contains vitamins A and C, antioxidants that help prevent the cell damage scientists believe eventually leads to cancer. But basil also contains a chemical (estragole) that produced liver tumors in mice, according to a report published in the *Journal of the National Cancer Institute*.

The cancer risk, if any, from basil remains unclear. Not even the most conservative herb critics advise caution when using basil.

No uterine stimulant has ever been identified in basil, but

given its pervasive multicultural use as a menstruation promoter and labor inducer, pregnant women should probably limit their consumption to culinary amounts. Other women might try it to trigger menstruation.

Despite its estragole content, basil is on the Food and Drug Administration's list of herbs generally regarded as safe. For otherwise healthy nonpregnant, nonnursing adults who do not have liver disease, basil is considered safe in amounts typically recommended.

Basil should be used in medicinal amounts only in consultation with your doctor. If basil causes minor discomforts, such as stomach upset or diarrhea, use less or stop using it. Let your doctor know if you experience unpleasant effects or if the symptoms for which the herb is being used do not improve significantly in two weeks.

Presto, Pesto!

An aromatic annual that reaches 2 feet, basil has the mint family's square stem but more branches than most mints, with toothed, pointed, oval leaves, and spikes of small white or purplish flowers that blossom in summer.

Basil grows easily from seeds planted after danger of frost has passed, when the soil has warmed to about 50°F. Plant seeds about 1/8 inch deep. Germination typically takes a week. Basil grows best in well-drained, manure- or compost-amended soil under full sun. Thin seedlings to 1-foot spacing.

After plants are established, mulch around them to conserve water and discourage weeds. Pinching promotes bushiness. After six weeks, cut the main stem above a node to produce twin-stem plants. Tim branches every few weeks. Use fresh leaves, or dry and store them in airtight opaque containers.

BAY

Beyond Bug Repellent

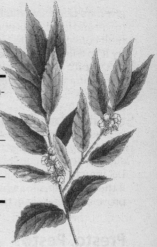

Family: Lauraceae; other members include avocado, cinnamon, nutmeg

Genus and species: *Laurus nobilis*

Also known as: Laurel, sweet bay, green bay, Grecian or Roman laurel

Parts used: Leaves

How ironic that the herb the ancients used to crown their poets and top athletes should turn out to be useful as a cockroach repellent. Most of the traditional uses for this once-glorious herb have not held up to scientific scrutiny, but don't toss it out just yet.

Some intriguing new research suggests that bay has yet to reveal its most potent secrets.

A Divine Heritage

Graduating medical students still recite the Hippocratic oath, which begins: "I swear by Apollo, the physician. . . ." Legend has it that we owe the bay laurel to Apollo, Greek god of medicine. It seems Apollo loved the beautiful nymph, Daphne, but Daphne loathed Apollo. When Daphne begged the gods to protect her from her amorous pursuer, they transformed her into the bay laurel.

97

Lovelorn Apollo declared the tree sacred. He bestowed laurel wreaths on distinguished poets and warriors. Mortals adopted the practice, and at the first Olympics in 776 B.C., winners were crowned with laurel wreaths. The Romans crowned their emperors with laurel. Today, distinguished poets are called "laureates," while the formerly noteworthy are said to be "resting on their laurels."

Soother for Sore Joints

The Roman physician Galen considered bay leaves and berries therapeutic for a great variety of ailments, particularly arthritis. He also used it as a menstruation promoter.

About 1,500 years later, 17th-century English herbalist Nicholas Culpeper recommended bay similarly, to treat "all griefs of the joints and womb . . . procure women's courses [menstruation] . . . and cause a speedy delivery in sore travail of childbirth." He also claimed the herb treated worms, cough, itching, shortness of breath, infectious diseases, and "all griefs of the nerves, arteries, and belly."

As time passed, herbalists backed away from Culpeper's exaggerations and used bay mostly to treat arthritis and women's health concerns. In the Middle East, a tincture of bay in brandy was rubbed on sore joints and taken internally to induce labor and abortion.

American Indians and early colonists used bay to promote labor and menstruation and to treat arthritis, headache, stomachache, urinary problems, insect bites and stings, and skin wounds.

But by the 19th century, bay fell out of favor as a healing herb. The Eclectic medical text, *King's American Dispensatory*, concluded: "All that remains of this ancient medication is the use of the oil for rheumatic [arthritis] pains."

HEALING with Bay

If all you do with bay is add a leaf or two to soups and stews, you're missing an opportunity to use a natural soother.

Bay will never replace sleeping pills, but it has a number of benefits, mainly in the area of mental health.

Stress Management. Low doses of bay oil have been found to sedate laboratory animals, and higher doses produce temporary stupor. The herb also reduces blood pressure in laboratory animals, but the effect is mild. Bay has never been shown to put people to sleep or lower their blood pressure, but these animal results are suggestive. Many people find that bay infusions are relaxing. Added to the bath, the herb seems to help some people relax and fall asleep.

Cockroach Repellent. On the subject of stress management, few household situations are more stressful than the sight of cockroaches scurrying around the kitchen. A chemical (cineole) in bay repels them, according to an article in *Science News*. If you're plagued by these pesky insects, spread some crushed bay leaves around your kitchen cupboards.

Infection. Like most aromatic spices, bay leaf oil kills disease-causing bacteria and fungi. Bay is not a powerful enough antiseptic to be used in place of appropriate medical treatment, but for minor household accidents, the fresh herb can be used externally.

Intriguing Possibility. In one recent study, laboratory animals were given a fatal dose of strychnine, then promptly treated with a bay oil preparation. They all lived, but scientists aren't sure why. Clearly bay has medical benefits that are yet to be explained.

Dead-End File. Several modern herbals continue to recommend rubbing bay oil into arthritic joints, but modern research has never demonstrated any anti-inflammatory action. Of course, even if bay has no effect on arthritis, the herb is applied by massaging it in, and massage itself is soothing.

R_x for Bay

For first aid, apply some freshly crushed leaves to minor cuts and scrapes.

For a relaxing aromatic infusion with a pleasantly sweet taste, use 1 to 2 teaspoons of crushed leaves per cup of boiling water. Strain the liquid before drinking (the leaves are quite sharp; swallowing a piece of leaf could prove harmful). Drink up to three cups a day. Or add 1 to 2 drops of bay oil to tea, brandy, or honey.

If you prefer a tincture, take ½ to 1 teaspoon up to three times a day.

Do not give medicinal preparations of bay to children under age 2. For older children and people over 65, start with low-strength preparations and increase strength if necessary.

The Safety Factor

No uterine stimulants have been found in bay, but the herb was used for thousands of years to stimulate menstruation and abortion. For that reason, pregnant women should stay away from medicinal doses.

Bay is on the Food and Drug Administration's list of herbs generally regarded as safe. For otherwise healthy nonpregnant, nonnursing adults, bay is considered safe in amounts typically recommended.

Bay should be used in medicinal amounts only in consultation with your doctor. If bay causes minor discomforts, such as stomach upset, use less or stop using it. Let your doctor know if you experience any unpleasant effects or if the symptoms for which the herb is being used do not improve significantly in two weeks.

You may want to avoid external use of bay if you have particularly sensitive skin, as it may cause a rash.

Challenge Your Green Thumb

Bay laurel is a small evergreen tree, which seldom grows taller than 20 feet in the United States. Its shiny, leathery, dark green leaves have wavy edges and grow on short stalks. Its spring-blooming flowers are inconspicuous and have no petals. Bay berries are dark purple or black, have one seed, and are about the size of small grapes.

Daphne played hard to get with Apollo, so perhaps it is fitting that the tree she became is so hard to grow. "Notoriously difficult to propagate" is how Gaea and Shandor Weiss put it in *Growing and Using the Healing Herbs*. "Seeds almost invariably grow moldy; cuttings are very difficult to root, and when successful, take up to six months."

The Weisses recommend purchasing saplings from nurseries. Bays cannot survive cold winters, but they do well in pots, reaching 6 to 8 feet. Grow them indoors and you'll have a wonderfully aromatic plant, not to mention fresh bay leaves all year long. Bays like moderately rich, well-drained soil and plenty of sun. Do not take potted bays outside again until danger of frost has passed.

Leaves may be harvested year-round.

BAYBERRY

All-American Fever Treatment

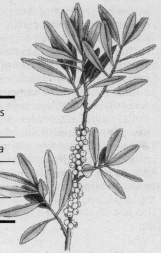

Family: Myricaceae; other members include myrtle

Genus and species: *Myrica cerifera*

Also known as: Wax myrtle, candleberry, tallow shrub

Parts used: Root bark

The early American colonists found the bayberry tree growing throughout the East, but they used it to make fragrant candles rather than medicines. Initially bayberry was used medicinally only in the South, where the Choctaw Indians boiled the leaves and drank the decoction as a treatment for fever. Later, Louisiana settlers adopted the plant and drank bayberry wax in hot water "as a certain cure for the most violent cases of dysentery," according to a medical account from 1722.

Second Only to Hot Pepper

During the early 19th century, bayberry was popularized by Samuel A. Thomson, a New England herbalist and creator of the first patent medicines. He touted it as second only to red pepper for producing "heat" within the body. Thomson recommended bayberry for colds, flu, and other infectious diseases in addition to diarrhea and fever.

Thomson's herbalism lost popularity after the Civil War, replaced by the more scientific Eclectic physicians, who prescribed the astringent herb topically for bleeding gums and internally for diarrhea, dysentery, sore throat, scarlet fever, menstrual difficulties, and even typhoid.

Although bayberry has since waned in popularity, some contemporary herbalists recommend using the herb externally for varicose veins and internally for diarrhea, dysentery, colds, flu, bleeding gums, and sore throat. One modern herbal calls it "one of the most useful herbs in botanical medicine" and goes so far as to advocate treating uterine bleeding by packing the vagina with cotton soaked in bayberry tea. (Do not do this. See a physician for unusual uterine bleeding.)

HEALING with Bayberry

Two hundred years ago bayberry was widely used medicinally. It's a shame it's been almost forgotten, because science has shown this native American herb may have some real benefits in treating fever and diarrhea.

Diarrhea. Bayberry root bark contains an antibiotic chemical (myricitrin), which may fight a broad range of bacteria and protozoa. Myricitrin's antibiotic action supports bayberry's traditional use against diarrhea and dysentery.

Bayberry also contains astringent tannins, which add to its value in treating diarrhea.

Fever. The antibiotic myricitrin also helps reduce fever, thus lending credence to bayberry's use among the Choctaw Indians.

Intriguing Possibility. Myricitrin promotes the flow of bile and might potentially be of value in liver and gallbladder ailments, but as yet no research demonstrates this.

Rx for Bayberry

For a decoction, boil 1 teaspoon of powdered root bark in a pint of water for 10 to 15 minutes. Add a bit of milk and drink cool, up to 2 cups a day. You'll find the taste bitter and astringent. A tincture might go down more easily.

In a tincture, take $1/2$ teaspoon up to twice a day.

Bayberry should not be given to children under age 2. For older children and people over 65, start with a low-strength preparation and increase strength if necessary.

The Safety Factor

The high tannin content of bayberry makes the herb of questionable value for anyone with a history of cancer. In various studies, tannins show both pro- and anti-cancer action. Their cancer-promoting action has received more publicity, notably from a study published in the *Journal of the National Cancer Institute*, which showed that tannins produce malignant tumors in laboratory animals. But tannins have also been shown to have an anti-cancer effect against some animal tumors.

Tannins' effects on human cancer remain unclear. Small quantities have never been implicated in human tumors, but Asians who drink large quantities of tea, which contains tannins, show unusually high rates of stomach cancer. Adding milk neutralizes the tannins, which may be why the tea-loving British have a low rate of stomach cancer. Those with a history of cancer, particularly stomach or colon cancer, should exercise caution and not use this herb. Others should drink no more than recommended amounts, and for extra safety, add milk.

Other Side Effects

In large doses, bayberry root bark may cause stomach distress, nausea, and vomiting. Those with chronic gastrointestinal conditions, such as colitis, for example, should use it cautiously.

Bayberry changes the way the body uses sodium and potassium. Those who must watch their sodium/potassium balance, such as people with kidney disease, high blood pressure, or congestive heart failure, for example, should consult their physicians before using it.

For otherwise healthy nonpregnant, nonnursing adults who need not pay special attention to their sodium/potassium balance, do not have gastrointestinal conditions, and have no history of stomach or colon cancer, bayberry root bark may be used cautiously in amounts typically recommended.

Bayberry should be used in medicinal amounts only in consultation with your doctor. If bayberry causes minor discomforts such as nausea or vomiting, use less or stop using it. Let your doctor know if you experience any unpleasant effects or if the symptoms for which the herb is being used do not improve significantly in two weeks.

Flourishes in Florida

Bayberry is native to the area from New Jersey to the Great Lakes and south to Florida and Texas. In the Southeast, it matures into an evergreen tree that reaches about 35 feet. Further north, the plant becomes smaller. Around the Great Lakes, mature plants rarely grow taller than 3 feet.

Bayberry has grayish bark, waxy branches, and dense, narrow, delicately toothed leaves dotted with resin glands, which produce a fragrant aroma when crushed. Yellow flowers appear in spring and produce nutlike fruits thickly covered with the wax once so highly valued in candlemaking.

Bayberry grows from seeds planted in spring or early fall. It prefers peaty soil under full sun but tolerates poorer sandy soil along streams and in swampy areas. Plants require little care other than pruning.

Harvest the root bark after a few years.

BLACKBERRY

Not Just Jam and Jelly

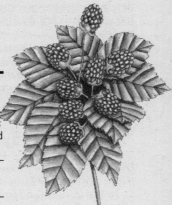

Family: Rosaceae; other members include rose, apple, almond, strawberry

Genus and species: *Rubus fruticosus* (European); *R. villosus* (American); and other species

Also known as: Bramble, dewberry, goutberry

Parts used: Leaves, bark, roots, fruit

If your acquaintance with the blackberry is confined to jam and jelly, it's time to branch out. You have to look to the whole bush to benefit from its full potential.

The blackberry bush was once as highly prized for its medicinal leaves, bark, and roots as it was for its sweet fruit. Today, however, blackberry has fallen from healing fashion, replaced by its close botanical relative, raspberry. It's time to bring back blackberry. Externally it may help treat wounds, and internally, it's a tasty treatment for mouth sores, sore throat, and diarrhea.

"Goutberry"

The ancient Greeks used blackberry to treat gout. They were the only people to use the herb as a treatment for this disorder, but Greek medicine was so influential in Europe that well into the 18th century, the herb was called goutberry.

The ancient Chinese used the unripe berries to treat kidney problems, urinary incontinence, and impotence.

The Romans chewed the leaves and bark for bleeding gums and drank a decoction for diarrhea.

Tenth-century Arab physicians considered the fruit an aphrodisiac (it isn't).

"An Excellent Syrup"

During the Middle Ages, blackberry leaves were applied to the skin to soothe burns and scalds.

In his influential *Herbal*, 17th-century English herbalist Nicholas Culpeper called the herb "very binding" and good for "fevers, ulcers, putrid sores of the mouth and secret parts [genitals], spitting blood [tuberculosis], piles [hemorrhoids], stones of the kidney, too much flowing of women's courses [menstruation], and hot distempers of the head, eyes, and body."

The 19th-century American Eclectic physicians recommended a preparation made from the fruit as "an excellent syrup which is of much service in dysentery, being pleasant to the taste, mitigating the sufferings of the patient, and ultimately effecting a cure." They also recommended blackberry leaves for gonorrhea, vaginal discharges, recovery from childbirth, and "cholera infantum"—an old term for infant infectious diarrhea, which, in the days before antibiotics, was often fatal (and still is in many parts of the world).

The few contemporary herbalists who discuss blackberry at all recommend it as an astringent for diarrhea.

HEALING with Blackberry

Contrary to the claims of Nicholas Culpeper, blackberry in any form doesn't do much for the genitals, but it is a tasty remedy for several common ills.

Diarrhea. Blackberry's high tannin content makes it quite astringent and supports its traditional use as a treatment for diarrhea and dysentery.

Wounds. Tannin's astringent action helps constrict blood vessels and stop minor bleeding. This action would tend to explain the traditional external use of the herb to treat wounds. Blackberry thorns often *cause* minor cuts, so it's nice to know first aid is close at hand.

Mouth Sores, Sore Throat. Enjoy some of the sweet, ripe berries. Their astringent tannins might help.

Hemorrhoids. The astringent nature of blackberry may explain its traditional use as a hemorrhoid treatment.

Intriguing Possibilities. One animal study shows that a strong infusion of blackberry leaves reduces blood sugar levels in diabetic rabbits, suggesting possible value in the management of diabetes.

Research has shown that blackberry's close relative, raspberry, relaxes the uterus. Women might try blackberry for painful menstrual cramps.

Rx for Blackberry

To treat diarrhea or soothe a sore throat, try an infusion, decoction, or tincture. For an infusion, use 2 to 3 teaspoons of dried leaves per cup of boiling water. Steep 10 to 20 minutes. Add a bit of milk. Drink up to 3 cups a day. You can also use a handful of crushed berries, either dried or fresh, or 1 to 2 teaspoons of dried powdered bark to make an infusion.

For a decoction, use 1 teaspoon of powdered root per cup of water. Boil for 30 minutes. Drink up to 1 cup a day. Enjoy it with a bit of milk.

In a tincture, take up to 2 teaspoons a day.

In commercial preparations, follow package directions.

To treat wounds or hemorrhoids, soak a clean cloth in a tincture or strong infusion and apply externally.

Medicinal doses of blackberry should not be given to children under age 2. For older children and people over 65, start with low-strength preparations and increase strength if necessary.

The Safety Factor

Safety questions have been raised about tannins. In various studies, they show both pro- and anti-cancer action. Their cancer-promoting action has received more publicity, notably from a study published in the *Journal of the National Cancer Institute*, which showed that tannins produce malignant tumors in laboratory animals. But tannins apparently also have an anti-cancer effect against some animal tumors.

Tannins' effects on human cancer remain unclear. Small quantities have never been implicated in human tumors, but Asians who drink large quantities of tea, which is high in tannins, show unusually high rates of stomach cancer. Adding milk neutralizes the tannins, which appears to be why the tea-loving British have a low rate of stomach cancer. People with a history of cancer, particularly stomach or colon cancer, should exercise caution and not use medicinal quantities of this herb. Other people should take no more than recommended amounts of infusions or decoctions, and for extra safety, add a bit of milk.

Distress Signals

In large amounts, tannins may cause stomach distress, nausea, and vomiting. Blackberry root bark contains the most tannins, followed by the leaves, and finally the fruit. People with chronic gastrointestinal conditions, such as colitis, for example, should probably not use the roots.

For otherwise healthy nonpregnant, nonnursing adults, blackberry is safe in amounts typically recommended.

Blackberry should be used in medicinal amounts only in consultation with your doctor. If blackberry causes minor discomforts such as nausea or vomiting, use less or stop using it. Let your doctor know if you experience any unpleasant effects or if the symptoms for which the herb is being used do not improve significantly in two weeks.

Go Wild in the Garden

Blackberry bushes grow wild around most of North America. They have long, tangled, thorny stems, lush foliage, and a profusion of berries that turn red as they ripen and become a juicy, purplish blue-black by midsummer.

Blackberry bushes are so vigorous and invasive, they quickly become a thick, thorny, impenetrable mass. Rooting them out is almost impossible—as any gardener who has tried can attest. Even when removed, stray root fragments continue to send up new shoots. To minimize problems, plant this shrub in containers or surround its roots with sheet metal.

Blackberries grow easily from ½-inch root cuttings taken in autumn and stored through the winter in cool sand (around 50°F). Plant cuttings vertically 1 to 3 feet apart in 3 to 4 inches of soil.

Blackberries adapt to many conditions but grow best in loose, moist, rich soil amended with manure or finished compost. The plants flower in spring and bear fruit throughout the summer.

Harvest the leaves and roots any time. For ease of harvesting the berries, train the branches along supports and prune them mercilessly.

BLACK COHOSH

The Indians Were Right

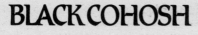

Family: Ranunculaceae; other members include buttercup, larkspur, peony

Genus and species: *Cimicifuga racemosa* or *Macrotys actaeoides*

Also known as: Squawroot, snakeroot

Parts used: Rhizome and root

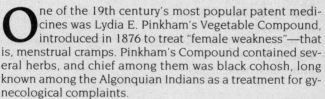

Root

One of the 19th century's most popular patent medicines was Lydia E. Pinkham's Vegetable Compound, introduced in 1876 to treat "female weakness"—that is, menstrual cramps. Pinkham's Compound contained several herbs, and chief among them was black cohosh, long known among the Algonquian Indians as a treatment for gynecological complaints.

Pinkham's product also contained an enormous amount of alcohol. During the 19th century, respectable ladies did not drink liquor. Many drank Lydia E. Pinkham's Vegetable Compound instead. A reformulated Vegetable Compound is still available today—minus most of the alcohol and, ironically, without any black cohosh, the ingredient that may have had the greatest effect on menstrual pain.

Medicine for Indian Women

This herb was named *black* because of its dark medicinal roots. *Cohosh* is Algonquian for "rough," another reference to its roots.

The Indians boiled black cohosh's gnarled roots in water and drank the decoction for fatigue, sore throat, arthritis, and rattlesnake bite—hence one popular name for this herb, "snakeroot." But black cohosh was used primarily by Indian women for gynecological problems and childbirth.

Wild black cohosh grew most profusely in the Ohio River Valley, which was fitting because the herb was championed by 19th-century Eclectic physicians, whose medical school was in Cincinnati on the banks of the Ohio. The Eclectics recommended black cohosh for fever, rashes, insomnia, malaria, yellow fever, and all "hysterical" (gynecological) ailments. The Eclectic medical text, *King's American Dispensatory*, stated: "In dysmenorrhea [menstrual cramps], it is of greatest utility, being surpassed by no other drug."

Non-Eclectic ("regular") physicians remained unimpressed, but Lydia Pinkham sided with the Eclectics and included it in her Vegetable Compound.

Many Modern Uses

Black cohosh does not grow in China, but Chinese physicians use several related plants to treat headache, measles, diarrhea, bleeding gums, and some gynecological problems.

Homeopaths recommend microdoses of black cohosh for menstrual problems and childbirth.

Contemporary herbalists prescribe it to relieve spasms, as a diuretic to treat water retention, as an expectorant to help clear mucus from the respiratory system, and as an astringent, sedative, and menstruation promoter. Several modern herbals, in fact, call it "one of our best" menstruation promoters.

HEALING with Black Cohosh

When used safely, this herb may play a role in healing. Because of its possible side effects, however, it should be used only with the approval and supervision of your physician. Several studies show its early advocates may have been right about the herb's potential to treat gynecological problems.

Menstrual Discomforts. Black cohosh has estrogenic effects, meaning it acts like the female sex hormone estrogen. The herb's estrogenic action may lend support to its traditional use for menstrual complaints.

Estrogenic herbs must be used carefully, however. Estrogen is a key ingredient in birth control pills. Any woman whose physician advises her not to take the Pill may have to avoid using this herb as well. She should discuss black cohosh's estrogenic activity with her doctor before using this herb.

Menopausal Discomforts. Estrogen is also prescribed for menopausal symptoms, and herbs with estrogenic action can be expected to have a similar effect on these symptoms. Today in Germany, where herbal healing is more mainstream than it is in the United States, black cohosh is a key ingredient in three drugs prescribed for discomforts of menopause. The German text *Herbal Medicine* says the drugs "appear to be effective . . . We can, in many cases, manage without hormones, though . . . success is not instant. The drug has to be given over some time . . . " These drugs are not available in the United States, but the herb itself is.

When used to treat menopausal discomforts, estrogen by itself may increase a woman's risk of uterine cancer. Taking another female sex hormone, progesterone, minimizes this risk. Any woman considering using black cohosh for menopause should consult her physician about using the herb by itself or in conjunction with progesterone.

Prostate Cancer. Female sex hormones slow the growth of prostate tumors. Physicians often prescribe hormones similar to estrogen for men with prostate cancer. Black cohosh's estrogenic action may help manage this cancer, but men with prostate cancer should consult their physicians before using it.

High Blood Pressure. A study published in *Nature* shows black cohosh reduces blood pressure by opening the blood vessels in the limbs (peripheral vasodilation). The herb may help manage high blood pressure, but consult your physician before using it for this purpose.

Intriguing Possibilities. One study shows black cohosh has anti-inflammatory activity, possibly explaining its Indian use as a treatment for arthritis. Another report shows it reduces animal blood sugar levels, suggesting possible value in controlling diabetes.

More study needs to be done to determine whether the herb will prove useful in treating these conditions.

Other preliminary animal findings point to possible antibiotic, sedative, and stomach-soothing action.

Rx for Black Cohosh

For a decoction, boil ½ teaspoon of powdered root per cup of water for 30 minutes. Let cool. It has an unpleasant aroma and a sharp, bitter taste. Add lemon and honey, or mix with a beverage tea. Take 2 tablespoons every few hours, up to 1 cup a day.

In a tincture, take up to 1 teaspoon per day.

Children under age 2 and people over 65 should start with low-strength preparations and increase strength if necessary.

The Safety Factor

Physicians argued about black cohosh a century ago, and the debate continues today. A 1986 Food and Drug Administration report dismissed black cohosh as having "no therapeutic value" and warned of its possible side effects. Other experts say the herb has many potentially beneficial effects but consider it too toxic to use. The Germans, meanwhile, include the herb in several prescription drugs to relieve menopausal discomforts.

Black cohosh overdose may cause dizziness, light-headedness, nausea, diarrhea, abdominal pain, vomiting, visual dimness, headache, tremors, joint pains, and depressed heart rate. For some, these effects may develop at relatively low doses.

In addition to the side effects listed above, the estrogen-like component of the herb may act just like estrogen itself and contribute to liver problems and abnormal blood clotting, as well as promote the development of certain types of breast tumors. Finally, pregnant women should not use estrogenic herbs.

Black cohosh's possible effects on the heart are most worrisome. Anyone with heart disease, especially congestive heart failure, should not use it.

Potentially Potent

Black cohosh is a potentially hazardous herb that should be used cautiously. Otherwise healthy nonpregnant, nonnursing adults who do not have heart disease or estrogen-dependent cancers and are not taking sedatives, blood pressure medication, birth control pills, or postmenopausal estrogen, may use it for short periods in amounts typically recommended—but only with a physician's consent.

If any of the side effects listed above develop, use less or stop using it. Let your doctor know if you experience any unpleasant effects or if the symptoms for which the herb is being used do not improve significantly in two weeks.

Get to the Root

Black cohosh is a leafy perennial that reaches 9 feet. It has knotty black roots and a smooth stem with large, toothed, compound leaves and small, multiple white flowers that develop in midsummer on long projections called racemes.

Black cohosh grows from seeds sown in spring or root divisions taken in spring or fall.

Harvest the roots in fall after the fruits have ripened. Cut them lengthwise to dry.

BLACK HAW

Slave Owner's Herb

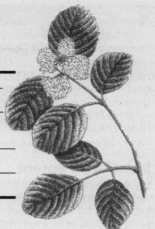

Family: Caprifoliaceae; other members include honeysuckle, elder

Genus and species: *Viburnum prunifolium*

Also known as: Viburnum

Parts used: Bark

B lack haw is an herb with a shadowy past. The reddish-brown bark of this native American shrub has a long history as a folk remedy for gynecological complaints—uses supported by some recent research. Before white people came to this continent, Indian women drank a decoction of black haw bark for menstrual cramps, childbirth recovery, and menopausal discomforts. But its special use was to prevent miscarriage.

It was left to southern slave owners to invent more nefarious uses for the bark—they used black haw coercively to prevent slave abortions. Slaves were a valuable asset, and slaveholders wanted slave women ("breeders") to bear as many children as possible. Slave owners often raped black women for pleasure and to increase their slave holdings. Many slave women attempted to abort the resulting pregnancies as a quiet protest against slavery.

A favorite means of inducing abortions on southern plantations was cotton root, an herb readily available to slaves. According to the 19th-century Eclectic medical text, King's American Dispensatory: "It was customary for planters to compel female slaves to drink an infusion of black haw daily whilst pregnant to prevent abortion from taking the cotton root."

Quiets the "Irritable Womb"

An Eclectic physician from Mississippi introduced black haw to the North, where it quickly became an herbal mainstay for gynecological complaints. The Eclectics valued it highly: "As a uterine tonic, it is unquestionably of great utility . . . for menstrual pains . . . and a good remedy for menopause. . . . But the condition for which black haw is most valued is threatened abortion. By its quieting effect upon the irritable womb, women who have been previously unable to go to term have been aided to pass through pregnancy without mishaps."

Modern herbalists continue to recommend black haw for menstrual cramps and threatened abortion. Some herbals encourage women to drink black haw tea throughout pregnancy.

HEALING with Black Haw

Here is another case where modern science supports folk wisdom—or at least some of it. It turns out that black haw may be a good treatment for some gynecological complaints. But pregnant women are advised against using it.

Menstrual Cramps. A report published in the British journal Nature shows that black haw contains a uterine relaxant (scopoletin), thus supporting its value in treating menstrual cramps. Today in Germany, where herbal medicine is more mainstream than it is in the United States, black haw preparations are widely used for menstrual cramps. These products are not available in the United States, but the herb itself is easily obtained.

Miscarriage Prevention. This herb has been used for centuries to prevent miscarriage. As a uterine relaxant, black haw may indeed do the job. Unfortunately, it also contains salicin, a close chemical relative of aspirin. Because aspirin has been linked to birth defects, pregnant women should not take black haw.

Fever, Headache, Arthritis, and Other Pain. The aspirin-like chemical in black haw may reduce fever and relieve pain.

R$_x$ for Black Haw

Use a decoction or infusion of black haw for relief of menstrual cramps, fever, headache, and general aches and pains.

For a decoction, use 2 teaspoons of dried bark per cup of water. Boil 10 minutes. Cool. Drink up to 3 cups a day. It has an extremely bitter taste, so you may want to take it with lemon and honey or even mix it with a beverage tea.

In a tincture, use up to 2 teaspoons three times a day.

The Safety Factor

Like aspirin, the salicin in black haw is a pain reliever (analgesic), which may contribute to the herb's ability to relieve menstrual cramping. However, aspirin has also been implicated as a cause of birth defects in the children of women who take it while pregnant.

Aspirin is most hazardous to the unborn early in the pregnancy. Recognizing this, the classic British herbal *Potter's New Cyclopaedia of Botanical Drugs and Preparations* says black haw should be used only during the final five weeks of pregnancy to prevent threatened prematurity.

Any woman facing possible premature birth should discuss her situation with her obstetrician. Most physicians advise bed rest for threatened prematurity, along with increased fluid intake and no breast or sexual stimulation. Drugs (including herbs) are a last resort and should only be used with the consent of a doctor.

Parents should not give black haw to children under 16

who are suffering fevers related to colds, flu, or chicken pox, because its salicin may increase the risk of Reye's syndrome, a rare but potentially fatal childhood disease.

Large doses of black haw may produce upset stomach, nausea, vomiting, and/or ringing in the ears (tinnitus), especially in those sensitive to aspirin.

For otherwise healthy nonpregnant, nonnursing adults, black haw is considered safe in amounts typically recommended.

Black haw should be used in medicinal amounts only in consultation with your doctor. If minor discomforts such as stomach upset or ringing in the ears develop, use less or stop using it. Let your doctor know if you experience any unpleasant effects or if menstrual cramps do not improve significantly after two months.

Harvest Branch Bark

In the North, black haw is a deciduous spreading shrub with reddish-brown bark. In the South, it becomes a small tree. The leaves are pointed, serrated ovals and resemble plum leaves. They turn red in fall. Black haw flowers are large, clustered, white, and showy. Depending on location, black haw blooms from early spring to summer.

Black haw grows best in rich, moist, well-drained soil under full sun, but tolerates poorer soil and partial shade as long as it gets adequate moisture. Branch bark may be collected in summer. The trunk bark should be collected in fall. Dry it in the shade.

BLUE COHOSH

Herbal Labor Inducer

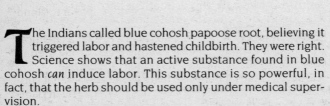

Family: Berberidaceae; other members include may apple, mandrake, barberry

Genus and species: *Caulophyllum thalictroides*

Also known as: Papoose root, blue berry

Parts used: Root

The Indians called blue cohosh papoose root, believing it triggered labor and hastened childbirth. They were right. Science shows that an active substance found in blue cohosh *can* induce labor. This substance is so powerful, in fact, that the herb should be used only under medical supervision.

Blue cohosh is not related to black cohosh—they belong to different botanical families. But the Indians used both as gynecological herbs and called them both *cohosh*, Algonquian for "rough," because they both have gnarled roots. The "blue" refers to this herb's bluish stem and dark blue berries.

Herb of Many Uses

In addition to using it to induce labor, menstruation, and abortion, the Indians also used blue cohosh to treat sore throat, hiccups, infant colic, epilepsy, and arthritis. Some Indian women even drank a strong decoction as a contraceptive.

Nineteenth-century American Eclectic physician John King popularized blue cohosh as a labor inducer and menstruation inducer in the first edition of his *King's American Dispensatory*. The Eclectics also prescribed it for menstrual cramps, breast pain, bladder and kidney infection, insomnia, bronchitis, and nausea.

Non-Eclectic ("regular") physicians never adopted blue cohosh, but it was listed in the U.S. *Pharmacopoeia* as a labor inducer from 1882 to 1905.

Modern herbals recommend blue cohosh as a labor inducer and menstruation promoter. Some herbalists also suggest it for asthma, anxiety, cough, arthritis, and high blood pressure.

HEALING with Blue Cohosh

Blue cohosh's traditional uses in gynecology appear to stand up to scientific scrutiny.

Labor Inducer. Researchers have discovered a chemical (caulosaponin) in blue cohosh that provokes strong uterine contractions, thus supporting its primary Indian use.

However, caulosaponin also narrows the arteries that supply blood to the heart. Blue cohosh has produced heart damage in laboratory animals, and human heart damage seems quite possible from overdose.

On the other hand, blue cohosh does not appear to be significantly more hazardous than Pitocin, the standard drug used to induce labor, which may also cause heart damage and other serious side effects, including even maternal and fetal death.

Pitocin requires constant professional monitoring. Blue cohosh should also be used under strict medical supervision. If you'd like to use it at term, discuss your desire with your obstetrician and/or midwife and use it only with your doctor's consent and supervision.

Menstruation Promotion. As a powerful uterine stimulant, blue cohosh could certainly trigger menstruation. But women should not use it for this purpose. It's too powerful, and its side effects are potentially too serious.

Intriguing Possibilities. Researchers in India have discovered tantalizing evidence that the American Indians may have been on the right track in using blue cohosh as a contraceptive. In animals, the herb inhibits ovulation, according to a report published in the *Journal of Reproduction and Fertility*.

European researchers have identified some antibiotic and immune-stimulating properties in blue cohosh, possibly explaining its use by Eclectic physicians for bladder and kidney infections.

Finally, blue cohosh also has anti-inflammatory activity, lending credence to its traditional use for arthritis.

Dead-End File. Despite its traditional reputation as a treatment for high blood pressure, studies show blue cohosh is more likely to *cause* this serious condition than treat it.

Rx for Blue Cohosh

Blue cohosh is a powerful herb that should be administered by a physician. The decoction tastes initially somewhat sweet, then bitter and unpleasant.

The Safety Factor

No one with high blood pressure, heart disease, diabetes, glaucoma, or a history of stroke should use blue cohosh.

When powdered, blue cohosh root irritates mucous membranes. Handle it with care. Take care not to inhale any or introduce it into your eyes.

Blue cohosh should be used only at term to induce labor, and then *only* under medical supervision.

Easy to Find

Blue cohosh is not a garden herb, but it's easy to recognize in early spring in forests from the Appalachians to the Mississippi. Before other forest-floor plants have shown signs of new life, blue cohosh's blue-purple stem and single large leaf have risen 2 to 3 feet. As spring turns to summer, blue cohosh produces three branches with three compound leaves each.

In summer, the plant produces small yellowish flowers and dark blue berries, which are poisonous and potentially fatal to children. Make sure children do not eat the berries.

BONESET

For Colds and Flu

Family: Compositae; other members include daisy, dandelion, marigold

Genus and species: *Eupatorium perfoliatum*

Also known as: Feverwort, sweat plant

Parts used: Leaves and flower tops

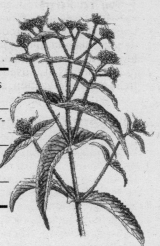

Let's clear up one matter right away: Boneset has nothing to do with mending broken bones. This herb helps treat minor viral and bacterial illnesses by possibly revving up the immune system's response to infection.

Breakbone Fever

Boneset's name comes from its traditional use as a treatment for "breakbone fever," an old term for dengue (pronounced DENG-*ee*) fever. Dengue is a mosquito-borne, viral disease that causes muscle pains so intense that people imagine their bones are breaking, hence its traditional name. Today, dengue is rare in the United States except among overseas travelers, who sometimes return from the tropics with it. Ironically, boneset has never been shown to provide significant relief from dengue fever.

The Indians introduced boneset to early colonists as a sweat-inducer, an old treatment for fevers. The Indians used boneset for all fever-producing illnesses: influenza, cholera, dengue, malaria, and typhoid, hence boneset's other names, feverwort and sweat plant.

The Indians also used boneset to relieve arthritis and to treat colds, indigestion, constipation, and loss of appetite.

In Every Attic and Woodshed

White settlers adopted boneset so enthusiastically, it was one of early America's most popular healing herbs. During the Civil War, soldiers used it not only to treat fever but also as a tonic to keep them healthy. (Modern science shows this is not a good idea. See "The Safety Factor" on page 127.)

In his classic book *American Medicinal Plants*, Dr. C. F. Millspaugh wrote: "There is probably no plant more extensively or frequently used than this. The attic or woodshed of almost every farm house has bunches hanging from the rafters, ready for immediate use should some family member or neighbor be taken with a cold."

Millspaugh also considered boneset excellent against malaria, a major problem in 19th-century America. He wrote he'd seen the herb cure malaria when it didn't respond to Peruvian cinchona bark, the source of the anti-malarial drug, quinine.

Herbal Aspirin

Boneset was listed as a treatment for fever in the U.S. *Pharmacopoeia* from 1820 through 1916, and in the *National Formulary*, the pharmacists' manual, from 1926 through 1950. But over time it fell from favor, replaced by another herbal fever-fighter, aspirin.

Contemporary herbalists continue to recommend boneset enthusiastically for fever. In his *Holistic Herbal*, David Hoffmann calls it "perhaps the best remedy for influenza."

HEALING with Boneset

Modern herbal critics tend to ridicule boneset as passionately as physicians a century ago praised it. One says, "It simply doesn't work." Another claims, "Boneset lacks therapeutic merit." A third writes, "In view of [boneset's] singular lack of effectiveness, it seems incredible that the plant held official status from 1820 to 1950."

Boneset's critics have a point. The herb has never been shown to suppress fever as well as aspirin. However, several recent studies seem to suggest that the herb has some therapeutic value, after all.

Colds and Flu. European studies show this herb helps treat minor viral and bacterial infections by stimulating white blood cells to destroy disease-causing microorganisms more effectively. In Germany, where herbal medicine is more mainstream than it is in the United States, physicians currently use boneset to treat viral infections, such as colds and flu.

Arthritis. One study shows boneset is mildly anti-inflammatory, lending some support to its traditional use in treating arthritis.

Intriguing Possibility. Recent studies conducted worldwide suggest the possible immune stimulants in boneset have anti-cancer effects, but more research is needed before boneset can be used to treat tumors.

Dead-End File. Traditional use notwithstanding, boneset has never been shown to be effective against dengue fever or malaria.

R$_x$ for Boneset

To treat colds, flu, and arthritis, and for minor inflammation, use an infusion or tincture. For an infusion, use 1 to 2 teaspoons of dried leaves per cup of boiling water. Steep 10 to 20 minutes. Drink up to 3 cups a day.

You'll find the taste very bitter and astringent. Add sugar or honey and lemon, or mix it with an herbal beverage tea.

In a tincture, use ¹/₂ to 1 teaspoon up to three times a day.

Boneset should not be given to children under age 2. For older children and people over 65, start with low-strength preparations and increase strength if necessary.

The Safety Factor

In large amounts, boneset may cause nausea, vomiting, and violent diarrhea.

Boneset contains chemicals (pyrrolizidines), which in large amounts cause liver damage and liver tumors in laboratory animals. Boneset's effect on human cancer, if any, is unclear because the plant also contains anti-cancer substances.

However, the pyrrolizidines in some healing herbs, such as comfrey (see page 194), have caused a few cases of liver damage in people who have taken more than recommended amounts for long periods of time. It's not a good idea to take boneset frequently as a tonic. And don't take more than recommended amounts. Anyone with a history of alcoholism, liver disease, or cancer should not use this herb without consulting his physician.

Toxic When Fresh

Do not eat fresh boneset. It contains a toxic chemical (tremerol), which causes nausea, vomiting, weakness, muscle tremors, increased respiration, and at high doses, possibly even coma and death. Drying the herb eliminates the tremerol and the possibility of poisoning.

The Food and Drug Administration lists boneset as an herb of "undefined safety." For otherwise healthy nonpregnant, nonnursing adults who have no history of alcoholism, cancer, or liver disease, boneset is considered safe in amounts typically recommended.

Boneset should be used in medicinal amounts only in consultation with your doctor. If boneset causes minor discomforts, such as stomach upset or a laxative effect, use less or stop using it. Let your doctor know if you experience any unpleasant effects or if the symptoms for which the herb is being used do not improve significantly in two weeks.

Do not take boneset for more than two weeks at a time, and do not exceed recommended amounts.

A Snap to Grow

Boneset is easy to identify because its long, narrow, pointed leaf pairs are not distinct, but rather connected and pierced by the stem.

The herb has round, erect, hairy, hollow stems which grow to 5 feet, then split into three branches, which produce tiny, densely clustered white to bluish florets from midsummer through fall.

A hardy perennial, boneset grows easily from seeds planted in spring or root divisions planted in spring or fall. It prefers rich, moist, well-drained soil under full sun but tolerates poorer soil and partial shade.

Harvest it as it flowers by cutting the entire plant a few inches above the ground.

BUCHU

A South African Water Pill

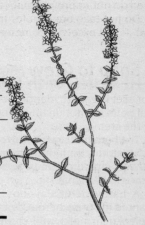

Family: Rutaceae; other members include orange, lemon, rue

Genus and species: *Barosma betulina, B. crenulata, B. serratifolia*

Also known as: Bookoo, buku, bucku, bucco

Parts used: Leaves

Buchu is Southern Africa's contribution to herbal healing.

The leaves of this 5-foot shrub contain an oil that increases urine production. The native peoples of what is now Namibia and South Africa used buchu for urinary problems long before they had any contact with Europeans. In the 17th century, when Dutch (Afrikaner) colonists settled the region, they adopted buchu for urinary tract infections, kidney stones, arthritis, cholera, and muscle aches.

Later English settlers also adopted buchu and used the herb to treat so many illnesses that medical botanists now claim it has been used for "almost every disease which afflicts mankind."

The Buchu King

In 1847, New York patent medicine entrepreneur Henry T. Helmbold introduced Helmbold's Compound Extract of

Buchu for urinary problems, kidney stones, and "diseases arising from imprudence [venereal diseases]." The American public responded as enthusiastically as the African colonists had. Helmbold grew rich and called himself Helmbold, the Buchu King.

HEALING with Buchu

The Buchu King is long forgotten, but herbalists have considered this herb a urinary antiseptic ever since.

Premenstrual Syndrome. Many women complain of "bloating" from water retention before their periods. Buchu is an ingredient in two over-the-counter diuretics (Fluidex and Odrinil) marketed to relieve the bloating of premenstrual syndrome (PMS).

High Blood Pressure and Congestive Heart Failure. Physicians prescribe diuretics to treat high blood pressure and congestive heart failure. These are serious conditions requiring professional care. Consult your physician about including buchu as part of your treatment plan.

Urinary Tract Infection. Most modern herbals continue to recommend buchu for urinary tract infections. One study of its effects on the bacteria that cause these infections showed no benefit, but herbal experts continue to stand behind it as an infection fighter.

Rx for Buchu

For relief of bloating due to PMS, try an infusion or tincture. You might also try these preparations for relief of chronic urinary tract infections.

For an infusion, use 1 to 2 teaspoons of dried, crumbled leaves per cup of boiling water. Steep 10 to 20 minutes. Drink up to 3 cups a day. Buchu has a minty aroma and a pleasant, minty taste.

In a tincture, take 1/2 to 1 teaspoon up to three times a day.

Do not give buchu to children under age 2. For older children and people over 65, start with low-strength preparations and increase strength if necessary.

The Safety Factor

Diuretics deplete body stores of potassium, an important nutrient. Anyone taking buchu should increase consumption of foods high in potassium, such as bananas and fresh vegetables.

Pregnant women should not take diuretics without a physician's approval.

The Food and Drug Administration considers buchu safe, and no harmful effects have been reported. For otherwise healthy nonpregnant, nonnursing adults who are not taking other diuretics, buchu is considered safe in amounts typically recommended.

Buchu should be used in medicinal amounts only in consultation with your doctor. If buchu causes minor discomforts, such as stomach upset or diarrhea, use less or stop using it. Let your doctor know if you experience any unpleasant symptoms or if the symptoms for which the herb is being used do not improve significantly in two weeks.

African Native

This 5-foot shrub with finely toothed opposite or alternative leaves is not grown in the United States.

BUCKTHORN

Relieves Constipation

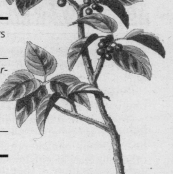

Family: Rhamnaceae; other members include cascara sagrada

Genus and species: *Rhamnus cathartica, R. frangula*

Also known as: Purging buckthorn, frangula, alder buckthorn

Parts used: Berries; bark

This herb's specific name, *cathartica*, is no joke. Buckthorn is a potent laxative—so powerful, in fact, that authorities advise using it only as a last resort, when other, gentler laxatives have failed.

Buckthorn became popular in herbal healing in Europe around the 13th century. At the time, they had few effective medicines to offer. And they believed the key to curing disease lay in purging the body of "foul humours." Not surprisingly, powerful laxatives were widely prescribed. Buckthorn was a favorite because it produced quick, reliable, dramatic results. Of course, it didn't cure any disease. All it did was send people running to their outhouses and leave them with intestinal cramps.

A Long History

Down through the ages, herbalists have also recommended buckthorn for jaundice, hemorrhoids, gout, arthritis, and menstruation promotion.

132

Buckthorn also has a long history as a cancer treatment. In America it was an ingredient in the popular—but highly controversial—Hoxsey Cancer Formula (see page 23).

HEALING with Buckthorn

Buckthorn doesn't treat jaundice or arthritis. And it's more likely to aggravate hemorrhoids than help them. But its laxative action is so powerful, it's considered a purgative.

Purgative. No one disputes buckthorn's laxative effect. It's an ingredient in the over-the-counter laxative Movicol.

Buckthorn contains chemicals (anthraquinones) that are dramatic purgatives—for most people, too dramatic. Buckthorn should be considered a last-resort treatment for constipation. First, eat a diet higher in fiber, drink more fluids, and exercise more. If that doesn't provide relief, try a bulk-forming laxative such as psyllium, for example (see page 423). If that doesn't help, try a gentler anthraquinone, cascara sagrada (see page 144). And if that doesn't work, try buckthorn in consultation with your physician.

Intriguing Possibility. Harry Hoxsey may have been on the right track. Buckthorn has an anti-tumor effect, according to research published in the *Journal of the National Cancer Institute*, but other studies must be conducted before this herb can be used to treat cancer.

Rx for Buckthorn

In Germany, physicians prescribe an infusion containing 1/2 teaspoon each of dried buckthorn bark, fennel seed, and chamomile flowers (which soothe the stomach) steeped in 1 cup of boiling water for 10 minutes. Drink it before bed. You'll find the taste initially sweet, then bitter.

If you prefer a decoction, boil 1 teaspoon of dried buckthorn in 3 cups of water and steep for 30 minutes. Drink cool, 1 tablespoon at a time before bed.

In a tincture, take 1/2 teaspoon before bed.

The Safety Factor

Because of buckthorn's powerful laxative action, it should not be used by people with chronic gastrointestinal problems, such as ulcers, colitis, or hemorrhoids. Pregnant women should not take buckthorn.

Don't use buckthorn for more than two weeks at a time. If you use it too long, it causes lazy bowel syndrome—an inability to move stool without chemical stimulation. If constipation persists, consult a physician.

If you use buckthorn, make sure it has been dried thoroughly. Otherwise, it causes vomiting, severe abdominal pain, and violent diarrhea. Most herbalists recommend drying the berries or bark for at least a year—some say two—before using them. Fresh buckthorn may also be artificially dried by baking at 250°F for several hours. If nausea and abdominal distress develop, seek professional medical attention immediately.

For otherwise healthy nonpregnant, nonnursing adults who do not have any chronic gastrointestinal conditions and are not taking other laxatives, buckthorn may be used very cautiously for short periods of time in amounts typically recommended.

Buckthorn should be used in medicinal amounts only in consultation with your doctor. If violent diarrhea occurs or if intestinal cramps develop, use less or stop using it. Let your doctor know if you experience any unpleasant effects or if constipation does not improve in a few days.

Not for the Garden

Buckthorn is a shrub or small tree which reaches about 20 feet. It has shiny, dark green leaves, and produces black, pea-size berries. It is not a garden herb.

BURDOCK

Likely to Stick Around

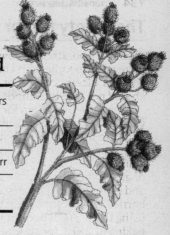

Family: Compositae; other members include daisy, dandelion, marigold

Genus and species: *Arctium lappa*

Also known as: Great burdock, burr

Parts used: Primarily roots, also leaves and seeds

Burdock—the name is a combination of *bur*, from its tenacious burrs, and *dock*, Old English for "plant"— seems to reach out and grab anything that comes near it. And the same could be said for its place in modern herbal healing. While many scientists have dismissed burdock as useless, it seems destined to hang on as a healing herb, particularly as a potential treatment for cancer.

Burdock has had its ups and downs in the past. When it wasn't being reviled as a pest, it was being recommended as a healing treatment for a surprising variety of conditions. The medieval German abbess/herbalist Hildegard of Bingen used it to treat cancerous tumors.

Early Chinese physicians considered burdock a remedy for colds, flu, throat infections, and pneumonia. India's traditional Ayurvedic healers used it similarly.

An Herb for All Reasons

During the 14th century in Europe, burdock leaves were pounded in wine and used to treat leprosy.

London's overly imaginative 17th-century herbalist Nicholas Culpeper recommended burdock for uterine prolapse, a condition in which the ligaments supporting the uterus weaken, causing it to fall into the vagina. Culpeper's bizarre prescription: Place burdock on the crown of the head to draw the womb back up.

Later European herbalists prescribed burdock root for fever, cancer, eczema, psoriasis, acne, dandruff, gout, ringworm, skin infections, syphilis, gonorrhea, and problems associated with childbirth.

America's 19th-century Eclectic physicians considered it an excellent diuretic and prescribed it for urinary tract infection, kidney problems, and painful urination, in addition to skin infections and arthritis.

The Cancer Controversy

Centuries after Hildegard recommended burdock for cancer, the herb's reputation as a tumor treatment spread to Russia, China, India, and the Americas.

From the 1930s to the 1950s, burdock was an ingredient in the alternative cancer treatment marketed by ex–coal miner Harry Hoxsey (see page 23).

Contemporary herbalists have abandoned burdock as a cancer treatment (perhaps prematurely) but continue to recommend it for skin problems, wound treatment, urinary tract infection, arthritis, sciatica, ulcers, and even anorexia nervosa.

HEALING with Burdock

Many modern herbal experts say thumbs down to burdock as a healing herb. In *Natural Product Medicine*, Ara Der Marderosian, Ph.D., and Lawrence Liberti write: "There is little evidence to suggest burdock is useful in treatment of any human disease." And in *The New Honest Herbal*, Varro Tyler, Ph.D., writes: "In spite of its long folkloric use, no solid evidence exists that burdock exhibits useful therapeutic activity."

Most traditional claims for burdock have not withstood scientific scrutiny. It does not treat leprosy, arthritis, uterine prolapse, or congestive heart failure. But several studies suggest the herb may prove to be therapeutic after all.

Infection. German researchers have discovered fresh burdock root contains chemicals (polyacetylenes) that kill disease-causing bacteria and fungi. Though dried burdock contains less of these chemicals, their presence may help explain the herb's traditional use against ringworm, a fungal infection, and several bacterial infections, including gonorrhea, skin infections, and urinary tract infections.

However, burdock is no substitute for professional medical treatment of fungal and bacterial infections.

Intriguing Possibilities. Burdock has been used extensively around the world as a cancer treatment, and several studies show that substances found in the herb do, in fact, have antitumor activity. An article published in *Chemotherapy* identified a chemical (arctigenin) in burdock as an "inhibitor of experimental tumor growth." And a study published in *Mutation Research* showed the herb decreases mutations in cells exposed to mutation-causing chemicals. (Most substances that cause genetic mutations also cause cancer.)

Of course, cancer requires professional care. If you'd like to try burdock in addition to standard therapy, discuss it with your physician.

Finally, burdock has an as-yet-unexplained anti-poisoning effect. Experimental animals fed the herb were somehow protected against several chemicals known to be toxic.

In view of these tantalizing findings, let's hope scientists cling to burdock research as tenaciously as the plant's burrs cling to just about anything.

R_x for Burdock

If your physician gives the okay, use burdock in conjunction with other cancer therapy. The herb may also be used as part of the treatment for certain infections, such as those that attack the urinary tract, and also for gonorrhea. Take it as a decoction or tincture.

For a decoction, boil 1 teaspoon of root in 3 cups of water for 30 minutes. Cool. Drink up to 3 cups a day. It has a sweet taste similar to celery root.

In a tincture, take $1/2$ to 1 teaspoon up to three times a day.

Do not give burdock to children under age 2. For older children and people over 65, start with low-strength preparations and increase strength if necessary.

The Safety Factor

No one questioned burdock's safety until the *Journal of the American Medical Association* linked it to one case of poisoning that could have proved fatal.

A woman who drank a strong decoction experienced blurred vision, dry mouth, and hallucinations—classic symptoms of atropine poisoning. Burdock does not contain atropine, but a plant that looks similar does—belladonna. Presumably, some belladonna accidentally adulterated the woman's burdock.

One case of adulteration is not cause for alarm, but if you use burdock, buy it from a reliable source, and if you develop any symptoms of atropine poisoning—dry mouth, blurred vision, and hallucinations—seek emergency medical treatment immediately.

The Toxicology of Botanical Medicines identifies burdock as a uterine stimulant. Pregnant women shouldn't use it.

The Food and Drug Administration lists burdock as an herb of "undefined safety," but except for that one case of atropine poisoning, it apparently never has caused problems. For otherwise healthy nonpregnant, nonnursing adults, burdock is considered safe in amounts typically recommended.

Burdock should be used in medicinal amounts only in consultation with your doctor. If burdock causes minor discomforts, such as stomach upset or diarrhea, use less or stop using it. Let your doctor know if you experience any unpleas-

ant effects or if the symptoms for which the herb is being used do not improve significantly in two weeks.

Medicine Is in the Roots

Burdock's medicinal root has brown bark and a white, spongy, fibrous interior, which becomes hard when dried. Its stem is multibranched, with long, egg-shaped leaves. Each branch is topped by a bristled "flower," actually a clump of many purplish flowers, which produces its infamous burrs.

Burdock grows easily from seeds planted in spring. Thin seedlings to 6-inch spacing. Burdock prefers moist, rich, deeply cultivated soil and full sun but tolerates poorer soils. Many herbalists mix wood chips and sawdust into burdock beds to keep the soil loose so roots are easier to harvest. Burdock roots deeply, so transplanting is not advised for established plants. Harvest the roots during the fall of the first year or the spring of the second.

CARAWAY

Digestive Aid Since Ancient Egypt

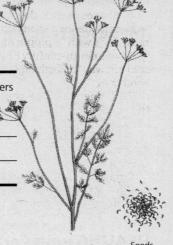

Family: Umbelliferae; other members include carrot, parsley

Genus and species: *Carum carvi*

Also known as: Carum

Parts used: Fruits ("seeds")

Seeds

araway is best known as the seed that flavors rye bread. The reason it's in rye bread, and many other foods, is that caraway has been used since ancient times to calm the digestive tract and expel gas.

Caraway seeds have been found in prehistoric food remains from 3500 B.C. The ancient Egyptians loved the aromatic seeds. They were recommended for digestive upsets in the E*bers Papyrus*, one of the world's oldest surviving medical documents, about 1500 B.C.

Unchanged for Centuries

Caraway is one of only a handful of herbs whose major medicinal use has remained unchanged throughout history. The ancient Greek physician Dioscorides mentioned the seeds to aid digestion, and herbals down through the ages have recommended them for indigestion, gas, and infant colic.

In Shakespeare's day, baked apples with caraway seeds were considered a stomach-soothing dessert. In *Henry IV*, a meal ends with "a pippin and a dish of caraway."

Seventeenth-century English herbalist Nicholas Culpeper said caraway "helpeth digestion . . . and easeth the pains of the wind colic."

And America's 19th-century Eclectic physicians believed the seeds "gently excite the digestive powers . . . [and are] used in flatulent colic, especially of children."

Throughout history, in Europe, the Middle East, and early America, caraway was a favorite addition to laxative herbs because it tempered their often violent effects.

Caraway's only other traditional uses relate to women's health—for menstrual cramps, menstruation promotion, and milk promotion in nursing mothers.

HEALING with Caraway

The Egyptians were right. It's amazing that a treatment used 3,500 years ago can still be effective today.

Digestive Aid. Modern researchers have discovered that two chemicals (carvol and carvene) in caraway seeds soothe the smooth muscle tissue of the digestive tract and help expel gas.

Women's Health. Antispasmodics, which appear to be present in caraway, soothe not only the digestive tract but other smooth muscles, such as the uterus, as well. Thus, caraway might relax the uterus, not stimulate it. Women may try it for relief of menstrual cramps.

Rx for Caraway

Fresh seeds may be mixed into any food or chewed a teaspoonful at a time.

Add caraway seeds to any dishes that benefit from their

unique flavor. They are often used in breads, soups, salads, stews, cheeses, sauerkraut, pickling brines, and meat dishes.

Caraway oil is also used to flavor two digestive-aid liqueurs, Scandinavian Aquavit and German Kummel.

For a pleasant-tasting infusion that might help aid digestion, relieve gas or menstrual cramping, use 2 to 3 teaspoons of bruised or crushed seeds per cup of boiling water. Steep 10 to 20 minutes. Drink up to 3 cups a day.

If you prefer a tincture, take $1/2$ to 1 teaspoon up to three times a day.

Low-strength caraway infusions may be given to infants for colic and gas.

The Safety Factor

There have been no reports of harm from caraway.

Although caraway appears to have antispasmodic properties, which means that it might *relax* the uterus, the herb has been used throughout history to promote menstruation. Pregnant women should exercise caution and not use the herb medicinally.

Caraway seed is on the Food and Drug Administration's list of herbs generally regarded as safe. For otherwise healthy nonpregnant, nonnursing adults, caraway is safe in amounts typically recommended.

Caraway should be used in medicinal amounts only in consultation with your doctor. Let your doctor know if you experience unpleasant effects or if stomach distress does not improve significantly in two weeks.

A Tasty Addition to the Garden

Caraway is an attractive biennial that reaches 2 feet. It has feathery leaves and umbrella-like clusters of tiny white flowers, which bloom in early summer.

Caraway grows easily from seeds planted in spring $1/2$ inch deep and 8 inches apart. Caraway likes rich, well-drained soil and full sun. Keep plants moist but not wet.

The first year, caraway produces a small rosette of leaves and a long taproot. Don't transplant it once it has become established. During the second year, caraway sends up its stem, reveals its feathery leaves, and produces its seeds.

Seeds appear in midsummer. Harvest them as soon as they ripen. Leave some seeds behind and the plants will self-sow.

CASCARA SAGRADA

World's Most Popular Laxative

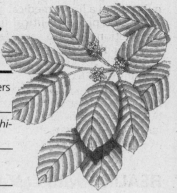

Family: Rhamnaceae; other members include buckthorn

Genus and species: *Rhamnus purshiana*

Also known as: Cascara, sacred bark, chittem bark

Parts used: Dried, aged bark

The 16th-century Spanish explorers who first visited northern California had a problem—constipation. The local Indians had the solution—a tea made from a healing herb they held sacred. The herb worked, and the Spanish named it *cascara sagrada*, "sacred bark." It has been the answer to millions of prayers ever since.

Wonder of the New World

The Spanish recognized cascara sagrada as a relative of buckthorn, the powerful laxative herb used in Europe since ancient times. But cascara sagrada was much gentler. The explorers sent some back to Spain, where its comparatively mild action was hailed as a wonder of the New World.

But the Spanish explorers were more interested in finding gold than in spreading laxatives around the newly discovered continent. For a long time cascara sagrada remained a West Coast folk remedy, known as "chittem bark," a polite variant of the Gold Rush '49ers' name, "sh—tin' bark."

In 1877, a Detroit Eclectic physician extolled cascara's mildness in a home medical guide, prompting Parke, Davis & Co., the pharmaceutical firm, to market a commercial preparation. Cascara sagrada has been one of the world's most popular herbal medicines ever since.

Cascara sagrada entered the U.S. *Pharmacopoeia* in 1890 and remains there to this day.

In Appalachian folk medicine, cascara sagrada has also been used to treat cancer. It was an ingredient in the popular— but highly controversial—Hoxsey Cancer Formula, an alternative therapy marketed from the 1930s to the 1950s by ex–coal miner Harry Hoxsey (see page 23).

HEALING with Cascara Sagrada

Modern herbals recommend cascara sagrada for constipation and endorse the Eclectic physicians' assertion that it "restores bowel tone."

Constipation. Cascara sagrada is an ingredient in dozens of over-the-counter laxatives, among them Comfolax Plus and Nature's Remedy. In addition, physicians write more than 2.5 million prescriptions a year for products that contain cascara.

Cascara sagrada contains chemicals (anthraquinones) that stimulate the intestinal contractions we know as "the urge." And the Spanish were right in believing that cascara sagrada is milder than the other anthraquinone laxatives, which include aloe, buckthorn, rhubarb, and senna. As a result, cascara is less likely to cause nausea, vomiting, and intestinal cramps. On the other hand, these reactions are possible. If they occur, use less or stop using it.

Research has also supported the Eclectics' observation that cascara sagrada restores bowel tone. According to the natural-product text, *Pharmacognosy*, "Cascara sagrada . . . not only acts as a laxative, but also restores natural tone to the colon."

Intriguing Possibility. Harry Hoxsey may have been on the right track. The herb contains aloe-emodin, which has been shown to have anti-leukemia action in laboratory animals, supporting its use as a cancer treatment. Unfortunately, aloe-emodin is also quite toxic, and scientists say more research is needed before it can be used to treat leukemia.

Rx for Cascara Sagrada

To benefit from the laxative action of cascara sagrada, use either a decoction or a tincture.

For a decoction, boil 1 teaspoon of well-dried bark in 3 cups of water for 30 minutes. Drink at room temperature, 1 to 2 cups a day before bed.

The taste is quite bitter. You may find that a tincture is more palatable. In a tincture, take ¹/₂ teaspoon at bedtime.

When using commercial preparations, follow package directions.

Do not give cascara sagrada to children under age 2. For older children and people over 65, start with low-strength preparations and increase strength if necessary.

The Safety Factor

Anthraquinone laxatives are considered a last resort for constipation. First, eat a diet higher in fiber, drink more fluids, and exercise more. If that doesn't work, try a bulk-forming laxative, such as psyllium, for example (see page 423). And if that doesn't provide relief, try cascara sagrada.

Cascara sagrada should never be used for more than two weeks. Over time, it causes lazy bowel syndrome, an inability to move stool without chemical stimulation. If constipation persists, consult a physician.

Cascara bark must be stored for at least a year before use. The fresh herb contains chemicals that can cause violent catharsis and severe intestinal cramps. Drying changes these chemicals and gives the herb milder action. Fresh bark may also be artificially dried by baking at 250°F for several hours.

Cascara sagrada should not be used by anyone with ulcers, ulcerative colitis, irritable bowel syndrome, hemorrhoids, or other gastrointestinal conditions.

Pregnant women should not use cascara sagrada.

For otherwise healthy nonpregnant, nonnursing adults who do not have digestive disorders and are not taking other laxatives, cascara sagrada is considered relatively safe when used cautiously in amounts typically recommended.

Cascara sagrada should be used in medicinal amounts only in consultation with your doctor. If cascara sagrada causes minor discomforts such as nausea, vomiting, diarrhea, or intestinal cramps, use less or stop using it. Let your doctor know if you experience any unpleasant effects or if constipation does not improve in a few days.

Not for the Backyard

Cascara sagrada is an unassuming, 20-foot tree with reddish-brown bark and thin, finely serrated leaves. It grows in the Northwest and is not a garden herb.

CATNIP

Enjoy It with Kitty

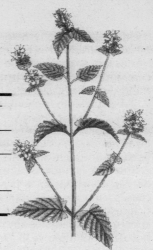

Family: Labiatae; other members include mint

Genus and species: *Nepeta cataria*

Also known as: Catmint, catnep, catswort, field balm

Parts used: Flowers and leaves

You don't have to be an herbalist to know this plant's effect on cats. But here's a case where one species' intoxicant is another's calmer. In people, catnip may help soothe the digestive tract. It may also help relieve menstrual cramps and soothe the nerves, and it might provide handy first aid for gardeners.

Healing Vapors

From Europe to China, catnip has been used medicinally for at least 2,000 years. In teas, its pleasant, lemon-minty vapors were considered a cold and cough remedy, relieving chest congestion and loosening phlegm. Old herbals also praised its ability to promote sweating, a traditional treatment for fever.

Catnip also has a long history of use as a tranquilizer, sedative, digestive aid, menstruation promoter, and treatment for menstrual cramps, flatulence, and infant colic. Parents used to give a weak catnip tea to colicky infants and even hang a small bag of the herb around their necks so they could inhale its soothing vapors.

Equal parts of catnip and saffron were once recommended for smallpox and scarlet fever.

The leaves were also chewed to relieve toothache, and as crazy as this sounds today, smoked to treat bronchitis and asthma.

Catnip was a popular beverage tea in pre-Elizabethan England. During the Age of Exploration, it was replaced by the more stimulating Chinese herb we call tea (*Camellia sinensis*). However, not all English catnip lovers switched to Chinese tea without regrets. In her book, *The Herb Garden*, a certain Miss Bardswell clucked, "Catmint Tea was . . . a good deal more wholesome."

Hangman's Root

Colonists introduced catnip into North America. It quickly went wild and now grows across the continent. The Indians adopted the herb and used it as the whites did, for indigestion and infant colic and as a beverage.

Early Americans also believed catnip roots made even the kindest person mean. Hangmen used to consume the roots before executions to get in the right mood for their work.

Catnip was listed as a stomach soother in the U.S. *Pharmacopoeia* from 1842 to 1882 and the *National Formulary*, the pharmacists' reference, from 1916 to 1950.

Contemporary herbalists continue to have great faith in catnip. One writes, "Surely a plant with such a powerful impact on our feline friends . . . could not be destitute of medicinal value in humans." Modern herbals recommend catnip as a tranquilizer, sedative, digestive aid, and treatment for colds, colic, diarrhea, flatulence, and fever.

Not a Hallucinogen

A report published in the *Journal of the American Medical Association* in 1969 claimed catnip produces marijuana-like intoxication. The wire services picked up the story, newspapers ran screaming headlines, and bewildered pet shop owners reported a sudden run on cat toys.

But the report was quickly discredited by correspondents who flooded the medical journal with letters pointing out that the "catnip" photos that ran with the article were actually marijuana. Catnip has no history as a human intoxicant, and authorities quickly dismissed the notion that smoking catnip caused anything but a sore throat.

Unfortunately, the same cannot be said for the popular press. As Varro Tyler, Ph.D., writes in *The New Honest Herbal*, "Once an erroneous statement has appeared in print, it is almost impossible to eradicate. Catnip continues to be listed in practically every book devoted to drugs of abuse as a mild intoxicant." For the record: It isn't.

Cat intoxication is another matter. All cats are attracted to catnip, but only about two-thirds exhibit strong "feline catnip euphoria," according to a report published in *Economic Botany*. Kitty euphoria is an inherited trait, and not all cats have the gene necessary for it.

HEALING with Catnip

Studies show catnip is definitely not just for cats. Modern herbalists tend to overstate its value, but scientists have confirmed several of its traditional uses.

Digestive Aid. Like the other mints, catnip may soothe the smooth muscles of the digestive tract (making it an antispasmodic). Have a cup of catnip tea after meals if you're prone to indigestion or heartburn.

Women's Health. Antispasmodics calm not only the digestive tract but other smooth muscles as well—the uterus, for example. Catnip's antispasmodic effect supports its traditional use for relieving menstrual cramps.

Catnip was also used traditionally as a menstruation promoter. Current research suggests it should not stimulate the uterus, but pregnant women should exercise caution and not use medicinal amounts.

Tranquilizer. German researchers report the chemicals

(nepetalactone isomers) responsible for cats' intoxication are similar to the natural sedatives (valepotriates) in valerian. This finding supports catnip's traditional use as a mild tranquilizer and sedative. Try a cup of tea when you feel tense or before bed and see if it works for you.

Infection Prevention. Catnip also has some antibiotic properties, which lends credence to its traditional use in some cases of diarrhea and fever. As an antibiotic, catnip is not particularly powerful, but it may help prevent infection after garden mishaps.

Rx for Catnip

Enjoy a pleasant, minty infusion of catnip as a digestive aid, as a mild tranquilizer, or to soothe menstrual cramps.

For an infusion, use 2 teaspoons of dried herb per cup of boiling water. Steep 10 to 20 minutes. Do not boil catnip; boiling dissipates its healing oil. Drink up to 3 cups a day.

If you prefer a tincture, take $1/2$ to 1 teaspoon up to three times a day.

Weak, cool catnip infusions may be given cautiously to colicky infants. For older children and people over 65, start with low-strength preparations and increase strength if necessary.

To treat minor garden mishaps, press some crushed catnip leaves into cuts and scrapes on your way to washing and bandaging them.

The Safety Factor

Catnip is considered nontoxic, but some people may experience upset stomach.

The Food and Drug Administration lists catnip as an herb of "undefined safety," but no significant toxic reactions have ever been reported. For otherwise healthy nonpregnant, nonnursing adults, catnip is considered safe in amounts typically recommended.

Catnip should be used in medicinal amounts only in consultation with your doctor. If catnip causes minor discomforts, such as stomach upset, use less or stop using it. Let your doctor know if you experience any unpleasant effects or if the symptoms for which the herb is being used do not improve significantly in two weeks.

Protect Plants from Cats

Catnip is a gray-green aromatic perennial that grows to 3 feet and bears all the hallmarks of the mint family: a square stem, fuzzy leaves, and twin-lipped flowers.

Catnip grows easily from seeds or root divisions planted in spring or fall. It thrives in almost any well-drained soil under full sun or partial shade. Some growers say keeping soil on the dry side produces more aromatic plants. Thin seedlings to 18-inch spacings.

Harvest the leaves and flower tops in late summer when the plants are in bloom. Dry and store in opaque, tightly sealed containers to preserve the volatile oil.

Gardeners' mythology holds that cats are not attracted to catnip in the ground. An old rhyme says: "If you set it/The cats will get it./But if you sow it/The cats won't know it." Don't you believe it. Cats often destroy sown plants. The current consensus is that sowing, per se, does not keep cats away. The key is to prevent bruising of the leaves. Carefully cultivated, completely unbruised plants reportedly hold little attraction for cats. But any bruising releases the plant's aromatic oil, and the cats come running.

CELERY SEED

A Natural Diuretic

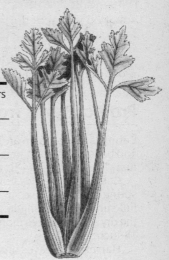

Family: Umbelliferae; other members include carrot, parsley

Genus and species: *Apium grave-olens*

Also known as: Marsh parsley, wild celery

Parts used: Fruit ("seeds")

Celery stalks don't do much but add crunch to salads. But scientists have discovered a surprising number of healing benefits in celery *seed*. They may help relieve insomnia and high blood pressure and may even help some people manage diabetes and congestive heart failure.

Elixir for Greek Athletes

The ancient Greeks gave celery wine to winning athletes, and celery elixirs have been used in healing throughout history. (A contemporary echo of this, minus any medicinal claims, is the celery-flavored soft drink, Dr. Brown's Cel-Ray Soda.)

India's traditional Ayurvedic physicians have prescribed celery seed since ancient times as a diuretic to treat water retention and as a treatment for colds, flu, indigestion, arthritis, and diseases of the liver and spleen.

153

The medieval German abbess/herbalist Hildegard of Bingen wrote: "Whoever is plagued by [the arthritis of] gout ... should powder celery seeds ... because this is the best remedy."

English herbalist John Gerard claimed celery "provoketh urine" as an aid to weight loss and expelled "phlegm out of the head."

Seventeenth-century England's Nicholas Culpeper also recommended celery seed as a diuretic for "dropsy" (congestive heart failure).

Later herbalists suggested it for insomnia, obesity, nervousness, and several cancers, as a menstruation promoter, and to bring on abortion. It has even been recommended as an aphrodisiac.

Oddly, America's 19th-century botanical physicians, the Eclectics, were not impressed. They considered celery a mere footnote under its close relative, parsley. If parsley were unavailable, the Eclectics grudgingly recommended celery as "a nerve tonic" and for arthritis and chest congestion.

Contemporary herbalists recommend celery as a diuretic, tranquilizer, sedative, and menstruation promoter, and as treatment for gout, arthritis, obesity, anxiety, and lack of appetite (gustatory, not sexual).

HEALING with Celery Seed

Several of celery seed's age-old uses in healing may be standing up to scientific examination.

Weight Loss. Celery seed contains a diuretic substance. This finding lends credence to its traditional use in treating obesity, because celery would tend to eliminate water weight. Keep in mind, however, that any water weight lost using diuretics invariably returns. The key to permanent weight control is a low-fat, high-complex-carbohydrate diet and regular aerobic exercise.

High Blood Pressure. Physicians prescribe diuretics for high blood pressure. In one study, celery oil injections significantly reduced blood pressure in rabbits and dogs. Of course, people don't take their celery by syringe, so Chinese researchers gave the herb to 16 people suffering from high blood pressure. Fourteen showed significant reductions.

If you want to use celery seed in your treatment plan, talk it over with your doctor.

Congestive Heart Failure. The fact that celery seed has been shown to contain a diuretic also supports its traditional use as a treatment for congestive heart failure, which involves serious fluid buildup. If you think you'd like to use celery seed for this purpose, discuss it with your doctor.

Anxiety and Insomnia. Celery seed oil contains chemicals (phthalides) that have sedative effects in animals. Animal findings don't always apply to humans, but if you're anxious, nervous, or wakeful, try this herb and see if it works for you.

Diabetes. Several studies have indicated that celery seed reduces blood sugar (glucose) levels, an important part of managing diabetes. Diabetes requires professional treatment. If you'd like to use celery seed as part of your treatment plan, discuss it with your physician.

Women's Health. Celery seed stimulates uterine contractions in animals, lending support to its traditional uses in menstruation promotion and abortion. Animal results don't always apply to people, but pregnant women should exercise caution and not use it. Celery stalks, however, are not harmful. Other women may try it to bring on their periods, but do not use celery seed to try to induce abortion.

Diuretics help relieve the bloated feeling caused by premenstrual fluid retention. Women bothered by premenstrual syndrome (PMS) might try some celery seed during the uncomfortable days right before their periods.

Intriguing Possibilities. Celery contains chemicals (psoralens), which have been used to treat psoriasis and more recently, one form of cancer, cutaneous T-cell lymphoma. But further research is needed before this herb can be used to treat these diseases.

R_x for Celery Seed

Celery seed may be used under the supervision of a physician as part of a program to treat high blood pressure, congestive heart failure, or diabetes.

Try a pleasant-tasting infusion as a mild relaxant or to bring on menstruation. Use 1 to 2 teaspoons of freshly crushed seeds per cup of boiling water. Steep 10 to 20 minutes. Drink up to 3 cups a day.

In a tincture, take $1/2$ to 1 teaspoon up to three times a day.

Celery seed preparations should not be given to children under age 2. For older children and people over 65, start with low-strength preparations and increase strength if necessary.

The Safety Factor

Diuretics should be used in consultation with a physician. They can deplete body stores of potassium, an essential nutrient. Those who use diuretics should also eat foods high in potassium, such as bananas and fresh vegetables, to replace lost electrolytes.

High blood pressure, congestive heart failure, and diabetes are serious conditions. Celery seed may help manage them, but it should be used in consultation with your physician as part of an overall treatment plan.

Pregnant women should not take diuretics without a physician's approval.

Celery seed and oil are considered nontoxic and are on the Food and Drug Administration's list of herbs generally regarded as safe. For otherwise healthy nonpregnant, nonnursing adults who are not taking other diuretics, celery seed is considered safe in amounts typically recommended.

Celery seed should be used in medicinal amounts only in consultation with your doctor. If celery seed causes minor discomforts, such as stomach upset or diarrhea, use less or stop using it. Let your doctor know if you experience any unpleas-

ant effects or if the symptoms for which the herb is being used do not improve significantly in two weeks.

Needs Rich Soil

Celery grows best in well-watered, richly organic soil. Less ideal conditions produce tougher, stringier, more bitter stalks.

In mild areas, celery grows virtually year-round. Elsewhere, start seeds indoors in January and bed seedlings in early spring after the danger of frost has passed. Soak seeds before planting. Germination typically takes about ten days. Transplant when seedlings are about 3 inches high at approximately three months. Space plants about 6 inches apart.

Water copiously. Stalk juiciness depends on how much water the plants receive.

Harvest seeds when they mature.

Certain chemicals (psoralens) in celery sometimes cause rashes in agricultural workers. Gardeners take note: Wearing sunscreen prevents the reaction.

CHAMOMILE

Pretty Flowers, Potent Medicine

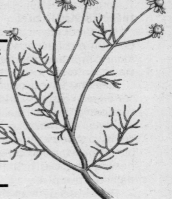

Family: Compositae; other members include daisy, dandelion, marigold

Genus and species: *Matricaria chamomilla* (German or Hungarian); *Anthemis nobilis* (Roman or English)

Also known as: Camomile, matricaria, anthemis, ground apple

Parts used: Flowers

I n *The Tale of Peter Rabbit*, Peter eats himself sick in Mr. McGregor's garden, then gets chased out at the wrong end of the angry man's hoe. When he gets home, his mother gives him chamomile tea.

Peter's mother was a wise herbalist. Chamomile is one of the best herbs for indigestion. It also soothes jangled nerves. Perhaps Peter's mother also feared his ordeal would give him an ulcer: Chamomile may help prevent and heal them. Or perhaps Mr. McGregor's hoe grazed Peter's tender bunny skin. A chamomile compress can help heal many wounds.

Unfortunately, few who sip chamomile tea know what a healer they hold in their paws. Sorry—*hands*.

Herb of the Sun

Actually, chamomile is not one herb, but two—German (or Hungarian) chamomile and Roman (or English) chamomile. The two plants are botanically unrelated, but they both produce the same light blue oil used in healing since ancient times.

Chamomile's daisylike flowers reminded the ancient Egyptians of the sun. They used it to treat fever, particularly the recurring fevers of malaria.

The Greek physician Dioscorides and the Roman naturalist Pliny recommended chamomile to treat headaches and kidney, liver, and bladder problems. India's ancient Ayurvedic physicians used it similarly.

Germans have used chamomile since the dawn of history for digestive upsets and as a menstruation promoter and treatment for menstrual cramps.

Seventeenth-century English herbalist Nicholas Culpeper recommended chamomile for fevers, digestive problems, aches, pains, jaundice, kidney stones, "dropsy" (congestive heart failure), and "to bring down women's courses" (promote menstruation).

British and German immigration introduced both chamomiles into North America, though most of the chamomile grown here today is the German variety.

America's 19th-century Eclectic physicians recommended chamomile poultices to speed wound healing and prevent gangrene. They prescribed infusions for digestive problems, malaria, typhus, menstrual cramps, menstruation promotion, and for all birth-related difficulties: to quiet fetal kicking, stop premature labor, relieve sore breasts and nipples, suppress milk production, and relieve infant colic.

Best-Seller

Today chamomile is one of the nation's best-selling herbs. It's a favorite tea, by itself or in blends. Its apple aroma is the fragrance in many herbal skin-care products. And it has been used in shampoos since the days of the Vikings because it adds luster to blond hair.

Contemporary herbalists recommend chamomile externally to spur wound healing and treat inflammation, and internally for fever, digestive upsets, anxiety, and insomnia.

HEALING with Chamomile

In Germany, where herbal healing is more mainstream than it is in the United States, one pharmaceutical company markets a popular chamomile product called Kamillosan, which Germans use externally to treat wounds and inflammations, and internally for indigestion and ulcers. (This product is not available in the United States.) Chamomile is so popular in Germany that many there call the herb *alles zutraut*—"capable of anything."

A slight exaggeration, perhaps, but chamomile does have a lot going for it.

Digestive Aid. Dozens of studies have supported chamomile's traditional use as a digestive aid. Several chemicals (primarily bisabolol) in chamomile oil appear to have relaxing action on the smooth muscle lining of the digestive tract (making it an antispasmodic). In fact, one study shows chamomile relaxes the digestive tract as well as the opium-based drug papaverine.

Ulcers. Chamomile also may help prevent stomach ulcers and speed their healing. In one experiment, two groups of animals were fed a chemical known to cause ulcers. Those also given chamomile developed significantly fewer. Then the animals who developed ulcers were divided into two groups. Those fed chamomile recovered more quickly.

Women's Health. Antispasmodics relax not only the digestive tract but other smooth muscles, such as the uterus, as well. Chamomile's antispasmodic properties support its age-old use to soothe menstrual cramps and to lessen the possibility of premature labor.

Oddly enough, chamomile was also used to stimulate menstruation. The apparent contradiction remains unresolved, but European researchers have isolated a substance in chamomile that stimulates uterine contractions.

Women should feel free to try chamomile both to soothe menstrual cramps and to promote the onset of menstruation, but pregnant women should steer clear of medicinal amounts.

Tranquilizer. Chamomile's long history as a tranquilizer also has a scientific basis according to researchers who showed that the herb depresses the central nervous system. Try an infusion when you feel anxious, or add a handful of chamomile flowers to a hot bath.

Arthritis. In animal studies, the herb successfully relieves arthritic joint inflammation. Animal findings don't necessarily apply to people, but chamomile has been used traditionally to treat arthritis. Try it and see if it works for you.

Infection Prevention. The Eclectic physicians of America were on the right track using chamomile compresses to prevent wound infections. Some studies show chamomile oil applied to the skin reduces the time it takes burns to heal. Other studies show the herb kills the yeast fungi (*Candida albicans*) that cause vaginal infections, as well as certain bacteria (*Staphylococcus*). Chamomile also impairs the replication of polio virus. For cuts, scrapes, or burns, brew a strong infusion, cool it, and apply in compresses.

Immune Stimulant. No one knew why chamomile prevented infections until British researchers discovered that the herb stimulated the immune system's infection-fighting white blood cells (macrophages and B-lymphocytes). Drink some when you have a cold or the flu. It does no harm, and it just might help.

Rx for Chamomile

Use an infusion or tincture to take advantage of chamomile's many proven healing benefits.

For a pleasant, refreshing infusion, use 2 to 3 heaping teaspoons of flowers per cup of boiling water. Steep 10 to 20 minutes. Drink up to 3 cups a day.

In a tincture, use 1/2 to 1 teaspoon up to three times a day.

When using commercial preparations, follow package directions.

Weak infusions of chamomile may be given cautiously to children under age 2 for colic. For older children and people over 65, start with low-strength preparations and increase strength if necessary.

For a relaxing herbal bath, tie a handful of chamomile flowers into a cloth and run your bathwater over it.

For cuts and scrapes or burns, brew a strong infusion. Soak a clean cloth in the liquid and apply it as a compress.

The Safety Factor

Controversy erupted when a report in the *Journal of Allergy and Clinical Immunology* claimed chamomile tea might cause a potentially fatal allergic reaction—anaphylactic shock—in people allergic to ragweed. Herb conservatives immediately urged the millions of people with ragweed allergy to shun chamomile. Outraged herb advocates insisted chamomile was villified unfairly.

To settle the issue, researchers compiled every report of chamomile-induced allergic reactions from the entire world medical literature for the 95-year period from 1887 to 1982. The grand total: No deaths and 50 reactions—45 from Roman chamomile and just 5 from the German variety, the one typically used in the United States. Chamomile poses no health hazard. The only people who should think twice about using this herb (and its close relative, yarrow) are those who have suffered previous anaphylactic reactions from ragweed.

That doesn't mean to say that reactions are impossible. Large amounts of highly concentrated preparations have caused some nausea and vomiting.

Chamomile is on the Food and Drug Administration's list of herbs generally regarded as safe. For otherwise healthy nonpregnant, nonnursing adults, chamomile is safe in amounts typically recommended.

Chamomile should be used in medicinal amounts only in consultation with your doctor. If chamomile causes minor discomforts, such as nausea or vomiting, use less or stop using it. Let your doctor know if you experience any unpleasant effects or if the symptoms for which the herb is being used do not improve significantly in two weeks.

Adds Fragrance to the Garden

German chamomile is an annual that reaches 3 feet. The Roman herb is a perennial groundcover that rarely exceeds 9 inches. Both have downy stems, feathery leaves, and daisy-like flowers with yellow centers and white rays.

Most chamomile seed available in the United States is the annual German variety. It grows easily when sown in spring after danger of frost has passed. Scatter the tiny seeds on well-prepared beds, then gently tamp down. Seedlings up to 2 inches tall transplant well. Taller plants do not.

German chamomile prefers sandy, well-drained soil in partially shaded gardens and tends to shrivel under full sun. It flowers at about six weeks and produces lush flowers even in the short summers of northern climes. The flowering lasts for several weeks, and if some flowers are left unharvested, the plant will sow itself. Don't leave too many. This herb may become a pest.

Perennial Roman chamomile comes in two subtypes, single-flower and double-flower. Herbalists prefer the double-flower variety, which adapts to almost any soil but favors moist, well-manured loam. The tiny seeds may be sown, but most gardeners prefer to propagate the plant from offshoots. Plant them about 18 inches apart in early spring.

Roman chamomile is quite hardy, but if your winters are particularly severe, protect the plants with mulch.

Oddly enough, Roman chamomile does best when it's stepped on. In Britain, the plant is often used as a groundcover on garden paths. Walking on it releases the herb's lovely apple fragrance and does not hurt the plant.

After harvesting, dry the flowers and store them in sealed containers to preserve their volatile oil.

CHAPARRAL

Cavity-Preventive Mouthwash

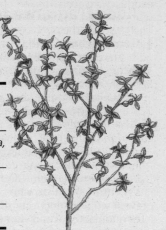

Family: Zygophyllaceae; other members include caltrop, star thistle, bean caper

Genus and species: *Larrea divaricata, L. tridentata*

Also known as: Stinkweed, greasewood, creosote bush

Parts used: Twigs and leaflets

Chaparral stinks. Literally. And it tastes downright unpleasant. So the herb's major healing benefit comes as something of a surprise—it's a mouthwash.

We're not talking minty fresh here. You wouldn't want to reach for it before puckering up for your morning kiss. But don't let that stop you—the unassuming chaparral shrub, native to the American Southwest, contains a chemical that may spell death to some of the germs that cause tooth decay. It owes its use in healing to a chemical called NDGA (nordihydroguaiaretic acid), which kills the bacteria and other microorganisms that turn fats and oils rancid.

Stinkweed

If, as some people believe, effective medicine smells foul and tastes terrible, chaparral should be a terrific healer. Its leaves

164

exude a waxy resin that smells like creosote and is the source of its popular names: stinkweed, greasewood, and creosote bush (though the plant contains no creosote). The Southwest Indians rubbed chaparral resin on burns. They used chaparral tea to treat colds, bronchitis, chicken pox, snakebite, and arthritis. And they heated the tips of its twigs and applied the hot resin to painful teeth.

White settlers adopted the plant and used it externally for bruises, rashes, dandruff, and wounds, and internally for diarrhea, stomach upset, menstrual problems, venereal diseases, and cancers of the liver, kidney, and stomach.

Chaparral was listed as an expectorant (to clear mucus from the respiratory system) and bronchial antiseptic in the U.S. *Pharmacopoeia* from 1842 to 1942. But today, few herbalists mention it. Those who do suggest using it externally to prevent wound infections, and internally for intestinal parasites and bacterial and viral illnesses.

HEALING with Chaparral

Chaparral is an intriguing and controversial herb. The chemical it contains, NGDA, is approved by the U.S. Department of Agriculture as a preservative in lard and animal shortenings.

Tooth Decay, Gum Disease. NGDA's antiseptic action, combined with its traditional use for toothache, prompted scientists to test it against the bacteria that cause tooth decay. A study in the *Journal of Dental Research* shows chaparral mouthwash reduces cavities by 75 percent. Oral microorganisms also cause gum disease, the leading cause of tooth loss in adults. Chaparral mouthwash is no substitute for regular brushing and flossing, but it may provide added protection. And you don't have to worry about the smell lingering either.

Cancer. NGDA is a powerful antioxidant, meaning it helps prevent the cell damage scientists believe eventually causes cancer.

For more than 100 years, chaparral has been a popular folk treatment for cancer. The National Cancer Institute has received many testimonials from people claiming the herb cured their cancers. Some laboratory studies agree chaparral has antitumor effects.

The medical literature contains several case reports of tumor shrinkage in people who used chaparral. One published in *Cancer Chemotherapy Reports* tells of a man diagnosed by University of Utah physicians with malignant melanoma, the most serious skin cancer. The doctors urged surgery, but the man refused, saying he intended to treat himself with chaparral tea. The Utah medical team was aghast, but eight months later, the man returned with "marked regression" of his cancer.

Melanoma is a life-threatening disease that requires professional treatment. Do not rely solely on chaparral as a treatment. Cancer patients might decide—in consultation with their physician—to use the herb in addition to other treatments.

Arthritis. Some animal studies agree chaparral has anti-inflammatory action, lending credence to its traditional use in treating arthritis. Try it and see if it helps your stiffness.

Life Extension. Life-extension advocates say antioxidants like NGDA help slow the aging process and might even extend the human life span. One French study shows NGDA significantly extends the average life span of laboratory animals. Other scientists claim the chemical almost doubles the average life span of laboratory insects. Scientists have not been able to extend the human life span, but these antioxidant results are certainly intriguing.

R$_x$ for Chaparral

For a mouthwash or infusion, use 1 tablespoon of dried leaves and stems per quart of boiling water. Steep 1 hour. Gargle or drink up to 3 cups a day. Because of its unpleasant taste, you might want to add honey and lemon to the infusion, or else mix it with a beverage tea.

Chaparral should not be given to children under age 2. Older children and people over 65 may use a full-strength gargle, but for internal use, they should start with a low-strength preparation and increase strength if necessary.

The Safety Factor

Although NGDA is a food preservative approved by the U.S. Department of Agriculture, the Food and Drug Administration removed it from the list of substances generally regarded as safe in 1968 because experimental animals fed large amounts for long periods developed kidney and lymph-system problems. No human kidney or lymphatic disease has ever been documented in chaparral users, but to be prudent, those with kidney and lymph conditions should not use this herb.

For otherwise healthy nonpregnant, nonnursing adults who do not have kidney or lymph-system conditions, chaparral is considered safe in amounts typically recommended.

Chaparral should be used in medicinal amounts only in consultation with your doctor. If urinary difficulties or swollen glands develop, stop using it, and consult a doctor for possible kidney or lymphatic problems. If chaparral causes minor discomforts, such as stomach upset or diarrhea, use less or stop using it. Let your doctor know if you experience any unpleasant effects or if the symptoms for which the herb is being used do not improve significantly in two weeks.

Flourishes in the Southwest

Chaparral is not a garden herb. It's a woody, olive green or yellow shrub that dominates the Southwest's arid landscape. Chaparral grows to about 10 feet and resembles a dwarf oak.

CINNAMON

Spice with a Punch

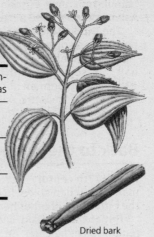

Family: Lauraceae; other members include bay, avocado, nutmeg, sassafras

Genus and species: *Cinnamomum zeylanicum, C. cassia, C. saigonicum*

Also known as: Cassia, Ceylon cinnamon, Saigon cinnamon

Parts used: Dried inner bark

Dried bark

We sprinkle it on toast, add it to cookie batter, stir it into hot apple cider, and find it in toothpastes and candies. But cinnamon is more than a sweet treat. It's one of the world's oldest healers. And modern science has confirmed its value for prevention of infection and indigestion.

Asian Prize

Cinnamon grew originally in southern Asia. Ancient Chinese herbals mention it as early as 2700 B.C. as a treatment for fever, diarrhea, and menstrual problems. India's ancient Ayurvedic healers used it similarly.

When ancient travelers introduced the aromatic herb to the Egyptians, they added it enthusiastically to their embalming mixtures. Egyptian demand for cinnamon (and other Asian spices) played a major role in ancient trade.

The Biblical Hebrews, Greeks, and Romans adopted cinnamon as a spice, perfume, and treatment for indigestion.

After the fall of Rome, trade with Asia came to a virtual halt, but somehow cinnamon still made it to Europe. The 12th-century German abbess/herbalist Hildegard of Bingen recommended it as "the universal spice for sinuses," and to treat colds, flu, cancer, and "inner decay and slime."

Back to the Kitchen

By the 17th century, Europeans considered cinnamon primarily a kitchen spice. In healing, they used it only to mask the bitterness of other healing herbs.

But as time passed, cinnamon slowly regained its former reputation as a healer. America's 19th-century Eclectic physicians prescribed it for stomach cramps, flatulence, nausea, vomiting, diarrhea, infant colic, and especially for uterine problems: "[Cinnamon's] most direct action is on the uterine muscle fibers, causing contraction and arresting bleeding. For postpartum and other uterine hemorrhages, it is one of the most prompt and efficient remedies."

Modern herbalists recommend cinnamon to relieve nausea, vomiting, diarrhea, and indigestion, and as a flavoring agent for bitter-tasting healing-herb preparations. They can't quite agree about how it affects the uterus. Some say it stimulates uterine contractions. Others say it calms the uterus.

HEALING with Cinnamon

Of course, cinnamon delights the taste buds. But it benefits other parts of the body as well.

Infection Prevention. A sound scientific reason for "flavoring" toothpastes and mouthwash with cinnamon does exist. Like many culinary spices, it's a powerful antiseptic. It kills many decay- and disease-causing bacteria, fungi, and viruses. Try sprinkling some on minor cuts and scrapes after they've been thoroughly washed.

Perhaps toilet paper should be impregnated with cinnamon. One German study showed it "suppresses completely" the cause of most urinary tract infections (*Escherichia coli* bacteria) and the fungus (*Candida albicans*) responsible for vaginal yeast infections.

Pain Relief. There's another reason to dust a bit of cinnamon on cuts and scrapes—it contains the natural anesthetic oil eugenol, which might help relieve the pain of household mishaps.

Digestive Aid. Cinnamon does more than add flavor to cakes, cookies, ice creams, and other high-fat desserts. Once you've consumed these delicacies, the herb helps break down fats in your digestive system, possibly by boosting the activity of some digestive enzymes.

Women's Health. Despite some modern herbalists' contention that cinnamon helps calm the uterus, the weight of historical evidence suggests the opposite. Pregnant women should limit their use to culinary amounts. Other women might try it to bring on menstruation or after delivery.

Intriguing Possibility. Japanese researchers report that cinnamon helps reduce blood pressure. If yours is high, it won't hurt to use more.

R$_x$ for Cinnamon

For a warm, sweet, spicy infusion, use $1/2$ to $3/4$ teaspoon of powdered herb per cup of boiling water. Drink up to 3 cups a day.

Cinnamon infusions should not be given to children under age 2. For older children and people over 65, start with low-strength preparations and increase strength if necessary.

To treat minor cuts and scrapes, wash the affected area thoroughly, then sprinkle on a little powdered cinnamon.

The Safety Factor

In powdered form, culinary amounts of cinnamon are non-toxic, though allergic reactions are possible.

Cinnamon *oil* is a different story. On the skin, it may cause redness and burning. Used internally, it can cause nausea, vomiting, and possibly even kidney damage. Don't ingest cinnamon oil.

Cinnamon is on the Food and Drug Administration's list of herbs generally regarded as safe. For otherwise healthy nonpregnant, nonnursing adults, cinnamon is considered safe in amounts typically recommended.

Cinnamon should be used in medicinal amounts only in consultation with your doctor. If cinnamon causes minor discomforts, such as stomach upset or diarrhea, use less or stop using it. Let your doctor know if you experience any unpleasant effects or if the symptoms for which the herb is being used do not improve significantly in two weeks.

Exotic Tree

Cinnamon is not grown in the United States. Most comes from Asia and the West Indies. The trees reach a height of 30 feet. Collectors strip the aromatic bark from young branches no more than three years old.

CLOVE

Your Dentist Loves It

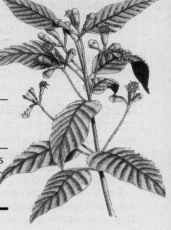

Family: Myrtaceae; other members include myrtle, eucalyptus

Genus and species: *Eugenia caryophyllata* or *Syzygium aromaticum*

Also known as: Clavos, caryophyllus

Parts used: Dried, powdered flower buds

Step into any spice shop, take a deep breath, and enjoy the rich, warm aroma that fills the air. Chances are the dominant fragrance is clove, one of the world's most aromatic healing herbs.

Step into your dentist's supply room, though, and things smell quite different. But chances are clove oil is one of the items on the shelf. It's a dental anesthetic—and more.

Ancient Breath Freshener

Clove is the bud of a highly aromatic tropical evergreen tree. During the Han dynasty (207 B.C. to A.D. 220) those who addressed the Chinese emperor were required to hold cloves in their mouths to mask bad breath. Traditional Chinese physicians have long used the herb to treat indigestion, diarrhea, hernia, and ringworm, as well as athlete's foot and other fungal infections.

India's traditional Ayurvedic healers have used clove since ancient times to treat respiratory and digestive ailments.

Clove first arrived in Europe around the 4th century A.D. as a highly coveted luxury. The medieval German abbess/herbalist Hildegard of Bingen recommended the rare herb in her antigout mixture.

Magellan's Voyage

Demand for clove (and other Asian herbs) helped launch the Age of Exploration. Magellan's flotilla brought some back to Spain in 1512 when the explorers completed their first voyage around the world.

Once clove became easily available in Europe, it was prized as a treatment for indigestion, flatulence, nausea, vomiting, and diarrhea. It was also used to treat cough, infertility, warts, worms, wounds, and toothache.

America's 19th-century Eclectic physicians used clove to treat digestive complaints and added it to bitter herb-medicine preparations to make them more palatable. The Eclectics were also the first to extract clove oil from the herbal buds. They used it on the gums to relieve toothache.

Contemporary herbalists recommend clove for digestive complaints and its oil for toothache.

HEALING with Clove

Clove oil, like allspice (see page 58), is 60 to 90 percent eugenol, which is the source of its anesthetic and antiseptic properties.

Toothache, Oral Hygiene. Dentists use clove oil as an oral anesthetic. They also use it to disinfect root canals.

Clove oil is the active ingredient in Lavoris mouthwash and a number of over-the-counter toothache pain-relief preparations, including Benzodent and Numzident.

Toothaches require professional care. Clove oil may provide temporary relief, but see a dentist promptly.

Digestive Aid. Like many culinary spices, clove may help relax the smooth muscle lining of the digestive tract, supporting its age-old use as a digestive aid.

Infection Fighter. Clove kills intestinal parasites and "exhibits broad antimicrobial properties against fungi and bacteria," according to one of many reports supporting its traditional use as a treatment for diarrhea, intestinal worms, and other digestive ailments.

Rx for Clove

For temporary relief of toothache prior to professional care, dip a cotton swab in clove oil and apply it to the affected tooth and surrounding gum.

For a warm, pleasant-tasting infusion, use 1 teaspoon of powdered herb per cup of boiling water. Steep 10 to 20 minutes. Drink up to 3 cups a day.

Medicinal amounts of clove should not be given to children under age 2. For older children and people over 65, start with low-strength preparations and increase strength if necessary.

The Safety Factor

Japanese researchers have discovered that like many spices, clove contains antioxidants. Antioxidants help prevent the cell damage that scientists believe eventually causes cancer.

On the other hand, in laboratory tests, the chemical eugenol, has been found to be a weak tumor promoter, making clove one of many healing herbs with both pro- and anticancer effects. At this point, scientists aren't sure which way the balance tilts. Until they are, anyone with a history of cancer should not use medicinal amounts of clove.

For otherwise healthy nonpregnant, nonnursing adults, powdered clove is considered nontoxic. However, high doses of its oil may cause stomach upset when ingested and rash when used externally.

Clove or clove oil should be used in medicinal amounts only in consultation with your doctor. If clove or clove oil causes minor discomforts, such as stomach upset or diarrhea, use less or stop using it. Let your doctor know if you experience any unpleasant effects or if the symptoms for which the herb is being used do not improve significantly in two weeks.

Some smokers switch to clove cigarettes, believing they're safer than tobacco. They aren't. Most clove cigarettes are 50 to 60 percent tobacco. And when clove burns, it releases many carcinogens. The *Journal of the American Medical Association* has reported many toxic reactions to clove cigarettes.

Grown in Far Places

Clove does not grow in the United States. The aromatic clove evergreen reaches 25 feet. Tanzania produces about 80 percent of the world's supply. Clove also grows in Indonesia, Sri Lanka, Brazil, and the West Indies.

COCOA (CHOCOLATE)

Yes! It's Good for You!

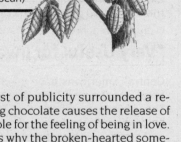

Family: Sterculiaceae; other members include kola

Genus and species: *Theobroma cacao*

Also known as: Chocolate, cacao

Parts used: Seed (often called bean)

Just a few years ago a burst of publicity surrounded a report suggesting that eating chocolate causes the release of brain chemicals responsible for the feeling of being in love. Researchers theorized this is why the broken-hearted sometimes seek solace in a box of chocolates.

Though this research is yet to be confirmed, there is still reason for chocoholics to rejoice! Your favorite vice may be just what the doctor ordered. Cocoa and its derivative, chocolate, may aid digestion, boost blood flow to the heart, and help anyone with chest congestion breathe easier. Unwrap a chocolate kiss and read on.

Aztec Treat

Imagine a world without chocolate. That would be a desolate world indeed. But that's how it was until 1519, when Spanish conquistador Hernando Cortez saw Mexico's Aztec ruler, Montezuma, sip a drink called *chocolatl* from a golden goblet. Cortez was more interested in the goblet than its contents until the Aztecs informed him the drink was made from beans so valuable that 100 could buy a healthy human slave.

Cortez introduced the Aztec treat to the Spanish court, where it became an instant sensation. The Spanish tried to keep chocolate a secret and succeeded for more than 100 years, but by the 1660s it had spread throughout Europe. Chocolate became especially popular in England and Holland, where the bitter drink was enriched and sweetened with milk and sugar.

Oddly, until the 19th century, chocolate was solely a beverage, sometimes bitter, sometimes sweet, but always a liquid. It was only about 150 years ago that it was fashioned into the blocks and candies we so love today.

"Very Useful for Invalids"

Central Americans have used cocoa for centuries to treat fever, coughs, and complaints of pregnancy and childbirth. They have also rubbed cocoa butter on burns, chapped lips, balding heads, and the sore nipples of nursing mothers.

America's 19th-century Eclectics recommended cocoa butter externally as a wound dressing and salve. For internal use, they prescribed hot cocoa for asthma, as a substitute for coffee, and as "a very useful nutritive for invalids and persons convalescing from acute illness."

Few contemporary herbalists recommended cocoa or chocolate as a healing herb. It's their loss.

Devil's Food?

Chocolate cake is called "devil's food." And no wonder. The product of this herb has long been villified as a cause of obesity, acne, heart disease, kidney stones, tooth decay, headaches, heartburn, and infant colic. Much of this reputation is undeserved.

Chocolate's fat content may contribute to obesity and heart disease, but the chocolate used in confections is rarely as much of a problem as their high-fat, high-cholesterol butter and cream. Cocoa and chocolate contain no cholesterol (except milk chocolate, whose dairy ingredients contain a small amount). However, they are high in saturated fat, the kind of fat that can raise cholesterol levels and contributes to heart disease. But a good deal of cocoa's saturated fat is in the form of stearic acid, which does *not* raise cholesterol. For the record, here's how the various kinds of chocolate stack up.

Type	Calories (1 oz.)	Calories from Fat (%)
Cocoa	75	65
Bittersweet	135	75
Baker's	143	93
Milk	147	56

Bad Rumors

Chocolate's contribution to tooth decay has been blown out of proportion. Some research even suggests that cocoa contains substances that *inhibit* the growth of bacteria that cause tooth decay. Again the problem with chocolate candy is not its cocoa content but rather the other sugary, gooey ingredients.

There is no evidence that chocolate causes acne, kidney stones, or infant colic. However, chocolate does contain chemicals (tyramines) that trigger headaches in some people, particularly those prone to migraines.

HEALING with Cocoa

Cocoa contains two chemicals that account for its uses in herbal healing—caffeine and theobromine.

Pick-Me-Up. Cocoa has only 10 to 20 percent of coffee's caffeine content—about 13 milligrams per cup compared with instant coffee's 65 milligrams and drip coffee's 100 to 150 milligrams. As a result, cocoa and chocolate may relieve drowsiness and provide mild stimulation without causing as much jitteriness, insomnia, and irritability as coffee. Try some when you feel lethargic—purely as herbal medicine, of course.

Digestive Aid. The theobromine in cocoa relaxes the smooth muscle lining of the digestive tract, which may be why many people have room for chocolate after a heavy meal. Try some to soothe your stomach after meals.

Asthma. Theobromine and caffeine are close chemical relatives of a standard treatment for asthma (theophylline), which opens the bronchial passages of the lungs. Theobromine and caffeine have similar effects. Even if you don't have asthma, try cocoa or chocolate for the chest congestion of colds and flu.

Rx for Cocoa

Kiss guilt good-bye. Now there are some genuine, good-for-you reasons to brew yourself a heavenly cup of cocoa. Try it as a pick-me-up or digestive aid. Anyone with asthma should be under a doctor's care, but there's no harm in a cup of cocoa for possible relief.

To make cocoa, use 1 to 2 heaping teaspoons per cup of hot water or low-fat or skim milk.

Some children and adults are extrasensitive to the stimulants in cocoa and chocolate. If insomnia, irritability, or hyperactivity become a problem, reduce consumption.

The Safety Factor

The real safety issues have to do with this herb's caffeine content. Caffeine is a powerfully stimulating, classically addictive drug. It is associated with insomnia, irritability, and anxiety attacks; increased blood pressure, cholesterol, and blood sugar (glucose) levels; and increased risk of birth defects. (See "Coffee" on page 182 for a complete discussion of caffeine's many effects.)

Cocoa and chocolate contain only 10 to 20 percent as much caffeine as coffee, but large amounts can produce classic caffeine effects. Anyone with insomnia, anxiety problems, high cholesterol, high blood pressure, diabetes, or heart disease should limit caffeine consumption.

Watch for the Burn

Many people find a cup of hot chocolate soothes their stomachs after meals. The only glitch here is that cocoa and chocolate may cause heartburn. The herb relaxes the valve between the stomach and the esophagus, the tube that carries food down to it. When this valve (the lower esophageal sphincter) does not shut tightly, stomach acids splash up into the esophagus, causing heartburn. If cocoa or chocolate gives you heartburn, use less or stop using it.

Cocoa and chocolate are on the Food and Drug Administration's list of herbs generally regarded as safe. For otherwise healthy nonpregnant, nonnursing adults with no history of insomnia, anxiety problems, high cholesterol, high blood pressure, diabetes, or heart disease, cocoa and chocolate are safe in amounts typically consumed.

Cocoa should be used in medicinal amounts only in consultation with your doctor. If heartburn, headache, or caffeine effects develop, use less or stop using it. Let your doctor know if you experience any unpleasant effects or if the symptoms for which the herb is being used do not improve significantly in two weeks.

Where Does Chocolate Come From?

Cocoa (or cacao) should not be confused with coconut, or with coca, the source of cocaine. Trees grow in the tropics, not in the United States.

Once harvested, cocoa beans are roasted and ground into a liquid known as cocoa liquor. Cocoa liquor then undergoes Dutching, the addition of a minute amount of lye to enhance its flavor. (The amount is so small, it poses no health hazard.) The liquor is then further processed to remove its fat, known as cocoa butter. The final product, chocolate, is a combination of the defatted cocoa powder with some cocoa butter added back.

The powder we call cocoa is simply dried cocoa liquor, with perhaps a little sugar added. Baker's chocolate is processed cocoa liquor with no sugar added. Bittersweet chocolate has some sugar added. Semi-sweet chocolate contains more sugar. And milk chocolate has the most sugar, plus milk to make it creamy.

COFFEE

Beyond the Boost

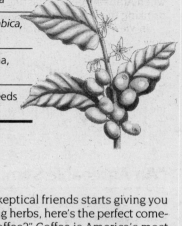

Family: Rubiaceae; other members include gardenia, ipecac, cinchona

Genus and species: *Coffea arabica, C. liberica, C. robusta*

Also known as: Arabica, mocha, java, espresso, capuccino, latté

Parts used: Roasted, ground seeds ("beans")

Next time one of your skeptical friends starts giving you a hard time about using herbs, here's the perfect comeback: "Do you drink coffee?" Coffee is America's most widely used herbal infusion. The average American drinks 28 gallons a year. But coffee does more than help us "take a break." It may help prevent asthma attacks. It may boost physical stamina. And it may help people lose weight and overcome jet lag.

Coffee can also cause significant health problems. Few Americans appreciate just how potent it is. Coffee should be used as carefully as any other healing herb. Its active constituent (caffeine) is an addictive drug.

Tribal War Tonic

Our word *coffee* comes from Caffa, the region of Ethiopia where the fabled beans were first discovered. Archeological evidence suggests that prehistoric East Africans loved coffee's remarkable stimulant properties. They ate the red, unroasted beans ("cherries") before tribal wars, extended hunts, and other activities requiring alertness, strength, and stamina.

The beverage we know as coffee emerged around A.D. 1000, when Arabians began roasting and grinding coffee beans and drinking the hot beverage as we do today.

In view of coffee's enormous popularity, it's surprising how slowly the habit spread. For 500 years, coffee remained in the Middle East. Around 1500, spice traders introduced it into Italy, and within 150 years, it had spread throughout Europe.

Until the 17th century, Arabia supplied all the world's coffee through the port of Mocha, which became one of coffee's names. Then the Dutch introduced the plant into Java, and the island quickly became synonymous with coffee.

"An Agreeable Stimulant"

Coffee has always been more popular as a beverage than as a healing herb. But European herbalists prescribed its stimulant effect to treat opium and alcohol sedation.

America's 19th-century Eclectics prescribed coffee as "an agreeable stimulant . . . that frequently overcomes the soporific [sedative] effects of opium, morphine, and alcohol." They also recommended it to treat asthma, constipation, menstrual cramps, and dropsy (congestive heart failure).

The Eclectics also recognized coffee's downside: "If taken too freely, [coffee causes] irritability, trembling, confusion, ringing in the ears, and disorders of the bowel. On the other hand, if one is accustomed to moderate amounts, headache will result if the coffee be withdrawn."

Folk healers have used coffee for centuries to treat asthma, fever, headache, colds, and flu. But few modern herbalists include it among healing herbs. How odd. Coffee is America's most popular herb.

HEALING with Coffee

Caffeine, the stimulant in coffee (and cocoa, tea, maté, and cola drinks) is also an ingredient in many cold, flu, sleep-prevention, and menstrual remedies—uses that are direct outgrowths of its role in traditional herbal healing.

Coffee's caffeine content depends on how it's prepared. A cup of instant contains about 65 milligrams. Drip or percolated coffee has 100 to 150 milligrams. A cup of espresso contains about 350 milligrams.

Caffeine is such an integral part of our culture, we seldom realize how much of a drug it is. The fact is, caffeine is classically addictive. Regular users develop a tolerance and require more to obtain the expected effect. Deprived of caffeine, regular users usually develop withdrawal symptoms, primarily headache.

The media regularly report health problems linked to coffee, but they never discuss its many possible healing benefits.

Pick-Me-Up. No doubt about it: Coffee is a powerful central nervous system stimulant. For those who drive long distances, it helps prevent dozing at the wheel. And it counteracts the sedative effects of antihistamines, which is one reason it's included in many cold remedies. It does not, however, help people sober up after overindulging in alcohol.

Increased Stamina. Attention, athletes: Coffee may improve physical stamina, according to a report in *The Physician and Sportsmedicine*. The International Olympic Committee forbids the use of more than seven cups within 3 hours before Olympic events.

Asthma. A few studies show coffee helps prevent asthma attacks. The caffeine opens the bronchial passages in the lungs, thus supporting one of the herb's traditional uses.

Weight Loss. Coffee may help some people lose weight. It may boost the number of calories you burn per hour—your metabolic rate—by about 4 percent. In people with weight problems, that translates to a significant increase in calories burned after a meal, according to one study.

Jet Lag. Jet lag is the disorientation, insomnia, and fatigue that develop after flying across time zones. Coffee may help shift the body's natural time cycle (circadian rhythm) after abrupt time-zone changes. Some jet-lag authorities recommend drinking coffee in the morning when traveling west and in the late afternoon when traveling east.

Rx for Coffee

Coffee has a wonderful, pleasantly bitter taste. Americans have more than proven that that's sufficient incentive to drink it regularly. You might also enjoy coffee as a pick-me-up for its stimulating effects, to possibly help increase stamina, prevent asthma attacks and jet lag, or with meals as a possible weight-loss aid.

For an infusion (otherwise known as a cup of java), use 1 heaping tablespoon of ground beans per cup of water. Brew it using your favorite method—or buy instant and follow directions on the label. Drink up to 3 cups a day.

Coffee-flavored food items (yogurt, ice cream, etc.) also contain caffeine. If you use them, adjust your coffee consumption downward.

Coffee should not be given to children under age 2. For older children and people over 65, start with low-strength brews and increase strength if necessary.

The Safety Factor

Coffee may increase anxiety, blood pressure, cholesterol, heart and respiration rate, and secretion of stomach acid. It may cause insomnia, irritability, and nervousness. Caffeine has also been implicated in cancer, heart disease, anxiety neuroses, and birth defects. One recent report noted: "If caffeine were a newly synthesized drug, its manufacturer would almost certainly have great difficulty getting it licensed under current [Food and Drug Administration] regulations. If it were licensed, it would almost certainly be available only by prescription."

More Than the Jitters

When you drink more coffee than you're used to, what happens? As every coffee drinker knows, you get jittery and impatient and have trouble falling asleep. Individual reactions to caffeine vary, but over time, large amounts cause "caffeinism," a condition with the same symptoms as anxiety neurosis: nervousness and irritability, chronic muscle tension, insomnia, heart palpitations, diarrhea, heartburn, and stomach upset. In fact, many people are misdiagnosed with "anxiety neurosis" when the problem is actually caffeinism, according to a report in the *American Journal of Psychiatry*.

Not everyone who quits or cuts back develops withdrawal symptoms, but most do. The throbbing headache usually begins within 18 to 24 hours and lasts a few days. Constipation is also possible for a day or two.

Special Orders for Special Conditions

- Coffee increases secretion of stomach acid. Those with ulcers or other chronic digestive disorders should use it sparingly, if at all.
- Three cups of brewed coffee can boost blood pressure as much as 15 percent. If you have this risk factor for heart disease and stroke, discuss your coffee consumption with your physician.
- Even a moderate coffee habit, a cup or two each morning, may boost blood cholesterol levels by about 5 percent. Five to 10 cups a day may boost it by as much as 10 percent.

But recently, researchers discovered that only *boiled* coffee appears to raise cholesterol. Drip and instant apparently do not, for reasons that remain a mystery.

If your cholesterol level is high enough to put you at increased risk of heart disease, discuss your coffee consumption with your physician. If you don't stop drinking it, make sure you use only drip or instant.

- Independent of coffee's action on cholesterol and blood pressure, it also increases risk of heart attack. Drinking five cups a day almost doubles heart attack risk, and ten cups almost triples it, according to a study published in the *American Journal of Epidemiology*.

If you have heart disease or a history of stroke, discuss your coffee consumption with your physician.

- Many animal studies link caffeine with an increased risk of birth defects. The doses given to the experimental animals were much higher than what even heavy coffee drinkers consume. But prudence suggests that pregnant women limit their consumption.
- Coffee has been linked to cancers of the breast, bladder, ovaries, pancreas, and prostate gland. All of these reports have subsequently been disputed. Several have been thoroughly debunked. Coffee's contribution to human cancer, if any, remains unclear. However, the roasting process introduces pro-cancer chemicals into coffee beans. People with a history of cancer might want to limit their consumption.
- Some studies link caffeine to painful, noncancerous breast lumps (fibrocysts), a normal but annoying condition. Women bothered by a fibrocystic breast condition might try cutting out *all* caffeine—in coffee, tea, cocoa, chocolate, soft drinks, and over-the-counter drugs—and seeing if their condition improves.
- In one study, women who drank two to four cups of brewed coffee a day suffered five times the rate of bloating and other premenstrual symptoms of those who abstained.
- Coffee interferes with iron absorption, a potential problem for people with iron-deficiency anemia, or for women who experience heavy menstrual flow.

Coffee and Conception

Women who drink 1 cup of brewed coffee a day are only about half as likely to get pregnant as those who don't, according to a study conducted by the National Institute of Environmental Health. Women attempting to conceive, especially those with a history of infertility, are advised to limit their intake of beverages or drugs containing caffeine.

On the other hand, researchers agree caffeine should not be used as a contraceptive, because its fertility-reducing effect is highly unreliable. You'd be foolish to use it as a contraceptive.

How Safe Is It?

Until recently, the Food and Drug Administration listed coffee among the herbs generally regarded as safe, but publicity concerning caffeine's many health hazards has prompted the agency to reconsider coffee's status.

For otherwise healthy nonpregnant, nonnursing adults who have no history of ulcers, hypertension, diabetes, high cholesterol, anxiety, fertility problems, or heart disease and are not taking other medications containing caffeine, coffee is considered relatively safe in amounts of up to three brewed cups per day.

Coffee should be used in medicinal amounts only in consultation with your doctor. If coffee causes insomnia, stomach distress, anxiety or any of the other problems discussed above, use less or stop using it. Let your doctor know if you experience any unpleasant effects or if the symptoms for which the herb is being used do not improve significantly in two weeks.

Pretty as a Houseplant

Coffee grows in tropical areas around the world. The plant is an evergreen shrub or small tree with two-seeded, bright crimson fruits. The green seeds (beans) are extracted and roasted to produce the dark brown, oily beans recognized the world over. (Most of the world's supply consists of the Arabian *arabica* species. But *liberica*, from Liberia, and *robusta*, from the Congo, are also cultivated worldwide.)

You can, however, grow a coffee plant purely as an ornamental if you live in a sunny, humid area where the temperature does not dip below 60°F. The plant requires full sun, moist air, moist soil, good drainage, and regular feeding. Coffee plants are also available as house plants. Again, they require full sun and high humidity. They grow well in greenhouses, but not in homes with forced-air heating, which tend to be too dry. Consult your local nursery or plant store.

COLTSFOOT

World's Oldest Cough Remedy

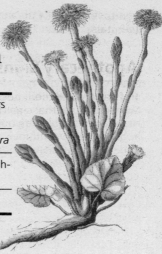

Family: Compositae; other members include daisy, dandelion, marigold

Genus and species: *Tussilago farfara*

Also known as: Cough plant, coughwort, horse hoof, horse foot

Parts used: Leaves, flowers

Coltsfoot has been a cough-suppressing mainstay of Asian and European herbal medicine for 2,000 years. And it's still widely used today.

In addition to using the herb to treat cough, Chinese physicians have long prescribed it for asthma, colds, flu, bronchial congestion, and even lung cancer.

India's traditional Ayurvedic doctors prescribed powdered coltsfoot in the form of snuff to treat cough, headache, and nasal congestion.

For cough and asthma, the ancient Greek physician Dioscorides and the Romans Pliny and Galen recommended a coltsfoot treatment that today sounds ridiculous—smoking the herb. But this approach continued for more than 1,500 years.

With characteristic exaggeration, 17th-century English herbalist Nicholas Culpeper touted coltsfoot not only for "wheezings, shortness of breath, and coughing," but also for fevers, inflammations, and burning in the "privy parts" (genitals).

Apothecary Signs

In Paris around the time of the French Revolution, coltsfoot was so popular that signs bearing its golden flowers were the standard symbol hung outside apothecary shops.

Colonists introduced coltsfoot into North America, and the Indians adopted it as a cough remedy. For whooping cough, the colonists soaked blankets in buckets of hot coltsfoot infusion and wrapped them around the ill person. The 19th-century American Eclectic physicians prescribed coltsfoot for all respiratory problems and digestive upsets.

Contemporary herbalists recommend the herb for respiratory problems. Some say poultices of the fresh, bruised leaf may be applied to burns, swellings, and inflammations.

Healing with Coltsfoot

Scientists are sharply divided on coltsfoot. The German medical text *Herbal Medicine* calls it "the remedy of choice" for cough, adding, "coltsfoot tea has proved particularly effective in emphysema." But herb conservative Varro Tyler, Ph.D., calls it carcinogenic and "no longer appropriate therapy" (see "The Safety Factor" on page 192).

Cough and Asthma. Coltsfoot may help treat respiratory problems in several ways. It contains a substance (mucilage) that may soothe the respiratory tract.

A German study using experimental animals showed the herb increases the activity of the microscopic hairs in the breathing tubes that move mucus out of the respiratory tract.

Another experiment shows that the herb suppresses a substance (platelet activating factor or PAF) in the body that is involved in triggering asthma attacks.

Rx for Coltsfoot

If you want to put coltsfoot's traditional cough-suppressing powers to the test, you should consult with your physician. Use of this particular herb continues to be somewhat controversial in the United States. Coltsfoot (and comfrey) have been banned in Canada and herb critics in the United States are pressing for a similar ban.

In European countries where coltsfoot is routinely used, the herb is taken as an infusion or tincture. As the taste is somewhat bitter, it is often taken with a little honey.

Coltsfoot should not be given to children under the age of 2.

Herb conservatives in this country recommend slippery elm (see page 496) as a safe herb to calm coughs.

The Safety Factor

Coltsfoot contains chemicals (pyrrolizidines) that in large amounts can cause serious liver damage in the form of hepatic veno-occlusive disease (HVOD). This is a condition in which the liver's blood vessels narrow, impairing its function. In addition, experimental animals fed diets containing large amounts of coltsfoot developed liver cancer, according to a report published in the *Journal of the National Cancer Institute*.

The discovery of hazardous substances in coltsfoot spurred several authorities to condemn the herb as dangerous, even "carcinogenic." But in Germany, where herbal medicine is considerably more mainstream than it is in the United States, it continues to be widely prescribed, and physicians consider short-term use safe.

A recent laboratory investigation shows that coltsfoot does not cause damage to human chromosomes, which suggests it is not carcinogenic. Carcinogens almost always cause chromosome damage.

On the other hand, pyrrolizidines can cause liver damage.

Anyone with a history of alcoholism or liver disease should not use coltsfoot.

Use with Caution

The Food and Drug Administration lists coltsfoot as an herb of "undefined safety." For otherwise healthy nonpregnant, nonnursing adults who have no history of alcoholism or liver disease and are not taking other drugs with potential liver toxicity, coltsfoot is considered relatively safe in amounts typically recommended.

Coltsfoot should be used in medicinal amounts only in consultation with your doctor. If coltsfoot causes minor discomforts, such as stomach upset or diarrhea, use less or stop using it. Let your doctor know if you experience any unpleasant effects, if a cough does not improve significantly in two weeks, if fever develops, or if you cough up brown or bloody phlegm.

Unusual Leaves

Unique among healing herbs, coltsfoot's flowers precede its leaves. The golden blossoms are among the first wildflowers to appear in spring. But the plant's broad, hoof-shaped leaves do not appear until after the flowers have withered.

Coltsfoot is a low-growing perennial with flowers resembling marigolds. It's so easy to grow, it may overrun a garden. But it works well in containers.

Coltsfoot is best propagated from root cuttings planted in spring or fall. It likes a moist, clay soil under full sun or partial shade. Flowers should be gathered in full bloom and dried. Leaves should be harvested when mature.

COMFREY

Controversial Wound Treatment

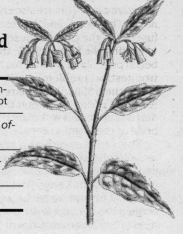

Family: Boraginaceae; other members include borage, forget-me-not

Genus and species: *Symphytum officinale*

Also known as: Bruisewort, knitbone, boneset, healing herb

Parts used: Roots and leaves

For years herbalists have touted comfrey as "an absolute must," an herb with "a healing and soothing effect on every organ," "ideal for the amateur herbalist," "perfectly safe and harmless." But ever since liver-damaging, cancer-causing chemicals were discovered in it, scientists have blasted it as "definitely hazardous to health."

Healer or hazard? The truth lies somewhere in between.

Battlefield Casts

The early Greeks first used juicy comfrey root externally to treat wounds, believing it encouraged torn flesh to grow back together. The Roman naturalist Pliny "verified" this practice with the observation that boiling comfrey in water produces a sticky paste capable of binding chunks of meat together.

Comfrey paste hardens like plaster, and cloths soaked in it were often wrapped around broken bones on ancient battlefields. When the paste dried, the result was a primitive but effective cast. This treatment earned comfrey the popular names "knitbone" and "boneset." (Comfrey should not be confused with the other Boneset; see page 124.)

During the first century, the Greek physician Dioscorides began prescribing comfrey tea internally for respiratory and gastrointestinal problems.

By the 1500s, herbalists were recommending comfrey tea—not paste—to mend broken bones. One early English herbal suggested it "helpeth [people who have] broken the bone of the legge."

The 17th-century English herbalist Nicholas Culpeper recommended comfrey roots, "full of glutinous and clammy juice," for "all inward hurts . . . and for outward wounds and sores in [all] fleshy or sinewy parts of the body . . . [It] is especially good for ruptures and broken bones." Culpeper also prescribed the herb for fever, gout, hemorrhoids, gangrene, and respiratory and menstrual problems.

Internal Soothing

As plaster replaced comfrey paste for casting broken bones, names like knitbone were discarded. Comfrey came to be used internally to soothe inflamed mucous membranes. America's 19th-century Eclectic physicians prescribed it for diarrhea, dysentery, cough, bronchitis, and "female debility" (menstrual discomfort).

Mexican midwives still apply comfrey to vaginal tears. In the Philippines, the herb is used to treat arthritis, diabetes, anemia, lung infections, and even leukemia.

Not many modern herbalists have been daunted by the discovery of cancer-causing chemicals in comfrey. A few herbalists, such as Michael Weiner in *Weiner's Herbal*, recommend using comfrey only externally, because of its cancer taint. But most modern herbalists pooh-pooh any association with cancer. They continue to tout it enthusiastically for ulcers, ulcerative colitis, internal hemorrhages, bronchitis, bleeding gums, hoarseness, and digestive complaints.

HEALING with Comfrey

The ancient Greeks and Romans were right about comfrey aiding wound healing, but the herb's stickiness has nothing to do with it.

Wound Healing. Comfrey contains a chemical (allantoin), that promotes the growth of new cells, thus validating its more than 2,500 years of external use on everything from minor cuts and burns to major battle wounds. Studies show comfrey also helps relieve inflammation, adding to its wound-treating effect.

Allantoin is the active ingredient in several over-the-counter skin creams, such as Unicare Lotion, for example. Two prescription skin preparations also contain it, Herpecin-L Cold Sore Lip Balm for relief of oral herpes, and Vagimide Cream for irritation associated with vaginal infections.

Comfrey is not absorbed through the skin, and even its harshest critics have never questioned its safety for external use. However, be sure to wash wounds thoroughly with soap and water before applying comfrey.

For wound treatment, comfrey roots are preferable to the leaves. Roots contain more than twice as much allantoin.

Digestive Aid. Some animal research suggests comfrey calms the digestive tract, lending support to its traditional use as a digestive aid.

Dead-End File. Despite the assertions in some recent herbals, one of which calls comfrey "one of the best healers of the respiratory system," no research to date shows any benefit for the lungs.

R_x for Comfrey

To use comfrey externally, sprinkle some dried, powdered root on clean cuts and scrapes.

Internal use of comfrey continues to be controversial in the United States. If you'd like to put its stomach-soothing powers to the test, ask your physician about using it for a short time. Herbalists traditionally took it in the form of an infusion or a tincture. Comfrey tastes earthy and slightly sweet.

If you'd like to use an herbal stomach soother on a regular basis, try peppermint, ginger, or any of the other herbs listed as Digestive Aids in chapter 6.

Comfrey should not be given to children under age 2.

The Safety Factor

Comfrey has been found to contain chemicals (pyrrolizidines) that in large amounts cause serious liver damage and cancer in laboratory animals. As a result, Canada banned comfrey (and coltsfoot), and herb critics are pressing for similar bans in the United States.

The Liver Scare

Comfrey has also been known to cause liver damage in humans. Excessive amounts of the herb can cause a disorder known as hepatic veno-occlusive disease (HVOD), or Budd-Chiari syndrome, in which the liver's blood vessels narrow, impairing its function.

In one case, a woman developed HVOD after four months of taking six comfrey/pepsin digestive capsules daily and drinking a quart of comfrey tea a day. According to a published report in the *New England Journal of Medicine*, six comfrey/pepsin tablets a day could cause HVOD within a few months.

In another case, the parents of a boy with Crohn's disease, a chronic intestinal disorder similar to ulcerative colitis, took him off standard treatment and gave him comfrey tea instead. After two years, he developed HVOD.

Both of these cases involved unusually high doses of comfrey for unusually long periods. HVOD has never been reported in people taking recommended amounts of the herb for brief periods.

The Cancer Question

Experimental animals fed large amounts of comfrey for almost two years developed liver cancer, according to the *Journal of the National Cancer Institute.* Roots caused more cancer in the animals than did leaves.

Comfrey also contains tumor-fighting substances, making it one of many healing herbs that contain both pro- and anti-cancer chemicals. Comfrey contains appreciable amounts of antioxidant nutrients—vitamins C and E and beta-carotene, which the body converts to vitamin A. The American Cancer Society recommends a diet high in antioxidant nutrients to help prevent cancer.

Safety Issue Unresolved

Today, authorities are divided on comfrey's safety for internal use. Critics continue to villify the herb. A study published in the *Lancet* estimated a single cup of comfrey root tea might constitute a "significant health risk."

But Britain's National Institute of Medical Herbalists says, "No man, woman, or child has been recorded as suffering toxic effects from taking [recommended doses] of comfrey leaf or root as medicine."

In a landmark study published in *Science*, cancer authority Bruce Ames, Ph.D., chairman of the Biochemistry Department at the University of California at Berkeley, attempted to estimate the average person's lifetime cancer risk from exposure to hundreds of man-made and naturally occuring carcinogens. He estimated one cup of comfrey tea posed:

- About the same cancer risk as one peanut butter sandwich, which contains traces of the natural carcinogen aflatoxin.
- About one-third the risk of eating one raw mushroom, which contains traces of the natural carcinogen hydrazine.
- About half the risk of one diet soda containing saccharin.
- And about one-hundredth the risk of a standard beer or glass of wine, which contains the natural carcinogen ethyl alcohol.

Dr. Ames also estimated that comfrey/pepsin tablets carry up to 200 times the risk of comfrey tea.

The lesson is clear: Don't use comfrey/pepsin tablets. Many other herbs aid digestion without any risk of liver damage.

Anyone with a history of liver disease, alcoholism, or cancer should steer clear of the herb altogether. But Dr. Ames's work strongly suggests that for the occasional user, comfrey's hazards have been blown out of proportion. Comfrey has never been implicated in any case of human liver cancer, and the two cases of comfrey-induced HVOD do not constitute a major public-health threat.

A Safe Path

The Food and Drug Administration lists comfrey as an herb of "undefined safety." For otherwise healthy nonpregnant, nonnursing adults who are not taking other medications and have no history of liver disease, alcoholism, or cancer, comfrey may be considered relatively safe for short-term occasional use in amounts typically recommended.

Comfrey should be used in medicinal amounts only in consultation with your doctor. If comfrey causes minor discomforts, such as stomach upset or diarrhea, use less or stop using it. Let your doctor know if you experience any unpleasant effects or if the symptoms for which the herb is being used do not improve significantly in two weeks.

Easy to Grow

Comfrey is a hardy 5-foot perennial with large, hairy, lance-shaped leaves, thick, spreading roots, a hollow, bristly stem, and bell-like flowers, which may be white, blue, or purple.

Comfrey can be started from seeds, but it grows best from root cuttings taken in spring or fall. An inch-long piece of root planted in 3 inches of soil almost always produces a plant. Set cuttings 3 feet apart. The herb grows in any well-drained soil and tolerates full sun or partial shade.

Comfrey spreads vigorously. Contain it in a pot, or border it with sheet metal to a depth of 12 inches.

Leaves may be harvested when the flowers begin to bud. Gather the roots in autumn, after the first frost, or in spring before the first leaves appear. Wash harvested roots thoroughly and cut them into slices to dry. Then powder them in a blender or coffee grinder. Store in a sealed container.

Just as necessity is the mother of invention, safety scares are often the mother of hybridization. University of Minnesota scientists report growing comfrey with no detectable pyrrolizidines. Even the herb's harshest critics may soon be able to give their blessings to new varieties of the herb.

CORIANDER (CILANTRO)

Healer from Heaven

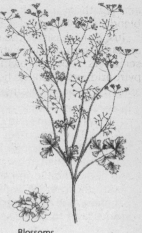

Family: Umbelliferae; other members include carrot, parsley

Genus and species: *Coriandrum sativum*

Also known as: The fruits (actually seeds) are coriander; the leaves are known as cilantro or Chinese parsley

Parts used: Seeds, leaves

Blossoms

Seeds

After the Exodus, when the Hebrews were starving in the Sinai wilderness, God fed them manna from heaven, which the Bible says tasted "like coriander." If manna did what coriander does, chances are none of the children of Israel had indigestion. Warm, spicy coriander, a flavor combination of sage and citrus, has been used as an herbal digestive aid for thousands of years. Science has lent support to the ancients.

Pharaohs' Favorite

The Hebrews adopted coriander from their former masters, the Egyptians, who used it as a spice, perfume, and digestive aid. The Egyptians considered coriander such a basic necessity that seeds have been found in several Pharaoh's tombs, presumably to prevent indigestion in the afterlife.

Hippocrates and other noted Greek and Roman physicians prescribed coriander as a digestive aid and gas remedy. The Romans also used the spice as a meat preservative.

In India, coriander became an ingredient in curry spice blends and gained a reputation as an aphrodisiac. India's traditional Ayurvedic healers used it to treat digestive complaints, allergies, and urinary problems, and as an ingredient in eyewashes used to prevent blindness.

Coriander arrived in China from India during the Han dynasty (207 B.C. to A.D. 220). At the time it was reputed to enhance lovemaking and confer immortality. Today, Chinese physicians use the herb more modestly to treat dysentery, measles, and hemorrhoids, and as a gargle for toothache.

Around the 8th century, the mythic Arabian princess Scheherazade described coriander as an aphrodisiac in the stories later collected as *The Thousand and One Arabian Nights*.

Today's Jawbreakers

Coriander was never a major healing herb in Europe, but it has always been considered a digestive aid, not only in foods but also in candies. In 16th-century England, coriander seeds were used as the centers of hard candies. Queen Elizabeth I loved the candies, which evolved into today's jawbreakers.

Early American herbalists added coriander to bitter laxative herbs, such as buckthorn, so they would taste better and have less violent action.

Contemporary herbalists recommend coriander internally for indigestion, flatulence, and diarrhea, and externally in salves for muscle and joint pains.

HEALING with Coriander

Coriander is no wonder herb, but who can argue with manna from heaven?

Digestive Aid. Some studies indicate coriander helps settle the stomach, but it's not as soothing as other herbs—

peppermint, chamomile, and caraway, for example. Still, it helps.

Infection Prevention. The ancient Roman use of coriander as a meat preservative has been supported by some Japanese and Russian research. The herb contains substances that kill certain bacteria, fungi, and insect larvae, which attack meats. These same microorganisms can cause human wound infections. Sprinkle some coriander on minor cuts and scrapes after they have been thoroughly washed with soap and water.

Intriguing Possibilities. One animal study shows coriander has anti-inflammatory action, suggesting it might help relieve arthritis. If you have arthritis, try it and see if it helps.

Another study shows it reduces blood sugar (glucose) levels, hinting at possible value in the management of diabetes. Diabetes requires professional treatment, but it can't hurt to try coriander in consultation with your physician.

Rx for Coriander

Coriander might not be the most potent digestive aid around, but there is one good excuse to select it over the alternatives—its taste. You'll find it a warm, fragrant combination of sage and citrus. For an infusion, use 1 teaspoon of bruised seeds (or 1/2 teaspoon of powder) per cup of boiling water. Steep 5 minutes. Drink up to 3 cups a day before or after meals.

Weak coriander infusions may be given cautiously to children under age 2 for colic. For older children and people over 65, start with low-strength preparations and increase strength if necessary.

To use coriander externally, sprinkle some of the powdered herb on freshly washed cuts and scrapes.

The Safety Factor

The Food and Drug Administration includes coriander in its list of herbs generally regarded as safe. For otherwise healthy nonpregnant, nonnursing adults, coriander is considered safe in amounts typically recommended.

Coriander should be used in medicinal amounts only in consultation with your doctor. If coriander causes minor discomforts, such as stomach upset or diarrhea, use less or stop using it. Let your doctor know if you experience any unpleasant effects or if the symptoms for which the herb is being used do not improve significantly in two weeks.

Great for the Garden

Coriander is a bright green, 3-foot annual with lobed lower leaves and lacy upper leaves. Its seeds are small, spherical, ribbed, and brownish. They develop in clusters and when fresh emit an odor that has been compared to burned rubber. As they ripen, however, they develop their characteristic spicy fragrance.

Coriander grows easily from seeds sown ½ inch deep in April or May in most parts of the United States. Germination takes up to three weeks, and the plant produces seeds in about three months.

Coriander grows best in moist, well-drained, moderately rich soil under full sun, but it tolerates some shade. Thin plants to 9-inch spacing. Do not overfertilize. Excess nitrogen impairs the herb's flavor and aroma.

An extra bonus from growing coriander is the leaves— which are known in their own right as cilantro, a tasty seasoning herb. To harvest cilantro, cut the small, immature leaves for best flavor.

To harvest coriander seeds, wait until a majority have turned from green to brownish, around the time their aroma stops being unpleasant. Dry and store in airtight jars. The flavor of whole coriander improves with age. Let some seeds fall, and the plant will self-sow.

CRANBERRY

Prevents Bladder Problems

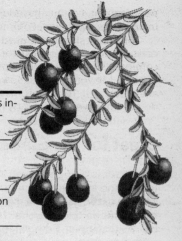

Family: Ericaceae; other members include azalea, rhododendron, blueberry

Genus and species: *Vaccinium macrocarpon* or *Oxycoccus quadripetalus*

Also known as: No other common names

Parts used: Juice from the berries

Many women drink cranberry juice, believing it helps prevent urinary tract infection (UTI). Herbalists and some physicians encourage the practice, but other physicians say the herb doesn't help. The scientific studies have gone both ways, but the latest research shows cranberry probably works.

Thanks to the Pilgrims

Cranberries were eaten for their tangy, refreshing taste long before anyone thought of them as a healing herb. The Pilgrims supposedly dined on cranberry dishes at the first Thanksgiving in 1621, but cranberry sauce did not become a national tradition until after the Civil War. General Ulysses S. Grant considered cranberry sauce an essential part of Thanksgiving, and he ordered it served to Union troops during the siege of Petersburg in 1864. Soldiers unfamiliar with the tart berries liked them, and the custom stuck.

The colonists were unaware of cranberries' high vitamin C content, but cranberries became a favorite among New England sailors because those who ate the bright red berries did not develop scurvy.

America's 19th-century Eclectic physicians did not consider cranberry particularly beneficial, but their text, *King's American Dispensatory*, contained this curious prescription: "A split cranberry, held in position by a daub of starch paste, will quickly relieve the pain and inflammation attending boils on the tip of the nose."

HEALING with Cranberry

Unique among healing herbs, cranberry's claim to fame as a UTI-preventive comes not from herbal tradition but rather from 19th-century German chemists.

Urinary Tract Infection. During the 1840s, German researchers discovered that after eating cranberries, people pass urine that contains a bacteria-fighting chemical known as hippuric acid. Sixty years later, American researchers speculated that urine acidified by a steady diet of cranberries might prevent UTI—a common, recurrent, and often chronic women's health problem.

Women adopted cranberry juice enthusiastically, and several studies endorsed it. But by the late 1960s, naysayers claimed the tart berries did not significantly acidify urine and therefore could not prevent UTI.

But the latest research lends support to the herb once again. An experiment reported in the *Journal of the American Medical Association* shows 73 percent of sufferers of recurrent UTI report "significant improvement" after drinking a pint a day of commercial cranberry juice cocktail for three weeks. The researchers suggest that urinary acidity has nothing to do with the herb's effectiveness. Instead, they wrote, the juice prevents UTI germs from adhering to the lining of the urinary tract, thus reducing the likelihood of infection.

Incontinence. Cranberry juice also helps deodorize urine. A report in the *Journal of Psychiatric Nursing* suggests incorporating the juice into the diet of anyone troubled by urinary incontinence to reduce the embarrassing odor of this problem.

Rx for Cranberry

Cranberry juice cocktail is available at most supermarkets. Pure cranberry juice is highly acidic and too sour to drink, which is why water and sugar are added to the juice sold commercially. If you suffer from UTI, try drinking a couple glasses of the commercial cocktail every day and see if it helps prevent recurrence.

The Safety Factor

For otherwise healthy nonpregnant, nonnursing adults who are not taking other medications affecting the kidney or urinary tract, cranberry juice is considered safe in any amount. No problems have been reported from drinking cranberry juice; however, some people may be allergic or sensitive to it.

Cranberry should be used in medicinal amounts only in consultation with your doctor. If UTI symptoms develop, let your doctor know. Antibiotic treatment is usually necessary.

Grows in Bogs

Cranberry is a small evergreen shrub, which grows in mountain forests and damp bogs from Alaska to Tennessee. Its pink or purple flowers bloom from late spring to late summer and produce bright red fruits in fall.

Few gardeners have the conditions necessary to grow this herb. It requires wet, boggy, acidic soil, amended with peat moss or leaf mold. Check with your local nursery to see if it can grow in your area.

DANDELION

Much More Than a Weed

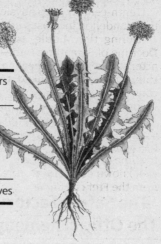

Family: Compositae; other members include daisy, marigold

Genus and species: *Taraxacum officinale*

Also known as: Lion's tooth, wild endive, piss-in-bed

Parts used: Root primarily; also leaves

Dandelion is so widely despised as a weed, it's sometimes difficult to see this plant for what it really is—a nutritious healing herb with a medicinal reputation dating back more than 1,000 years.

Dandelion may help treat premenstrual syndrome, high blood pressure, and congestive heart failure. It may also help prevent gallstones and may have other medically intriguing possibilities as well.

Chinese Cold Remedy

Chinese physicians have prescribed dandelion since ancient times to treat colds, bronchitis, pneumonia, hepatitis, boils, ulcers, obesity, dental problems, itching, and internal injuries. They also used a poultice of chopped dandelion to treat breast cancer. India's traditional Ayurvedic physicians used the herb similarly.

Tenth-century Arab physicians were the first to recognize that dandelion increases urine production.

During the Middle Ages, Europeans believed in the Doctrine of Signatures—the idea that plants' physical characteristics reveal their healing value. Under this doctrine, anything yellow was linked to the liver's yellow bile and considered a liver remedy. That's why dandelion gained a reputation in Europe as a treatment for jaundice and gallstones.

The Doctrine of Signatures was also used to explain dandelion's use as a diuretic to treat water retention. Dandelion has a juicy root, stem, and leaves. Anything juicy was linked to urine production. By the 17th century, dandelion was so well known as a diuretic, the English called it "piss-a-bed," from the French *pissenlit*.

The Official Remedy

Thanks to such herbal exaggerators as 17th-century English herbalist Nicholas Culpeper, dandelion's medicinal reputation spread as widely as dandelions across an untended lawn. Culpeper recommended the herb for every "evil disposition of the body." In fact, dandelion was used for so many ailments, it became known as "the official remedy for disorders."

Early colonists introduced dandelion to North America, and the Indians quickly adopted it as a tonic.

Dandelion root was an ingredient in Lydia E. Pinkham's Vegetable Compound, a popular 19th-century patent medicine for menstrual discomforts. As a diuretic, the dandelion no doubt helped relieve the bloating many women experience before they menstruate. (There is no dandelion in the Pinkham's Compound marketed today.)

Despite dandelion's incorporation into the U.S. *Pharmacopoeia* from 1831 to 1926, many 19th-century herbalists despised it for the weed it had become. The American Eclectic physicians' text, *King's American Dispensatory*, called it "overrated. . . . Dandelion root possesses little medicinal virtue [except] slightly diuretic action."

Contemporary herbalists recommend dandelion almost exclusively as a diuretic for weight loss, premenstrual syndrome, menstrual discomforts, swollen feet, high blood pressure, and congestive heart failure.

HEALING with Dandelion

The Food and Drug Administration (FDA) continues to treat dandelion as a weed. Here's the agency's official position: "There is no convincing reason for believing it possesses any therapeutic virtues."

The FDA forgot to read their Ralph Waldo Emerson. "What is a weed?" Emerson wrote. "A plant whose virtues have not yet been discovered." As far as dandelion is concerned, truer words were never penned, though its virtues *have* been well documented.

Premenstrual Syndrome. Animal studies show that dandelion does indeed have diuretic action. Animal findings don't always apply to people, but this one appears to. Diuretics may help relieve the bloated feeling of premenstrual syndrome. Try some before your period and see if it works for you.

Weight Loss. In one study, animals fed dandelion lost up to 30 percent of their weight. Diuretics can help eliminate water weight, but authorities do not recommend diuretics for permanent weight control. They advocate a low-fat, high-fiber diet and regular aerobic exercise.

High Blood Pressure. Physicians often prescribe diuretics to treat high blood pressure. Dandelion might help. Of course, high blood pressure is a serious condition requiring professional treatment. Use dandelion in consultation with your physician.

Congestive Heart Failure. Physicians often prescribe diuretics to treat this condition. Dandelion might be appropriate in conjunction with other medications and therapies prescribed by your physician.

Like high blood pressure, congestive heart failure is a serious condition that cannot be self-treated. If you'd like to try dandelion, discuss it with your physician and use it in addition to standard medication.

Cancer Prevention. A 1-cup serving of raw dandelion leaves contains 7,000 international units of vitamin A—that's 1½ times the Recommended Dietary Allowance and more than you'd find in a carrot. Dandelion also contains some vitamin C. Vitamins A and C are antioxidants that help prevent the cell damage scientists believe eventually causes cancer. Dandelion leaves are a zesty addition to salads, soups, and stews.

Yeast Infection. One study shows dandelion inhibits the growth of the fungus responsible for vaginal yeast infections (*Candida albicans*).

Digestive Aid. Score one for the Doctrine of Signatures. Two German studies suggest that dandelion stimulates the flow of bile, which helps digest fats.

In Germany, where herbal medicine is more mainstream than it is in the United States, physicians routinely use dandelion to help stimulate bile flow and prevent gallstones. The German preparation Chol-Grandelat, a combination of dandelion, milk thistle, and rhubarb, is prescribed for gallbladder disease. (This product is not available in the United States.)

Intriguing Possibilities. Dandelion also may help reduce the amount of sugar in the blood. As a result, the herb may help manage diabetes. Diabetes is a serious condition that requires professional treatment, but try dandelion in consultation with your physician.

Some studies suggest dandelion root has anti-inflammatory properties, suggesting possible value in treating arthritis. And a Japanese study suggests some antitumor activity as well, though it's much too early to consider it a cancer treatment.

Think twice before using dandelion as a diuretic to promote weight loss. Weight lost using diuretics almost always returns, because the body, which is largely water, eventually senses a lack of fluid and adjusts by decreasing urine output.

In addition, long-term use of diuretics can be hazardous. Diuretics deplete the body of potassium, an essential nutrient. People taking diuretics should be sure to eat foods high in potassium, such as bananas and fresh vegetables.

Fortunately, dandelion causes less potassium loss than other diuretics because the herb itself is high in potassium. Nonetheless, if you use dandelion for long periods, be sure to eat foods high in potassium.

Pregnant and nursing women should not take diuretics.

Rx for Dandelion

Eat fresh leaves as a salad item or vegetable.

If you're using dandelion as a diuretic (for premenstrual syndrome, high blood pressure, or congestive heart failure) or digestive aid, take it as a leaf infusion, root decoction, or tincture. The taste is reasonably pleasant with a slightly bitter sharpness.

To make a leaf infusion, use 1/2 ounce of dried leaves per cup of boiling water. Steep 10 minutes. Drink up to 3 cups a day.

For a root decoction, gently boil 2 to 3 teaspoons of powdered root per cup of water for 15 minutes. Cool. Drink up to 3 cups a day.

In a tincture, take 1 to 2 teaspoons up to three times a day.

As a potential aid to help keep vaginal yeast infections at bay, add a couple of handfuls of dried leaves and flowers to the bathwater.

Dandelion should not be given to children under age 2. For older children and people over 65, start with a low-strength preparation and increase strength if necessary.

The Safety Factor

Dandelion may cause skin rash in sensitive individuals.

Dandelion is included in the Food and Drug Administration's list of herbs generally regarded as safe. For otherwise healthy nonpregnant, nonnursing adults who are not taking other diuretics, dandelion is considered safe in amounts typically recommended.

Dandelion should be used only in consultation with your doctor. If dandelion causes minor discomforts, such as stomach upset or diarrhea, use less or stop using it. Let your doctor know if you experience any unpleasant effects or if the symptoms for which the herb is being used do not improve significantly in two weeks.

Don't Tell Your Neighbors

If you cultivate dandelions, be careful whom you tell. You might end up with some unhappy neighbors.

As every gardener knows, dandelions grow like weeds. Dandelion is a low-growing perennial with deep taproot, a rosette of jaggedly toothed leaves that radiate from its base, and a smooth, hollow, 6- to 12-inch stem capped by a single yellow flower, which gives rise to hundreds of tufted single-seed fruits. The root, leaves, and stem contain a milky fluid. Harvest young leaves as they develop. As the leaves mature, they become unpleasantly bitter. Herbalists generally recommend harvesting the root at the end of the second growing season. To prevent spreading, clip the flowers before seed tufts form.

Dandelion seeds may not be readily available, but check seed catalogs. Better yet, check nearby lawns or vacant lots. It's unlikely that anyone will mind if you take a few. Plant seeds in early spring. They grow in almost any soil but prefer moist, well-drained loam.

DILL

The Seed That Soothes the Stomach

Family: Umbelliferae; other members include carrot, parsley

Genus and species: *Anethum graveolens*

Also known as: No other common names

Parts used: Fruit ("seeds"); leaves are used in cooking

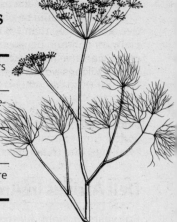

Dill does more for pickles than provide flavor. It's also a natural preservative, and food preservation was the original purpose of pickling.

Dill has been used in herbal healing since the dawn of Egyptian civilization—and for good reason. In addition to its preservative action, dill is an infection fighter and soothing digestive aid.

Deli Comes to the Nile

Records found in 3,000-year-old Egyptian tombs show that ancient physicians used fragrant dill as a digestive aid and intestinal gas remedy.

The first-century Greek physician Dioscorides prescribed dill so frequently it was known for centuries as the herb of Dioscorides.

214

The Romans chewed dill seeds to promote digestion, and they hung dill garlands in their dining halls, believing the herb would prevent stomach upset.

Traditional Chinese physicians have used dill as a digestive aid for more than 1,000 years. They recommend it especially for children because its action was milder than that of other digestive herbs such as caraway, anise, and fennel.

The Vikings were well aware of dill's digestive benefits. In fact, our word *dill* comes from the Old Norse *dilla*, meaning to lull or soothe.

The 17th-century English herbalist Nicholas Culpeper claimed dill "stayeth the belly . . . and is a gallant expeller of wind." Culpeper also recommended the herb for hiccups, swellings, and to "strengthen the brain."

Deli Arrives in America

Colonists brought dill to North America. Its seed infusion, known as dillwater, became a favorite among American folk healers for such childhood ailments as colic, cough, indigestion, gas, stomachache, and insomnia. In adults, the herb was used to treat hemorrhoids, jaundice, scurvy, and "dropsy" (congestive heart failure).

Contemporary herbalists call dill "the herb of choice" for infant colic. They recommend chewing the seeds for bad breath and drinking dill tea both as a digestive aid and to stimulate milk production in nursing mothers.

HEALING with Dill

If you use dill only in your pickling spices, you're missing out on a marvelous healer. It won't cure hemorrhoids or increase milk production, but science has supported several of its traditional uses.

Digestive Aid and Gas Remedy. Research supports dill's 3,000 years of use as a digestive aid. The herb helps relax the smooth muscles of the digestive tract. One study shows it's also an antifoaming agent, meaning it helps prevent the formation of intestinal gas bubbles.

Dill seed oil inhibits the growth of several bacteria that attack the intestinal tract, suggesting that it may help prevent infectious diarrhea caused by these microorganisms.

Women's Health. Urinary tract infections (UTI) are usually caused by one of the bacteria inhibited by dill (E. *coli*). If you suffer recurrent UTI, try adding a cloth full of dill or some dill seed oil to your bath. It just might help.

Intriguing Possibilities. When injected into laboratory animals, dill extract stimulates respiration, slows heart rate, and opens blood vessels, all of which reduce blood pressure. Of course, people don't inject dill preparations, but these effects suggest there's more to learn about this herb's healing potential.

R~x~ for Dill

As a breath freshener, chew 1/2 to 1 teaspoon of seeds. As a digestive aid, take an infusion or tincture. To make a pleasant-tasting infusion, use 2 teaspoons of bruised seeds per cup of boiling water. Steep 10 minutes. Drink up to 3 cups a day.

In a tincture, take 1/2 to 1 teaspoon up to three times a day.

For colic or gas in children under age 2, give small amounts of a weak infusion. For older children and people over 65, start with low-strength preparations and increase strength if necessary.

To discourage urinary tract infections, tie some dill seeds in a cheese-cloth bag and add it to your bath. You can also use up to a teaspoonful of dill seed oil in the bath.

The Safety Factor

In sensitive individuals, dill might cause skin rash, but the leaf, seed, and seed oil are generally considered nontoxic.

Dill is included in the Food and Drug Administration's list

of herbs generally regarded as safe. For otherwise healthy nonpregnant, nonnursing adults, dill is considered safe in amounts typically recommended.

Dill should be used in medicinal amounts only in consultation with your doctor. If dill causes minor discomforts, such as stomach upset or diarrhea, use less or stop using it. Let your doctor know if you experience unpleasant effects or if the symptoms for which the herb is being used do not improve significantly in two weeks.

Deli Comes to the Garden

Dill is an annual with a long taproot like its close relative, carrot. It has a delicate, fast-growing, spindly stem with lacy leaves. Yellow flowers appear in summer and produce great quantities of tiny ridged fruits ("seeds").

Dill grows vigorously from seeds sown ¼ inch deep in early spring. Germination takes about two weeks. Thin seedlings to 12-inch spacing.

Dill grows to 3 feet in rich, moist, slightly acidic soil under full sun, or in the South in partial shade. Shelter plants from the wind.

Dill leaves may be harvested once plants have established themselves. Fresh dill leaves are much more aromatic than dried. To guarantee a supply of fresh leaves from late spring to late fall, plant seeds periodically throughout your growing season.

Seeds mature in about two months. Harvest them when they begin to turn brown.

Dill self-sows. Leave a few plants unharvested and you'll have this tasty healing herb every year.

ECHINACEA

Antibiotic and Immune System Stimulant

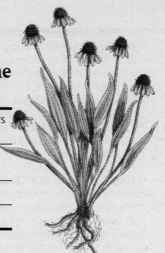

Family: Compositae; other members include daisy, dandelion, marigold

Genus and species: *Echinacea angustifolia, E. purpurea*

Also known as: Purple coneflower

Parts used: Roots

E chinacea is the best-kept secret among native American healing herbs. Few other plants are so potentially beneficial as immune-boosting infection fighters. Yet, like the prophet ignored in his native land, no healing herb has been dismissed as thoroughly by this country's orthodox medical authorities. Echinacea (pronounced *eh-kin-AY-sha*) was once quite popular here, but since the 1930s its many benefits have been enjoyed almost entirely by Europeans. Fortunately, the situation is changing as echinacea regains its former—and well-deserved—prominence on this side of the Atlantic.

The Original "Snake Oil"

Echinacea was the Plains Indians' primary medicine. They applied root poultices to all manner of wounds, insect bites and stings, and snakebites. They used echinacea mouthwash for painful teeth and gums and drank echinacea tea to treat colds, smallpox, measles, mumps, and arthritis.

Plains settlers adopted the plant, but it remained a folk remedy until 1870, when a patent-medicine purveyor, Dr. H. C. F. Meyer of Pawnee City, Nebraska, used it in his Meyer's Blood Purifier. He promoted the remedy as "an absolute cure" for rattlesnake bite, blood poisoning, and a host of other ills. Claims like Dr. Meyer's gave patent medicines the name "snake oil."

But Dr. Meyer *truly believed* echinacea could cure rattlesnake bite, and he set out to prove it. In 1885, he sent a sample to John Uri Lloyd, professor at the Eclectic Medical Institute in Cincinnati, cofounder (with his brothers) of Lloyd Brothers Pharmacists, and later president of the American Pharmaceutical Association. Lloyd identified the plant as echinacea. But after one look at Dr. Meyer's label with its claim of "absolute cure" for rattlesnake bite, Lloyd dismissed Dr. Meyer as a crackpot.

Dr. Meyer wrote back insisting echinacea was a cure for rattlesnake bite. He was so confident, he offered to bring a live rattlesnake to Cincinnati and let it bite him in Lloyd's presence to demonstrate his Blood Purifier's effectiveness. Lloyd declined the offer.

Undaunted, Dr. Meyer shipped some echinacea to Lloyd's Eclectic colleague, John King, who had mentioned the plant's Indian uses in the first edition of his Eclectic text, *King's American Dispensatory*. King tested the herb, and after successfully using it to treat bee stings, chronic nasal congestion, leg ulcers, and infant cholera, he extolled the plant and included it in subsequent editions of his *Dispensatory*.

In Every Medicine Cabinet

Eventually, John Uri Lloyd accepted echinacea, declaring it useful in treating wounds, venomous bites and stings, blood poisoning (septicemia), diphtheria, meningitis, measles, chicken pox, malaria, scarlet fever, influenza, syphilis, and gangrene.

Lloyd's enthusiasm was not simply academic. His family business, Lloyd Brothers Pharmacists, developed several echinacea products, which enjoyed tremendous popularity nationally as infection treatments from the 1890s well into the 1920s. During the early 20th century it was a rare home medicine cabinet that didn't contain tincture of echinacea. (The Lloyd brothers founded the Lloyd Library in Cincinnati. Today the library houses one of the world's largest collections of botanical information.)

Eclectics Versus the "Regulars"

Unfortunately, echinacea became a casualty of the war between orthodox physicians (known prior to World War I as "regulars") and the alternative Eclectic physicians. Each side was hostile to the medicines touted by the other. In 1909 the following appeared in the *Journal of the American Medical Association*: "Echinacea . . . has failed to sustain the reputation given it by its enthusiasts . . . [who] make use of early unverified reports to endow their nostrums with remarkable therapeutic properties."

By the 1930s, as antibiotics became available, echinacea's popularity waned. It was listed in the *National Formulary*, the pharmacists' reference, from 1916 until 1950, but from the 1940s on, it was largely forgotten—that is, until the herbal revival of the 1970s.

Contemporary herbalists are as enthusiastic about echinacea as the Eclectics were. They tout it as a botanical antibiotic and immune system stimulant for boils, colds and flu, bladder infections, tonsillitis, and other infectious diseases. Many recommend taking the herb daily as a tonic, infection preventive, and immune-system enhancer.

HEALING with Echinacea

Old Dr. Meyer would be tickled to learn how potent his favorite herb actually is. Echinacea has never been shown to cure rattlesnake bite, but many European (mostly German) studies from the 1950s through the 1980s agree it has remarkable healing properties.

Infection Fighter. Echinacea kills a broad range of disease-causing viruses, bacteria, fungi, and protozoa, which tends to support its traditional uses in wound healing and treatment of many infectious diseases. German researchers report success using echinacea to treat colds, flu, tonsillitis, bronchitis, tuberculosis, meningitis, wounds, abscesses, psoriasis, whooping cough (pertussis), and ear infections.

The herb fights infection in several ways. It contains a natural antibiotic (echinacoside), which is comparable to penicillin in that it has broad-spectrum activity.

Echinacea strengthens tissues against assault by invading microorganisms. Tissues contain a chemical (hyaluronic acid or HA) that in part acts as a shield against germ attack. Many germs produce an enzyme (hyaluronidase) that dissolves this chemical shield, allowing them to penetrate tissues and cause infection. But echinacea contains a substance (echinacein) that counteracts the germs' tissue-dissolving enzyme, keeping them out of the body's tissues.

Immune System. Echinacea may also prevent infection by revving up the immune system. When disease-causing microorganisms attack, cells secrete chemicals that attract infection-fighting white blood cells (macrophages) to the area. The macrophages (literally, "big eaters") engulf and digest the invaders. A study published in *Infection and Immunology* showed that a substance derived from echinacea boosts the macrophages' ability to destroy germs.

Another study at the University of Munich showed echinacea extracts increase production of infection-fighting T-cells (T-lymphocytes) up to 30 percent more than other immune-boosting drugs.

Colds and Flu. In addition, echinacea may behave like the body's own virus-fighting chemical, interferon. Before a virus-infected cell dies, it releases a tiny amount of interferon, which boosts the ability of surrounding cells to resist infection. Echinacea may do essentially the same thing. Researchers bathed cells in echinacea extract, then exposed them to two potent viruses, influenza and herpes. Compared with untreated cells, only a small proportion became infected. These findings have led herb conservative Varro Tyler, Ph.D., to write that echinacea "may result in . . . clear improvement in such conditions as the common cold." It may also help fight other infectious diseases, such as flu, urinary tract infection, and bronchitis.

Yeast Infection. Tests of echinacea in people have produced dramatically positive results. In a recent German study, 203 women with recurrent vaginal yeast infections were treated with either an anti-yeast cream or the cream plus an oral echinacea preparation. After six months, 60 percent of the women treated with just the antifungal cream had experienced recurrences, but among those also treated with echinacea, the figure was only 16 percent, a highly significant difference.

Radiation Therapy. Cancer patients undergoing radiation therapy typically suffer reduced white blood cell counts, increasing their risk of infection. Echinacea may help preserve white blood cells and thus protect radiation patients from infection.

If you're in radiation therapy, use echinacea only in consultation with your physician.

Wound Healing. Science has confirmed echinacea's traditional use in wound treatment. The same chemical (echinacein) that prevents germs from penetrating tissues also spurs broken skin to knit faster by spurring cells that form new tissue (fibroblasts) to work more efficiently.

Echinacea preparations can be applied to cuts, burns, psoriasis, eczema, genital herpes, and cold sores.

Arthritis. The same chemical (HA) that helps shield tissues against germs also lubricates the joints. Joint inflammation (arthritis) breaks down HA, but echinacea's HA-protective action may have an anti-inflammatory effect, thus lending credence to the herb's traditional use in treating arthritis.

German researchers have successfully treated rheumatoid arthritis with echinacea preparations. If you have arthritis or another inflammatory condition, use echinacea only in consultation with your physician.

Intriguing Possibility. Echinacea shows promising anticancer activity against leukemia and a few animal tumors. It's too early to call the herb a cancer treatment, but one day it might be.

Rx for Echinacea

Use either a tincture or decoction to take advantage of echinacea's infection-fighting potential or as a possible treatment for arthritis. To make a decoction, bring 2 teaspoons of root material per cup of water to a boil, then simmer 15 minutes. Drink up to 3 cups a day. You'll find the taste initially sweet, then bitter.

In a tincture, take 1 teaspoon up to three times a day.

If you're using a commercial preparation, follow package directions.

Echinacea should not be given to children under age 2. For older children and people over 65, start with a low-strength preparation and increase strength if necessary.

The Safety Factor

Echinacea often causes a tingling sensation on the tongue. This is normal and not harmful. The medical literature contains no reports of echinacea toxicity.

However, there have been a few reports of bulk echinacea root being adulterated by other herbs. Any adulteration would reduce the herb's effectiveness, and depending on the adulterant, might cause adverse reactions.

Fortunately, many U.S. herb companies market prepackaged echinacea preparations under Food and Drug Administration (FDA) purity regulations. These may be used with confidence.

The FDA lists echinacea as an herb of "undefined safety," but available evidence suggests it's safe. For otherwise healthy nonpregnant, nonnursing adults, echinacea is considered safe in amounts typically recommended.

Echinacea should be used only in consultation with your doctor. If echinacea causes minor discomforts, such as stom-

ach upset or diarrhea, use less or stop using it. Let your doctor know if you experience any unpleasant effects or if the
symptoms for which the herb is being used do not improve
significantly in two weeks.

Pretty Flowers

Echinacea is a 2- to 5-foot perennial whose flowers resemble
black-eyed Susan, with purple rays radiating from a cone-
shaped center—hence its common name, purple coneflower.
Echinacea has black roots, a single stem covered with bristly
hairs, and narrow leaves.

Echinacea grows from seeds or root cuttings taken in
spring or fall. Don't cover seeds. When the temperature is in
the 70s, simply tamp them into moist, sandy soil.

Echinacea grows in poor, rocky, slightly acidic soil under
full sun, but it also thrives in richer soils.

It takes three or four years for roots to grow large enough
to harvest. Pull them in autumn after the plant has gone to
seed. Roots greater than 1/2 inch in diameter should be split
before drying.

ELECAMPANE

Good-bye, Intestinal Parasites

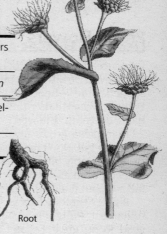

Family: Compositae; other members include daisy, dandelion, marigold

Genus and species: *Inula helenium*

Also known as: Wild sunflower, velvet dock, scabwort, horseheal

Parts used: Root

Root

Legend has it that Helen of Troy carried a handful of elecampane on the fateful day the Trojan prince, Paris, abducted her from Sparta, igniting the Trojan War. Perhaps the woman whose face launched 1,000 ships had amoebic dysentery, pinworms, hookworms, or giardiasis. We'll probably never know. But we do know the herb with the Latin name that memorializes the Greek beauty may help expel parasites from the intestine.

"Let No Day Pass"

Hippocrates said elecampane stimulated the brain, kidneys, stomach, and uterus. The ancient Romans used it to treat indigestion. The Roman naturalist Pliny wrote: "Let no day pass without eating some roots of elecampane to help digestion, expel melancholy, and cause mirth." And the Roman physician Galen recommended the herb as "good for passion of the hucklebone [sciatica]."

Traditional Chinese and Indian Ayurvedic physicians used elecampane to treat respiratory problems, particularly bronchitis and asthma.

Used on Horses and Sheep

During the Middle Ages, European herbalists prescribed elecampane to treat coughs, bronchitis, and asthma, but the herb was more popular as a veterinary medicine. It was reputed to cure scab disease in sheep, hence one popular name, scabwort. It was also considered a panacea for horses, and for that reason it was also known as horseheal.

As time passed, elecampane regained its reputation as a human digestive aid. It was the main ingredient in a medieval elixir known as *potio Paulina*, an allusion to St. Paul.

Seventeenth-century London herbalist Nicholas Culpeper touted elecampane "to relieve cough, shortness of breath, and wheezing in the lungs." Echoing Galen, he also suggested the herb for sciatica, and claimed it restored vision and cured gout, sores, and "worms in the stomach."

Elecampane root was also candied and eaten as a confection. Lozenges combining elecampane and honey were used to treat whooping cough (pertussis).

Popular in the New World

Early American colonists naturalized elecampane and used it as an expectorant, digestive aid, menstruation promoter, and diuretic for treatment of the water retention associated with "dropsy" (congestive heart failure). Indian tribes in the Northeast adopted the plant for respiratory problems.

America's 19th-century Eclectic physicians also used elecampane as a diuretic and menstruation promoter, but prescribed it primarily for "asthma, bronchial and chronic pulmonary [lung] affections, weakness of the digestive or-

gans, itching, dyspepsia [indigestion], night sweats, and severe colds."

Present-day herbalists generally recommend elecampane
only for respiratory ailments: cough, asthma, bronchitis, and
emphysema. Some recommend it as a digestive aid, as a
treatment for menstrual and skin problems, and to banish intestinal parasites.

HEALING with Elecampane

The Food and Drug Administration says elecampane "was em-
ployed by the ancients for diseases in which it was probably
of no service." This herb has not been well researched, but
the few scientific studies to date suggest that for once,
Nicholas Culpeper wasn't completely off the deep end.

Intestinal Parasites. European scientists have discovered
elecampane contains a chemical (alantolactone) that really does
help expel intestinal parasites, as Culpeper claimed for the
herb. The herb also kills some bacteria and fungi, adding to its
potential therapeutic action in the intestine.

Intestinal parasites, especially pinworms and giardiasis
(caused by the protozoan *Giardia lamblia*) are a growing problem in the United States. Families with children in day care
are particularly susceptible.

Intestinal parasites are quite common in the tropics. If you
travel overseas, do what Helen of Troy did—take some elecampane with you.

Women's Health. Elecampane has not been shown to
stimulate uterine contractions, but because of its long tradition as a menstruation promoter, women may want to try
some to help bring on their periods.

Intriguing Possibilities. In animal tests conducted in
Europe, elecampane reduces blood pressure. People with
high blood pressure might try it in consultation with their
physicians.

Elecampane has been shown to have a sedative effect in experimental animals. Those with insomnia might try some before bed.

Rx for Elecampane

Elecampane's main use is to help prevent and fight intestinal parasites. To use it for this purpose or (in consultation with your physician) to keep your blood pressure down, use either a decoction or a tincture. For a decoction, gently boil 1 to 2 teaspoons of dried, powdered root in 3 cups of water for 30 minutes. The taste is bitter. Take 1 or 2 tablespoons at a time with honey, up to 2 cups a day.

In a tincture, use $1/4$ to $1/2$ teaspoon up to three times a day.

Elecampane should not be given to children under age 2. For older children and people over 65, start with low-strength preparations and increase strength if necessary.

The Safety Factor

Although elecampane has never been proven to stimulate the uterus, it has been used traditionally to promote menstruation. For that reason, pregnant women should not use it. Animal studies show that small doses of the herb lower blood sugar levels, but higher doses raise them. These studies have not been replicated in humans, but diabetics should steer clear of the herb.

Sensitive individuals may develop a rash from skin contact with elecampane or its oil. Otherwise, no harmful effects have been reported.

Elecampane is included in the Food and Drug Administration's list of herbs generally regarded as safe. For otherwise healthy nonpregnant, nonnursing adults who do not have diabetes, elecampane is considered safe in amounts typically recommended.

If elecampane causes minor discomforts, such as stomach upset or diarrhea, use less or stop using it. Elecampane should be used only in consultation with your doctor. Let your doctor know if you experience any unpleasant effects or if the symptoms for which the herb is being used do not improve significantly in two weeks.

A Beauty of a Plant

Elecampane is a striking perennial that reaches 5 feet and produces a large flower, hence its common name, wild sunflower. The entire plant is covered with woolly hairs. The medicinal roots are large, branching, and fleshy.

Elecampane may be started from seeds sown indoors in late winter, then transplanted. But once plants have been established, the herb is best propagated from 2-inch root cuttings taken in autumn from the buds ("eyes") of two-year-old roots. Cover the cuttings with moist, sandy soil and store for the winter in a cool indoor room. Plant the cuttings 3 feet apart after danger of frost has passed. Deeply cultivated soil produces the biggest roots.

Elecampane likes rich, moist, well-drained, slightly acid loam and full sun or partial shade. Harvest the roots during the autumn of their second year. Older roots become too woody. To speed drying, slice roots into pieces.

EPHEDRA

The World's Original Healer

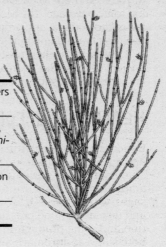

Family: Ephedraceae; other members include broom, horsetail

Genus and species: *Ephedra sinica, E. vulgaris, E. nevadensis, E. antisyphilitica,* and other species

Also known as: *Ma huang,* Mormon tea, whorehouse tea

Parts used: Stems, branches

Ephedra, a powerful bronchial decongestant, is generally considered the world's oldest medicine. Sadly, few people who take over-the-counter cold remedies containing this herb's laboratory analog (pseudoephedrine) have any idea they are part of an herbal healing tradition dating back 5,000 years.

Ma Huang and Mormon Tea

The origins of Chinese medicine are lost in legend, but authorities agree Chinese physicians began prescribing ephedra tea for colds, asthma, and hay fever around 3000 B.C. The Indian and Pakistani species of the herb have been used medicinally almost as long. Chinese ephedra (E. *sinica*) is known as *ma huang*.

When the Mormons reached Utah in 1847, local Indians

introduced them to native American ephedra, a piney-tasting tonic beverage. The Mormons adopted it as a substitute for coffee and tea, and around the West it became known as Mormon tea, a name that survives to this day.

Contemporary herbalists recommend ephedra just as the ancient Chinese did, to treat asthma, hay fever, and the nasal and chest congestion of colds and flu.

HEALING with Ephedra

Ephedra's active constituents (ephedrine, pseudoephedrine and norpseudoephedrine) are strong central nervous system stimulants, more powerful than caffeine but less potent than amphetamine. Ephedrine itself opens the bronchial passages, thus acting as a bronchodilator, stimulates the heart, and increases blood pressure, metabolic rate, and perspiration and urine production. It also reduces the secretion of both saliva and stomach acids.

Chinese ephedra contains significant amounts of ephedrine. The American species is richer in norpseudoephedrine.

Some herb marketers have mistakenly called American ephedra *ma huang*, and the Chinese herb "Mormon tea." Make sure any ephedra you purchase is identified by species. *E. sinica* has the greatest decongestant/bronchodilator potential. The other species of ephedra are generally less potent in this regard.

Decongestant. From the late 1920s through the 1940s, ephedrine was used in cold, asthma, and hay fever products as a decongestant and bronchodilator. Ephedrine was generally effective and reasonably safe, but it was also known to cause potentially hazardous side effects, including increased blood pressure and rapid heartbeat (palpitations). It was eventually replaced with a close chemical substitute, pseudoephedrine, which scientists consider equally effective but less problematic. Pseudoephedrine is the active ingredient in many over-the-counter cold and allergy products, notably Sudafed.

Weight Loss. As a central nervous system stimulant, the ephedrine in *ma huang* increases basal metabolic rate (BMR), meaning it spurs the body to burn calories faster. Laboratory animals given ephedrine show BMR increases, and as a result, significant weight loss, according to a study in the *American Journal of Clinical Nutrition*.

Caffeine (in coffee, tea, cocoa, chocolate, maté, and cola drinks) enhances ephedra's weight-loss-promoting effect. Both caffeine and ephedrine, however, are powerful stimulants. Taken at the same time, they cause insomnia, nervousness, irritability, and "speediness."

Weight-loss authorities say the key to permanent weight control is a low-fat, high-fiber diet and regular aerobic exercise.

Smoking Cessation. One study shows ephedrine helps smokers quit by decreasing cigarette cravings. If you're attempting to quit, try ephedra and see if it works for you.

Women's Health. Ephedrine causes uterine contractions in laboratory animals. Pregnant women should not use it. Other women may try it to initiate menstruation.

Dead-End File. In the Old West, American ephedra also developed a reputation as a cure for syphilis and gonorrhea. It was served at many brothels, hence the name whorehouse tea and the Latin name for one species, *E. antisyphilitica*.

It turns out that ephedra has no effect whatsoever on syphilis or gonorrhea. Anyone who develops a genital sore or discharge should consult a physician.

Rx for Ephedra

Use a decoction or tincture to take advantage of ephedra's potent healing benefits as a decongestant or weight-loss aid, to help quit smoking, or to promote menstruation. You'll find the taste pleasantly piney.

For a decoction, mix 1 teaspoon of dried *ma huang* per cup of water, bring to a boil, then simmer for 10 to 15 minutes. Drink up to 2 cups a day.

In a tincture, take ¼ to 1 teaspoon up to three times a day.

When using commercial preparations, follow package directions.

Ephedra should not be given to children under age 2. For older children and people over 65, start with low-strength preparations and increase strength if necessary.

The Safety Factor

Mainstream medical researchers insist pseudoephedrine, the related chemical used in commercial cold preparations, is safer than ephedrine. Scientific herbalists agree, but they insist *the whole ephedra plant* is safer than either ephedrine or psuedoephedrine. In *Herbal Medicine for Everyone*, British herbalist Michael McIntyre writes that pure ephedrine "markedly raises blood pressure. . . . But the whole [ephedra] plant actually reduces blood pressure." German medical herbalist Rudolph Fritz Weiss, M.D., maintains that the whole plant "has certain advantages [over psuedoephedrine]. Above all, it is better tolerated, causing fewer heart symptoms such as palpitations."

The ephedra/pseudoephedrine issue remains unresolved. Anyone who has high blood pressure should consult his physician before using this herb. Also, he should invest in a home blood pressure device to self-monitor his condition. If you have one, you can check ephedra's effects. If the herb lowers your blood pressure, your physician will probably give you the go-ahead to use it. If it raises your blood pressure, don't use it. Anyone with heart disease, diabetes, glaucoma, or an overactive thyroid gland (hyperthyroidism) should exercise caution and not use ephedra.

Ephedra often causes insomnia. People with sleep problems should not take it late in the day.

Finally, ephedra causes dry mouth. Increase your nonalcohol fluid intake when you use it.

The Food and Drug Administration considers ephedra an herb of "undefined safety." For otherwise healthy nonpregnant, nonnursing adults who do not have high blood pressure, heart disease, diabetes, glaucoma, or overactive thyroid, and who are not taking other medications that raise blood pressure or cause anxiety or insomnia, ephedra is considered relatively safe when used cautiously for short periods of time.

Ephedra should be used in medicinal amounts only in consultation with your doctor. If ephedra causes insomnia, nervousness, or stomach upset, use less or stop using it. Let your doctor know if you experience any unpleasant effects or if the symptoms for which the herb is being used do not improve significantly in two weeks.

Competitive athletes should be extremely cautious regarding the use of ephedra. For example, it is on the United States Olympic Committee's list of banned substances.

A Weird Plant

Ephedra is not a garden herb. It is an odd-looking, botanically primitive, almost leafless shrub that resembles horsetail. It has tough, jointed, barkless stems and branches, with small scale-like leaves and tiny yellow-green flowers that appear in summer. Male and female flowers appear on different plants. Seeds develop in cones.

EUCALYPTUS

The Australian Flu Remedy

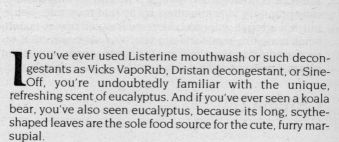

Family: Myrtaceae; other members include myrtle

Genus and species: *Eucalyptus globulus*

Also known as: Gum tree, blue gum, Australian fever tree

Parts used: Leaf oil

L f you've ever used Listerine mouthwash or such decongestants as Vicks VapoRub, Dristan decongestant, or Sine-Off, you're undoubtedly familiar with the unique, refreshing scent of eucalyptus. And if you've ever seen a koala bear, you've also seen eucalyptus, because its long, scythe-shaped leaves are the sole food source for the cute, furry marsupial.

The symbol of Australia is also Down Under's contribution to herbal healing. It's a Food and Drug Administration–approved cold and flu remedy.

Australian Fever Tree

Eucalyptus roots hold an astonishing amount of water. Australia's aborigines chewed them for water in the dry outback. They also drank eucalyptus leaf tea for fevers.

When England declared Australia a penal colony and started shipping convicts in the 1780s to what is now Sydney, it took a while for the new immigrants to catch on to eucalyptus as a water source. Many early outback explorers died of thirst within sight of eucalyptus stands.

Around 1840, crew members of a French freighter anchored off Sydney developed a disease involving high fever—and cured it with eucalyptus tea. Reports of similar incidents slowly made their way back to Europe, and the herb became known as "Australian fever tree." By the 1860s, eucalyptus leaves and oil were being used around the Mediterranean to treat the fever that had plagued the area since ancient times—"intermittent fever" or malaria. Some physicians reported malaria cures with eucalyptus, but others dismissed it as worthless.

We now know eucalyptus has no direct effect on the protozoan that causes malaria, but ironically, the tree virtually eradicated the devastating disease in much of Italy, Sicily, and Algeria, where it had raged unchecked for thousands of years. Malaria is transmitted by mosquitoes that live in swampy areas. Europeans planted eucalyptus in the marshlands bordering the Mediterranean, and as they grew, their roots soaked up water and drained the swamps, eliminating malarial mosquitoes' habitat—and the disease they carried.

Catheter Oil

Eucalyptus oil was used as an antiseptic on urinary catheters in 19th-century British hospitals, where it became known as catheter oil.

America's 19th-century Eclectic physicians used eucalyptus oil as an antiseptic on wounds and medical instruments. They also recommended inhaling the vapors in steam to treat bronchitis, asthma, whooping cough (pertussis), and emphysema.

Contemporary herbalists recommend eucalyptus as a topical antiseptic, a gargle for sore throat, and an inhalant for asthma, bronchitis, croup, and the nasal congestion of colds and flu.

HEALING with Eucalyptus

Eucalyptus leaf oil contains a chemical (eucalyptol) that gives the herb its pleasant aroma and healing value.

Colds and Flu. Eucalyptol loosens phlegm in the chest, making it easier to cough up. That's why so many cough lozenges are flavored with it.

Russian animal studies show eucalyptol kills influenza, a virus that causes the most serious form of flu. And eucalyptol kills some bacteria, meaning it may help prevent bacterial bronchitis, a common complication of colds and flu.

Wound Treatment. The antibacterial action of eucalyptol also makes it an effective treatment for minor cuts and scrapes.

Cockroach Repellent. Eucalyptol repels cockroaches, according to a report in *Science News*.

Rx for Eucalyptus

For an inhalant, boil a handful of leaves or a few drops of essential oil in water.

Rub a drop or two of eucalyptus oil into minor cuts and scrapes after they have been thoroughly washed with soap and water.

For an herbal bath, wrap a handful of leaves in a cloth and run bathwater over it.

For a cool, spicy, refreshing infusion to treat colds and flu, use 1 to 2 teaspoons of dried, crushed *leaves* per cup of boiling water. Steep 10 minutes. Drink up to 2 cups a day. If you use the essential oil to make an infusion, do not use more than one or two drops.

Do not give eucalyptus to children under age 2. For older children and people over 65, start with low-strength preparations and increase strength if necessary.

If your home is infested with cockroaches and you don't want to use insecticides, try soaking small cloths in eucalyptus oil and distributing them around your cabinets.

The Safety Factor

Used externally, eucalyptus oil is considered nonirritating, but sensitive individuals may develop a rash.

When taken internally, eucalyptus oil is highly poisonous. Fatalities have been reported from ingestion of as little as a teaspoon.

The FDA has approved eucalyptus oil for use in food and drugs. Anyone may use eucalyptus preparations externally, although infants and children may rebel against the pungent aroma. If you develop a rash, stop using it. For otherwise healthy nonpregnant, nonnursing adults, eucalyptus is considered relatively safe for *cautious* internal use in the very small amount typically recommended.

Eucalyptus should be used in medicinal amounts only in consultation with your doctor. If eucalyptus causes minor discomforts, such as stomach upset or diarrhea, use less or stop using it. Let your doctor know if you experience unpleasant effects or if the symptoms for which the herb is being used do not improve significantly in two weeks.

Think Twice Before Planting

The more than 500 species of eucalyptus account for three-quarters of the native vegetation in Australia. Eucalyptus vary from 5-foot shrubs to the tallest trees on earth, up to 475 feet, the size of a 40-story building.

Eucalyptus grows anywhere with loamy soil and adequate water where the temperature does not dip below freezing. Plant saplings obtained at a nursery. If leaves begin to blister, cut back on watering.

Eucalyptus often kills surrounding vegetation (except

other Australian plants), which is why the trees are usually found in stands with little between them.

Eucalyptus trees grow extremely rapidly, up to several feet per year, and their trunks eventually attain enormous girth. If you plant a eucalyptus, be prepared for it to dominate your yard. Horticulturists discourage planting eucalyptus because their roots break up water and sewage lines, their trunks buckle sidewalks, and their limbs have a tendency to break off in gusting winds, damaging property and endangering life.

FENNEL

Great for Digestion

Family: Umbelliferae; other members include carrot, parsley

Genus and species: *Foeniculum vulgare, F. vulgare dulce*

Also known as: Finocchio, carosella, Florence fennel

Parts used: Fruits ("seeds"); stalks and bulbs are used in cooking

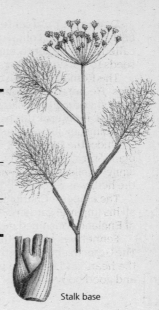

Stalk base

New England's Puritans called fennel "meeting seeds." The meetings were their endless church services. Some authorities say the Puritans used fennel as an appetite suppressant. Others say many Puritans steeled themselves for church with whiskey, then chewed fennel seeds to mask the odor. The Puritans also used fennel as a digestive aid, its major use in herbal healing from the time of the Pharaohs to the present day.

Part of Marathon History

The ancient Greeks called fennel *marathon*. It grew wild around the village of Marathon, about 25 miles from Athens, where the Athenians defeated the Persians in 490 B.C. A long-distance runner brought news of the victory back to Athens, and his athletic feat inspired today's marathon races.

During the third century B.C., Hippocrates prescribed fennel to treat infant colic. Four hundred years later, Dioscorides called it an appetite suppressant and recommended the seeds to nursing mothers to boost milk production.

The Roman naturalist Pliny included fennel in 22 remedies. He noted that some snakes rubbed against the plant after shedding their skins and soon after, their glazed eyes cleared. Pliny took this as a sign that fennel cured human eye problems, including blindness.

Under the Doctrine of Signatures, the medieval notion that plants' physical characteristics revealed their medicinal value, fennel's yellow flowers were linked to the liver's yellow bile, and the herb was recommended for jaundice.

The emperor Charlemagne ordered the herb cultivated in all his imperial gardens. And the household of King Edward I of England consumed more than 8 pounds a month.

Fennel was one of Hildegard of Bingen's favorite herbs. The German abbess/herbalist recommended it for colds, flu, the heart, and to "make us happy, [with] good digestion . . . and good body odor."

Witchcraft and Other Hocus-Pocus

The Anglo-Saxons who settled England around the 5th century used fennel both as a spice and digestive aid. They also hung fennel over their doors to protect against witchcraft.

By the 17th century, fennel was a mainstay of herbal healing and a standard seasoning for fish. Seventeenth-century English herbalist Nicholas Culpeper, apparently not a fish lover, wrote it "consumes the phlegmatic humour which fish . . . annoys the body with." Culpeper recommended fennel to "break wind, increase milk, cleanse the eyes from mists that hinder sight, and take away the loathings which oftentimes happen to stomachs of sick persons." He also claimed it "brought women's courses" (menstruation).

Folk healers mixed fennel with strong laxatives, such as buckthorn, senna, rhubarb, and aloe, to counteract the intestinal cramps they often caused.

Fennel Comes to America

Colonists brought fennel to North America. Henry Wadsworth Longfellow alluded to Pliny when he wrote:

> Above the lower plants it towers
> The Fennel with its yellow flowers;
> And in an earlier age than ours
> Was gifted with wondrous powers
> Lost vision to restore.

America's 19th-century Eclectic physicians prescribed fennel as a digestive aid, milk and menstruation promoter, and to "conceal the unpleasantness of other medicines."

Latin Americans still boil the seeds in milk as a milk promoter for nursing mothers. Jamaicans use it to treat colds. And Africans take fennel for diarrhea and indigestion.

Contemporary herbalists recommend fennel as a digestive aid, milk promoter, expectorant, eyewash, and buffer in herbal laxative blends.

HEALING with Fennel

Fennel won't cure blindness, but science has supported some of its traditional uses.

Digestive Aid. Like most other aromatic herbs, fennel appears to relax the smooth muscle lining of the digestive tract (making it an antispasmodic). It also helps expel gas. And European research shows it kills some bacteria, lending some support to its traditional use in treating diarrhea.

In Germany, where herbal medicine is more mainstream than it is in the United States, fennel is used like anise and caraway as a treatment for indigestion, gas pains, and infant colic.

Women's Health. Antispasmodics soothe not only the digestive tract but other smooth muscles, such as the uterus, as well. However, fennel was traditionally used not to relax the uterus but to stimulate it into menstruation. It is possible that high doses of fennel provide sufficient stimulation to promote menstruation.

One study suggests the herb has a mild estrogenic effect, meaning it acts like the female sex hormone estrogen. This action may have something to do with its traditional use as a milk and menstruation promoter.

Other women may try it to help begin their periods or increase milk production. Older women might give it a try to relieve the discomforts of menopause.

Prostate Cancer. Female sex hormones are often prescribed for prostate cancer. All forms of cancer require professional care. Try fennel in addition to standard therapies only with the supervision of your physician.

Rx for Fennel

As a digestive aid, either chew a handful of seeds or try an infusion or tincture. Use either an infusion or tincture to attempt to bring on menstruation or (while under the care of a physician) as a possible aid in the treatment of prostate cancer.

To make a pleasant, licorice-flavored infusion, use 1 to 2 teaspoons of bruised seeds per cup of boiling water. Steep 10 minutes. Drink up to 3 cups a day.

In a tincture, take 1/2 to 1 teaspoon up to three times a day.

Weak fennel preparations may be given cautiously to children under age 2 for colic. If the condition persists, consult your pediatrician. For older children and people over 65, start with low-strength preparations and increase strength if necessary.

The Safety Factor

Fennel has at best only a mild estrogenic effect, but estrogen, a key ingredient in birth control pills, has many effects on the body. Women advised by their doctors not to take the Pill should not use medicinal amounts of fennel, nor should anyone with a history of abnormal blood clotting or estrogen-dependent breast tumors.

Pregnant women should not use medicinal amounts of fennel.

Liver Questions

One study suggests fennel has oddly contradictory effects on the liver. It aggravates liver damage in experimental animals but spurs liver regeneration in animals with parts of their liver removed. Until its effects are clarified, people with a history of alcoholism, hepatitis, or liver disease should err on the side of caution and not take medicinal amounts of this herb.

Fennel seeds are safe, but fennel oil may cause skin rash in sensitive individuals. When taken internally, the oil may cause nausea, vomiting, and possibly seizures. *Don't ingest it*!

Other Cautions

Fennel is included in the Food and Drug Administration's list of herbs generally regarded as safe. For otherwise healthy nonpregnant, nonnursing adults, fennel is considered safe in amounts typically recommended.

Fennel should be used in medicinal amounts only in consultation with your doctor. If fennel causes minor discomforts, such as stomach upset or diarrhea, use less or stop using it. Let your doctor know if you experience unpleasant effects or if the symptoms for which the herb is being used do not improve significantly in two weeks.

Smells Like Licorice

Fennel is a striking, 6-foot perennial with feathery leaves and tall stalks capped by large umbrella-like clusters of tiny yellow flowers. The tiny oval-shaped fruits ("seeds") are ribbed and greenish gray. All parts of the plant have the herb's characteristic anise/licorice fragrance.

Fennel grows easily from seeds sown in rich, moist soil in fall or after danger of frost has passed. Germination takes about two weeks. Thin seedlings to 12-inch spacing. Do not over-water seedlings, but as plants develop, extra water increases stem succulence. Leaves may be harvested once plants are established.

When stems are about an inch thick, hill the soil over them to cause blanching, which results in milder flavor. Harvest about ten days after hilling.

Harvest seeds in late summer as they turn greenish gray.

Fennel may damage some neighboring plants: bush beans, tomatoes, caraway, and kohlrabi. If coriander is planted nearby, fennel will not fruit.

Alert: In the wild, fennel may be confused with poison hem-lock, which has caused fatalities. Don't gather wild fennel un-less you're sure you've identified it correctly.

FENUGREEK

Cholesterol-Controlling Hopeful

Family: Leguminosae; other members include beans, peas

Genus and species: *Trigonella foenum-graecum*

Also known as: Greek hay, foenugreek, fenigreek

Parts used: Seeds

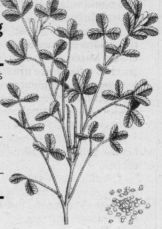

Seeds

From ancient times through the late 19th century, fenugreek played a major role in herbal healing. Then it fell by the wayside. Now things are looking up for the herb with a taste that is an odd combination of bitter celery and maple syrup. In animal studies, fenugreek helps reduce cholesterol levels, and it may well have similar benefits for people.

Greek Hay

Fenugreek plants were used to help sick animals long before its seeds became a popular remedy for human ills. Early Greeks mixed the plant into moldy or insect-damaged animal forage to make it more palatable, and in the process discovered that sick horses and cattle would eat fenugreek when they wouldn't eat anything else. The Egyptians and Romans adopted "Greek hay," a name that evolved into fenugreek.

Today the plant is widely used to flavor horse and cattle feed, and some veterinarians still use it to encourage sick horses and cattle to eat.

As fenugreek spread around the Mediterranean, ancient physicians learned that its seeds contain a great deal of mucilage. Mixed with water, mucilage becomes gelatinous and soothes inflamed or irritated tissue. Egyptian physicians used fenugreek in ointments to treat wounds and abscesses. They also recommended the herb internally to treat fevers and respiratory and intestinal complaints. Hippocrates and other ancient Greek and Roman physicians used it similarly.

Ancient Chinese healers used fenugreek to treat fevers, hernia, gallbladder problems, muscle aches, and even impotence.

In India, where the herb was incorporated into curry spice blends, Ayurvedic physicians used it to treat arthritis, bronchitis, and digestive upsets. Indian women ate the seeds to increase their milk production.

Arab women from Libya to Syria ate the roasted seeds to gain weight and attain the Rubenesque proportions synonymous with beauty from ancient times through the 19th century.

Military Weapon

Fenugreek is the only healing herb ever used as a weapon of war. During the Roman siege of Jerusalem (A.D. 66–70), general and future emperor Vespasian ordered his troops to scale the city's imposing walls. The standard defense against this was to pour boiling water or oil on the attackers and their ladders. According to *The History of the Jewish War* by Jewish traitor Flavius Josephus, Jerusalem's defenders added fenugreek to the oil they poured on the Romans, making it more slippery.

Those avid herb gardeners (and creators of fine liqueurs), the Benedictine monks, popularized fenugreek throughout Europe around the 9th century. From that time on, it was widely used in folk medicine as it had been by the ancients—

to treat wounds, fevers, and digestive and respiratory ailments.

Part of Pinkham's Compound

Early settlers brought fenugreek to North America and used it as forage and in folk medicine, where it gained a reputation as a potent menstruation promoter. As a result, the herb became a key ingredient in Lydia E. Pinkham's Vegetable Compound, one of 19th-century America's most popular patent medicines for "female weakness" (menstrual discomforts). The manufacturer proclaimed it "the greatest medical discovery since the dawn of history." Health authorities were outraged, and their outcry played a part in creating the Food and Drug Administration (FDA), which regulates drug claims. (A reformulated Pinkham's Compound is still available today—minus the fenugreek.)

Modern herbalists recommend fenugreek poultices and plasters to treat wounds, boils, and rashes. They say a warm fenugreek gargle soothes a sore throat. And they recommend the herb internally to treat coughs and bronchitis.

But fenugreek is most widely used in the United States today as a source of imitation maple flavor.

HEALING with Fenugreek

Some of fenugreek's traditional uses have been supported by modern science, but its most important potential use has only recently come to light.

Cholesterol Control. Studies show fenugreek reduces cholesterol in dogs. The herb has not yet been tested in humans, but this finding warrants that such studies be done.

Sore Throat. Fenugreek's soothing mucilage may help relieve sore throat pain, cough, and minor indigestion.

Women's Health. Almost a century after Lydia Pinkham's death, an animal experiment has lent some support to fenugreek's action as a uterine stimulant, especially during the late stages of pregnancy. Fenugreek seeds contain a chemical (diosgenin) similar to the female sex hormone estrogen. Estrogen encourages the body to retain water, and one side effect of the Pill is bloating. Water retention means increased weight, so perhaps those Arab women who ate fenugreek to gain weight were on the right track. It may help nonpregnant women bring on their periods, but this use has not been confirmed.

Arthritis. Belgian researchers have discovered that fenugreek has mild anti-inflammatory action, which lends some credence to its traditional use in treating wounds, arthritis, and other inflammations.

Intriguing Possibilities. Animal studies show fenugreek reduces blood sugar (glucose) levels. The effect has not been demonstrated in humans, and diabetics should get their doctor's approval before trying it to see if it helps control their glucose.

Rx for Fenugreek

Take fenugreek as a decoction to take advantage of its many potential healing benefits: to help soothe a sore throat, possibly bring on menstruation, or potentially help in the treatment of arthritis. In conjunction with regular treatment from your physician, you might also try it to lower your cholesterol or help control glucose levels. For a bitter, maple-flavored decoction, gently boil 2 teaspoons of bruised seeds per cup of water. Simmer 10 minutes. Drink up to 3 cups a day. To improve flavor, add sugar, honey, lemon, anise, or peppermint.

In a tincture, use 1/4 to 1/2 teaspoon up to three times a day.

Do not give medicinal preparations to children under age 2. For older children and people over 65, start with low-strength preparations and increase strength if necessary.

The Safety Factor

Because it may be a uterine stimulant, fenugreek should not be taken by pregnant women.

Fenugreek is included in the FDA's list of herbs generally regarded as safe. For otherwise healthy nonpregnant, non-nursing adults, fenugreek is considered safe in amounts typically recommended.

Fenugreek should be used in medicinal amounts only in consultation with your doctor. If the herb causes minor discomfort, such as stomach upset or diarrhea, use less or stop using it. Let your doctor know if you experience any unpleasant effects or if the symptoms for which the herb is being used do not improve significantly in two weeks.

As Easy as Beans

Fenugreek is an annual that reaches 18 inches and resembles a large clover. It has three-lobed leaves and white, triangular, pealike flowers, which produce the long seed pods characteristic of the bean family. Fenugreek's seed pod is sickle-shaped, 2 inches long, and contains 10 to 20 hard, smooth, oblong, somewhat flattened seeds.

After frost danger has passed and soil temperature has reached 55°F, plant seeds in almost any soil that receives full sun. Germination typically takes only a few days. Plants flower in about three weeks and produce seeds about three weeks later.

To prevent root rot, do not overwater.

Harvest the pods when fully formed, but before they begin to crack. Remove the seeds and dry them in the sun.

FEVERFEW

For Migraine Prevention

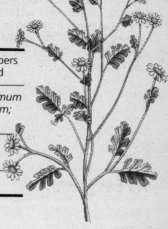

Family: Compositae; other members include daisy, dandelion, marigold

Genus and species: *Chrysanthemum parthenium; Matricaria parthenium; Tanacetum parthenium*

Also known as: Febrifuge plant, wild quinine, bachelor's button

Parts used: Leaves

Until the late 1970s, feverfew was discredited as a healing herb. In *The Herb Book*, John Lust summarized most herbalists' feelings: "Feverfew has fallen into considerable disuse. Its name no longer fits. It is also hard to find, even at herb outlets."

Now feverfew is hot. Recent studies show it's remarkably effective at preventing migraine headaches.

Fever a Misnomer

Many sources claim the name feverfew comes from the Latin *febrifugia*, meaning "driver out of fevers." They also say it's been used since ancient times to treat fever. They're wrong on both counts.

The plant was never called *febrifugia*. Ancient physicians including Dioscorides and Galen used its Greek name, *parthe-*

nion, and prescribed it for menstrual and birth-related problems, not fever. During the Middle Ages, the name *parthenion* faded, and the plant was renamed *featherfoil* because of its feathery leaf borders. *Featherfoil* became *featherfew* and eventually *feverfew*.

Once feverfew acquired its name, herbalists decided it was, in fact, a fever treatment. They planted the strong-smelling herb around their homes in hopes of purifying the air to ward off malaria, which they mistakenly believed was caused by bad air (hence malaria, from the Italian *mala*, "foul," and *aria*, "air").

Malaria had plagued Europe since prehistoric times, and it was untreatable until Spanish explorers returned from Peru with cinchona bark and early chemists isolated its anti-malarial constituent, quinine. Quinine proved so successful at treating malaria that for a brief period, other fever herbs basked in its reflected glow, and feverfew picked up the name "wild quinine." But the name didn't stick. Quinine proved so superior as a malaria treatment that feverfew fell by the wayside.

Headache Hints

For a while, some herbalists recommended feverfew for other ailments, particularly headache. In the 17th century, England's John Parkinson claimed feverfew "is very effectual for all paines in the head." And more than 100 years later, John Hill wrote, "In the worst headache, this herb exceeds whatever else is known."

But most herbalists stuck to feverfew's traditional gynecological uses. Seventeenth-century English herbalist Nicholas Culpeper called it a "general strengthener of wombs" and prescribed it in tea for colds and chest congestion. Culpeper also recognized the herb's decline, declaring it "not much used in present practice."

Early colonists introduced feverfew into North America, where malaria was also a major problem, but as it fell from fashion in England, it stopped being used here as well.

America's 19th-century Eclectics prescribed it mainly as a menstruation promoter and treatment for "female hysteria," (menstrual discomforts) and some fever-producing diseases.

HEALING with Feverfew

In the late 1970s a happy accident occurred that made earlier observations about feverfew's benefit for "paines in the head" appear prophetic.

Migraine Headaches. The wife of the chief medical officer of Britain's National Coal Board suffered chronic migraines. A miner heard about her problem and told her he'd also been a longtime migraine sufferer—until he started chewing a few feverfew leaves every day. The woman tried the herb, noticed immediate improvement, and after 14 months was free of her searing headaches.

Her husband brought his wife's experience to the attention of Dr. E. Stewart Johnson of the City of London Migraine Clinic. Dr. Johnson gave feverfew leaves to ten of his patients. Three pronounced themselves cured, and the other seven reported significant improvement.

Dr. Johnson then gave feverfew to 270 of his migraine patients, then surveyed their experiences. Seventy percent reported significant relief—and for many, standard medical treatment had provided no relief at all.

Next, Dr. Johnson arranged a scientifically rigorous trial. Some participants took feverfew. Others took a look-alike placebo. And neither the researchers nor the subjects knew who got what until the end of the trial period. Feverfew significantly outperformed the placebo.

Soon after, the results of an even more rigorous experiment were published in the British medical journal *Lancet*. Seventy-two migraine sufferers were randomly assigned to receive either a look-alike placebo or a capsule a day of powdered, freeze-dried feverfew (the equivalent of two medium-size leaves). Neither the volunteers nor the researchers knew who got what, and after two months, the groups were switched, so the initial placebo-takers tried the feverfew and vice versa. The results were striking: Feverfew cut migraines 24 percent, and the headaches the herb-takers experienced were comparatively mild, with significantly less nausea and vomiting.

High Blood Pressure. The feverfew/migraine studies also showed the herb may reduce blood pressure. High blood pressure is a serious condition that requires professional care, but there's no harm in taking feverfew in addition to standard medical treatment.

Digestive Aid. Like its close botanical relative, chamomile, feverfew contains chemicals that may calm the smooth muscles of the digestive tract, making it an antispasmodic. Try feverfew after meals.

Women's Health. Antispasmodic herbs soothe not only the digestive tract but other smooth muscles, such as the uterus, as well. In addition, part of the reason feverfew prevents migraines is possibly its ability to neutralize certain substances in the body (prostaglandins) linked to pain and inflammation. Prostaglandins also play a role in menstrual cramps. Feverfew's possible antispasmodic and anti-prostaglandin actions support its traditional use in treating menstrual discomforts.

Intriguing Possibilities. One animal study suggests feverfew has a mild tranquilizing effect. Taken before bedtime, it just might help bring on sleep.

Another report suggests tumor-fighting properties. It's much too early to call feverfew a cancer treatment, but one day it might be.

Rx for Feverfew

For migraine control, chew two fresh (or frozen) leaves a day, or take a pill or capsule containing 85 milligrams of leaf material. Feverfew is quite bitter. Most people prefer the pills or capsules to chewing the leaves. If feverfew capsules do not provide benefit after a few weeks, don't give up on the herb without changing brands. A report in *Lancet* showed some "feverfew" pills and capsules contain only trace amounts of the herb.

Take feverfew in the form of an infusion to enjoy its other possible healing benefits: to help lower blood pressure, as a digestive aid, or to help bring on menstruation.

For an infusion, use $1/2$ to 1 teaspoon per cup of boiling water. Steep 5 to 10 minutes. Drink up to 2 cups a day.

Do not give feverfew to children under age 2. For older children and people over 65, start with low-strength preparations and increase strength if necessary.

The Safety Factor

Feverfew has not been shown to cause uterine contractions, but it has a long folk history as a menstruation promoter. Pregnant women should err on the side of caution and not use it.

Feverfew may cause sores inside the mouth. Some people also report abdominal pain.

Feverfew may inhibit blood clotting. Those with clotting disorders and anyone taking anticoagulant medication should consult a physician before using it.

Feverfew suppresses migraines but does not cure them. When the herb is terminated, the headaches typically return, which means migraine sufferers might wind up taking feverfew for years. To date, long-term use of the herb has caused no problems, but there is no research on its long-term effects.

For otherwise healthy nonpregnant, nonnursing adults who do not have clotting disorders and are not taking anticoagulants, feverfew is considered safe in amounts typically recommended.

Feverfew should be used in medicinal amounts only in consultation with your doctor. If feverfew causes mouth sores or stomach upset, use less or stop using it. Let your doctor know if you experience any unpleasant effects or if the symptoms for which the herb is being used do not improve significantly in two weeks.

Grow Your Headache Medicine

Feverfew is a perennial that reaches 3 feet and has lovely daisylike flowers with yellow centers and up to 20 white rays.

For personal migraine prevention, a few plants should suffice. Feverfew grows from seeds, but most authorities recommend root cuttings planted when the temperature reaches 70°F. Space plants 18 inches apart. Feverfew does best in partial shade. Compost stimulates better growth. Pinch back flower buds to encourage bushiness. Harvest leaves when they become mature.

Bees dislike feverfew and generally avoid the plant. Don't plant this herb around other plants requiring bee pollination.

Feverfew can also be maintained indoors year-round as a houseplant.

GARLIC

The Wonder Drug

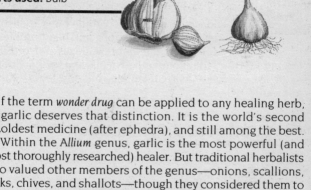

Family: Amaryllidacae; other members include onion, chives, shallots

Genus and species: *Allium sativum*

Also known as: Stinking rose, heal-all, rustic's or poor man's treacle

Parts used: Bulb

I f the term *wonder drug* can be applied to any healing herb, garlic deserves that distinction. It is the world's second oldest medicine (after ephedra), and still among the best.

Within the *Allium* genus, garlic is the most powerful (and most thoroughly researched) healer. But traditional herbalists also valued other members of the genus—onions, scallions, leeks, chives, and shallots—though they considered them to be less potent. Modern researchers have reached similar conclusions. Onions have almost as much medicinal value as garlic. Scallions, leeks, chives, and shallots have less.

Caves and Cuneiform

Garlic remains have been found in caves inhabited 10,000 years ago, but the first garlic prescription, chiseled in cuneiform on a Sumerian clay tablet, dates from 3000 B.C. The entire ancient world from Spain to China loved garlic, but no people enjoyed it more than the Egyptians, called "the stinking ones" because of their garlic breath. Egyptians taking solemn oaths swore on garlic in the same way that we swear on the Bible. The herb was found in the tomb of King Tut. And 15 pounds bought a healthy male slave.

Speaking of slavery, garlic played a major role in the lives of the slaves who built Egypt's pyramids. The Egyptians believed the herb prevented illness and increased strength and endurance. They gave their slaves a daily ration, and the slaves came to revere the herb as their masters did. Legend has it that during the construction of one pyramid, a garlic shortage forced the Egyptians to cut the slaves' ration. The result was the world's first recorded strike.

Garlic appeared prominently in the world's oldest surviving medical text, the *Ebers Papyrus*. It was an ingredient in 22 remedies for headache, insect and scorpion bites, menstrual discomforts, intestinal worms, tumors, and heart problems.

Soon after Moses led the Hebrew slaves out of Egypt around 1200 B.C., they complained of missing the finer things of life in bondage—"fish, cucumbers, melons, leeks, onions, and garlic."

For Combat and Competition

Greek athletes ate garlic before races, and Greek soldiers munched the herb before battle.

In Homer's *Odyssey*, Ulysses found strength from garlic against the sorceress, Circe.

Greek midwives hung garlic cloves around birthing rooms to safeguard newborns from disease and witchcraft. As the centuries passed, Europeans fastened braided garlic plants to their doorposts to keep evil spirits at bay, a custom which survives today in the garlic braids that hang in many kitchens.

The "Stinking Rose"

Greek and Roman physicians loved garlic. Hippocrates recommended it for infections, wounds, cancer, leprosy, and digestive problems. Dioscorides prescribed it for heart problems. And Pliny listed it in 61 remedies for ailments ranging from the common cold to epilepsy and from leprosy to tapeworm. Many of these uses have been supported by modern science.

But upper-class Greeks and Romans came to hate the "stinking rose." They viewed garlic breath as a sign of low birth, a belief that lasted well into the 20th century.

Like the Greeks, ancient India's Ayurvedic healers prescribed garlic for leprosy, a practice that continued for thousands of years. In fact, when India became a British colony and adopted English, leprosy became known as "peelgarlic" because lepers spent so much time peeling cloves and eating them. The Indians also used garlic to treat cancer. Modern research supports garlic's ability to treat leprosy and prevent certain cancers.

Ambivalence about garlic was rife in medieval Europe. The well-to-do shunned it, but the peasantry consumed huge amounts and viewed it as an all-purpose preventive medicine and cure-all. By the Elizabethan era, the Latin term for antidote, *theriaca*, had become the English word *treacle*, meaning panacea, and garlic was commonly called the "rustic's or poor man's treacle."

As the centuries passed, the upper class returned to garlic, but only medicinally, and even then sparingly. Seventeenth-century English herbalist Nicholas Culpeper endorsed it "as the poor man's treacle . . . a remedy for all diseases and hurts."

America's 19th-century Eclectic physicians shared the widespread prejudice against garlic's "strong, offensive smell . . . and acrimonious, almost caustic taste." But they conceded its effectiveness in treating colds, coughs, whooping cough, and other respiratory ailments. The Eclectics also believed fresh garlic juice applied to the ear could cure deafness, a recommendation echoed in some present-day herbals.

Russian Penicillin

During World War I, British, French, and Russian army physicians treated infected battle wounds with garlic juice. They also prescribed garlic to prevent and treat amoebic dysentery.

Alexander Fleming's discovery of penicillin in 1928 launched the Age of Antibiotics, and by World War II, penicillin and sulfa drugs had largely replaced garlic as the treatment of choice for infected wounds. But Russia's more than 20 million World War II casualties overwhelmed its antibiotic supply. Red Army physicians relied heavily on garlic, which came to be called Russian penicillin.

Modern herbalists recommend garlic (and the other *Alliums*) for colds, coughs, flu, fever, bronchitis, ringworm, intestinal worms, elevated cholesterol, and liver, gallbladder, and digestive problems.

HEALING with Garlic

Garlic does not cure epilepsy or deafness, but an enormous amount of scientific evidence shows beyond doubt that "the poor's man's treacle" is an herbal wonder drug.

A Powerful Antibiotic. During World War I, garlic's success in treating infected wounds and amoebic dysentery (caused by the protozoan E*ndameba histolytica*) clearly showed it had potent antibacterial and anti-protozoan effects, validating thousands of years of herbal tradition.

But garlic's antibiotic constituent remained a mystery until the 1920s, when researchers at Sandoz Pharmaceuticals in Switzerland isolated alliin (pronounced AL-*lee-in*) from the herb. Alliin by itself has no medicinal value, but when garlic is chewed, chopped, bruised, or crushed, the alliin comes in contact with a garlic enzyme (allinase), which transforms it into another chemical (allicin), which *is* a powerful antibiotic.

Since the 1920s, garlic's broad-spectrum antibiotic properties have been confirmed in literally dozens of animal and human studies. Garlic kills the bacteria that cause tuberculosis, food poisoning, and women's bladder infections. Garlic also may prevent infection by the influenza virus.

Chinese researchers report success using garlic to treat 21 cases of cryptococcal meningitis, an often fatal fungal infection. And several studies show the herb to be effective in treating the fungi that cause athlete's foot (*Trichophyton mentagrophytes*) and vaginal yeast infections (*Candida albicans*).

Heart Disease and Stroke. No standard medications can match garlic when it comes to acting on so many cardiovascular risk factors at the same time. Some drugs reduce blood pressure. Others decrease cholesterol. And some reduce the likelihood of internal blood clots, which trigger heart attacks and some strokes. But garlic does all these things—thanks to allicin and another chemical in the herb (ajoene).

Several studies dating back to the Sandoz experiments confirm garlic's ability to reduce blood pressure in animals and humans.

More than a dozen journal reports document garlic's ability to reduce cholesterol. In one experiment published in the British medical journal *Lancet*, researchers had volunteers eat a meal containing about 4 ounces of butter, which raises cholesterol. Half the group also ate about 9 cloves of garlic. After 3 hours, the average cholesterol level in the non-garlic group increased 7 percent. But in the garlic group, it *decreased* 7 percent. The researchers concluded: "Garlic has a very significant protective action [against high cholesterol]."

Finally, garlic helps prevent the blood clots that trigger heart attack. One researcher called the herb "at least as potent as aspirin," which has recently been promoted as an anticlotting heart-attack preventer.

Diabetes. Garlic reduces blood sugar levels in both laboratory animals and humans. Diabetes is a serious condition, requiring professional treatment, but if you have diabetes, there's no harm in upping your garlic consumption in addition to standard therapy.

Cancer. Tantalizing evidence suggests garlic plays a role in preventing and treating cancer. In a study reported in the journal *Science*, researchers separated mouse tumor cells into two groups. One group of tumor tissue was left alone. The other was treated with allicin. Then both batches of tumor cells were injected into mice. The mice who received the untreated cells quickly died, but there were no deaths among the mice that received the garlic-treated tumor cells. Since then, other animal studies have shown similar results.

Of course, animal findings don't necessarily apply to humans, but a study reported in the *Journal of the National Cancer Institute* suggests garlic may help prevent human stomach cancer. Researchers analyzed the diets of 1,800 Chinese, including 685 with stomach cancer. Those with the cancer ate considerably less garlic. The researchers concluded a diet high in garlic "can significantly reduce risk of stomach cancer."

Lead Poisoning. European studies show garlic helps eliminate lead and other toxic heavy metals from the body. Lead interferes with thinking and causes other serious medical problems. Exposure to leaded gasolines has introduced this metal into the body of everyone in North America. Children are particularly susceptible to lead's effects. Add garlic liberally to spaghetti sauces and other foods children enjoy.

Leprosy. Ancient Ayurvedic healers were onto something when they used garlic to treat leprosy (now called Hansen's disease). In one study, Indian researchers gave Hansen's sufferers a garlic ointment and food containing large amounts of the herb. Compared with others who did not receive the herb, those in the garlic group showed significant improvement.

AIDS. Studies that look at garlic as a treatment for AIDS are preliminary but exciting. In one study, seven AIDS patients who took a clove of garlic a day for three months experienced significant increases in immune functions usually destroyed by the disease. And while the patients were taking the garlic, chronic herpes sores cleared up in two of the seven, and in two others chronic diarrhea, a common AIDS symptom, also improved.

Rₓ for Garlic

You're undoubtedly anxious to put garlic's powerful infection-fighting action to the test. But how do you take it? For minor skin infections, garlic juice applied externally may prove sufficient, but unless you're an experienced herbalist, it's a mistake to rely exclusively on garlic to treat infectious diseases. No antibiotic, including garlic, kills *all* disease-causing microorganisms. The standard medical approach is to conduct what's known as a sensitivity test in which several antibiotics are tested against the germ. The doctor then prescribes the one that works best. You might ask your physician to include garlic in a sensitivity test. Or simply take the herb in addition to standard medication.

Researchers have found that 1 medium-size garlic clove packs the antibacterial punch of about 100,000 units of penicillin. Depending on the type of infection, oral penicillin doses typically range from 600,000 to 1.2 million units. The equivalent in garlic would be about 6 to 12 cloves. It's best to chew 3 cloves at a time, two to four times a day.

To help reduce blood pressure, cholesterol, and the likelihood of internal blood clots, 3 to 10 cloves of fresh garlic a day is recommended.

Garlic must be chewed, chopped, bruised, or crushed to transform its medicinally inert alliin into antibiotic allicin.

Using It in Cooking

Raw garlic has a sharp, biting flavor; some people experience a burning sensation on the tongue. Cooking eliminates the bite and softens the flavor.

In foods, season to taste. (The cloves' papery skins peel easily if you smash them with the flat side of a cleaver.)

For an infusion, chop 6 cloves per cup of cool water and steep 6 hours.

For a tincture, soak 1 cup of crushed cloves per quart of brandy, shake daily for two weeks, then take up to 3 tablespoons a day.

Garlic may be given cautiously to children under age 2.

What About the Smell?

Since 3000 B.C., the main problem with garlic has been its odor. The stinking rose continues to bother some people, but in recent decades, garlic-rich Italian and Asian cuisines have become increasingly popular, and some of the nation's finest restaurants now proudly serve dishes heavily flavored with garlic. We may well be entering the Age of Garlic Chic, but we're probably a long way from appreciating garlic breath.

To eliminate garlic breath, try chewing traditional herbal breath fresheners: parsley, fennel, or fenugreek.

The Safety Factor

Garlic's anticlotting action may help prevent heart attack and some kinds of stroke, but medicinal amounts could conceivably cause problems for those with clotting disorders. If you have a clotting disorder, consult your physician before using garlic in medicinal amounts.

Some people with allergies to garlic develop a rash from touching or eating the herb. If the herb gives you a rash, don't eat it. Garlic-induced upset stomach has also been reported.

Garlic enters the milk of nursing mothers and may cause colic in infants.

It has never been implicated in miscarriage or birth defects.

Other Cautions

For otherwise healthy nonpregnant, nonnursing adults who do not have clotting disorders, garlic is considered safe even in large amounts.

Garlic should be used in medicinal amounts only in consultation with your doctor. If garlic causes minor discomforts, such as stomach upset, use less or stop using it. Let your doctor know if you experience unpleasant effects or if the symptoms for which the herb is being used do not improve significantly in two weeks.

A Different Kind of Bulb

Garlic grows easily from seeds or cloves. It's easier to start with cloves. Plant them 2 inches deep and 6 inches apart in early spring for harvesting in fall.

Garlic is cold-tolerant and may be planted up to six weeks before the final frost date. It thrives best in rich, deeply cultivated, well-drained soil. Do not overwater. Full sun produces the largest bulbs, but garlic tolerates some shade. During summer, cut back the flower stalks so the plant devotes all its energy to producing fat, aromatic bulbs.

Harvest bulbs in late summer. Store them in cool darkness.

Take care not to bruise the bulbs. Bruising invites mold and insects. You can braid the leaves into a wreath or rope and display it in your kitchen, removing heads as needed.

GENTIAN

Feel Better with Bitter Moxie

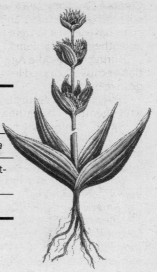

Family: Gentianaceae; other members include other gentians, marsh felwort

Genus and species: *Gentiana lutea*

Also known as: Yellow gentian, bitter root, bitterwort

Parts used: Roots

I n Depression-era slang, *moxie* meant courage tinged with recklessness. Teddy Roosevelt, Charles Lindberg, Al Capone—they all had moxie. The term comes from Moxie, a bitter soft drink available only in New England since the 1890s. Moxie owes its bitterness to gentian root, a healing herb with a 3,000-year history as a digestive "bitter." Modern research shows gentian may stimulate digestion.

For Whatever Ails You

Gentian was used by the ancient Egyptians, Greeks, and Romans as an appetite stimulant, antiseptic wound wash, and treatment for intestinal worms, digestive disorders, liver ailments, and "female hysteria" (menstrual discomforts).

Sixth-century Arab physicians adopted gentian from the Greeks and introduced its medicinal use to Asia. Since then,

Chinese physicians have used it to treat digestive disorders, sore throat, headache, and arthritis. India's Ayurvedic physicians have used it to treat fevers, venereal diseases, jaundice, and other liver problems.

During the Middle Ages, European herbalists prized gentian because it caused less intestinal irritation than other digestive bitters.

Seventeenth-century English herbalist Nicholas Culpeper wrote gentian "strengthens the stomach exceedingly, helps digestion, comforts the heart, helps agues [fevers] of all sorts, kills worms, and preserves against fainting and swooning. It provokes urine and terms [menstruation] exceedingly; therefore, let it not be given to women with child."

When colonists arrived in Virginia and the Carolinas, they were greeted by Indians who applied a root decoction of native American gentian (*G. puberula*) to treat back pain.

America's 19th-century Eclectics considered gentian "a powerful tonic," and prescribed it to "improve appetite and stimulate digestion." But their text, *King's American Dispensatory*, warned: "When taken in large doses, it is apt to oppress the stomach, irritate the bowels, and produce nausea, vomiting, and headache."

Gentian was listed in the U.S. *Pharmacopoeia* from 1820 to 1955 as a digestive stimulant.

Before the introduction of hops, gentian root was used in beer brewing, and the herb is still used in liqueurs, vermouths, and many digestive bitters popular in Europe.

Moxie Makes Money

Then came Moxie. In 1885, Augustin Thompson of Union, Maine, introduced it as Beverage Moxie Nerve Food. The original label proclaimed the bitter brew cured "brain and nervous exhaustion, loss of manhood, helplessness, imbecility, and insanity"—claims that took a lot of moxie even in the pre–Food and Drug Administration (FDA) heyday of patent medicines. Thompson peddled Moxie on the road in classic snake-oil style, and eventually it caught on—not as a medicine but as a beverage. That was fine with Thompson, who backed off from his medicinal claims and repositioned Moxie as a soft drink. For years, Moxie outsold Coca-Cola in New England. It's still available there, and gentian is still one of its ingredients.

In her *Modern Herbal*, Maude Grieve called gentian "one of our most useful bitter tonics, especially in general debility, weakness of the digestive organs, or want of appetite. It is one of the best strengtheners of the human system." Contemporary herbalists echo Grieve. One suggests chewing the root as a substitute for cigarettes.

HEALING with Gentian

Forget gentian for "loss of manhood, helplessness, imbecility, and insanity." But the bitter root may live up to its ancient reputation.

Digestion. Gentian contains a chemical (gentianine) that stimulates the secretion of stomach acid, lending some credence to its 3,000-year history as a digestive aid. Try it before meals.

Arthritis. One Chinese study showed gentian has strong anti-inflammatory properties, which suggests traditional Chinese physicians may have been on the right track when they prescribed the herb for arthritis. Try it if you have arthritis or any other inflammatory condition.

Women's Health. Gentian has never been shown to stimulate the uterus, but for hundreds of years, herbalists have considered it a powerful menstruation promoter. Pregnant women should err on the side of caution and not use it. Other women may try it to begin their periods.

Rx for Gentian

Use a decoction or tincture to stimulate digestion. You might give either a try to help treat arthritis or bring on menstruation.

For a decoction, boil 1 teaspoon of powdered root in 3

cups of water for 30 minutes. Cool. Drink 1 tablespoon before meals. Gentian tastes very bitter, so you might want to add sugar or honey.

In a tincture, use ¼ to 1 teaspoon before meals.

Gentian should not be given to children under age 2. For older children and people over 65, start with low-strength preparations and increase strength if necessary.

The Safety Factor

Gentian bitters are popular in Germany, where herbal medicine is considerably more mainstream than it is in the United States. German physicians discourage its use by people with high blood pressure. They also echo the Eclectics' warning that large amounts may cause stomach irritation with possible nausea and vomiting.

The FDA has approved gentian for use in foods and alcoholic beverages. For otherwise healthy nonpregnant, nonnursing adults, who do not have hypertension or chronic gastrointestinal conditions, gentian is considered safe in amounts typically recommended.

Gentian should be used in medicinal amounts only in consultation with your physician. If gentian causes minor discomforts, such as stomach upset or nausea, use less or stop using it. Let your doctor know if you experience any unpleasant effects or if the symptoms for which the herb is being used do not improve significantly in two weeks.

Hard to Start

Gentian is a striking 6-foot perennial with branching medicinal roots, deeply veined, pointed oval leaves, and large, beautiful yellow flowers.

Once established, gentian requires little care other than abundant water and shelter from wind and excessive sun. But establishing this herb can be a problem. The seeds need frost to germinate, and even with frost, germination may take a year, if it occurs at all. Most authorities recommend using root cuttings. Gentian prefers rich, loamy, slightly acidic soil. An annual dressing of peat moss helps.

Harvest the roots in late summer. Desirable roots are dark reddish brown, tough, and flexible with a strong, unpleasant odor. They should taste rather sweet initially, then very bitter. Dry the roots, then reduce them to powder.

GINGER

Put a Stop to Motion Sickness

Family: Zingiberaceae; other members include turmeric, cardamom

Genus and species: *Zingiber officinale*

Also known as: Jamaican ginger, African ginger, Cochin (Asian) ginger

Parts used: Roots

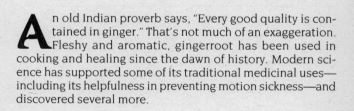

An old Indian proverb says, "Every good quality is contained in ginger." That's not much of an exaggeration. Fleshy and aromatic, gingerroot has been used in cooking and healing since the dawn of history. Modern science has supported some of its traditional medicinal uses—including its helpfulness in preventing motion sickness—and discovered several more.

Herb of the Gods

Ancient Indians used their native ginger in cooking, to preserve food and to treat digestive problems. They also considered it a physical and spiritual cleanser. Indians shunned strong-smelling garlic and onion before religious celebrations for fear of offending their deities, but they ate lots of ginger because it left them smelling sweet and therefore presentable to the gods.

Ginger appeared prominently in China's first great herbal, the *Pen Tsao Ching* (*Classic of Herbs*), compiled by legendary emperor/sage Shen Nung around 3000 B.C. As the story goes, this wise herbalist tested hundreds of medicinal herbs on himself—until he took a little too much of a poisonous herb and died. Shen Nung recommended ginger for colds, fever, chills, tetanus, and leprosy. The *Pen Tsao Ching* also echoed Indian practice, saying fresh ginger "eliminates body odor and puts a person in touch with the spiritual [realm]."

As time passed, Chinese sailors began chewing ginger to prevent seasickness, and Chinese physicians prescribed it to treat arthritis and kidney problems.

Chinese women still drink ginger tea for menstrual cramps, morning sickness, and other gynecological problems.

The Chinese also consider ginger an antidote to shellfish poisoning, which is why Chinese fish and seafood dishes are often seasoned with the herb.

Gingerbread and Ginger Ale

The ancient Greeks adopted ginger as a digestive aid. After big meals, they ate ginger wrapped in bread. Over time, the herb was incorporated into the bread, and this indigestion preventive evolved into gingerbread.

The Romans also used ginger as a digestive aid, but after the fall of Rome, it became scarce in Europe and quite costly.

Once renewed Asian trade made ginger more available, European demand proved almost insatiable. The ancient Greeks' modest gingerbread cakes evolved into sugary gingerbread men and such elaborate confections as the witch's gingerbread house in *Hansel and Gretel*. In England and her American colonies, ginger was incorporated into a stomach-soothing drink, ginger beer, forerunner of today's ginger ale, which is still a popular home remedy for diarrhea, nausea, and vomiting.

America's 19th-century Eclectics prescribed ginger powder, tea, wine, and beer for infant diarrhea, indigestion, nausea, dysentery, flatulence, fever, headache, toothache, and "female hysteria" (menstrual complaints).

Contemporary herbalists recommend ginger for colds, flu, and motion sickness, and as a digestive aid and menstruation promoter.

HEALING with Ginger

Break out the gingerbread and ginger ale. Science has lent support to some of ginger's traditional uses—and discovered several more.

Motion Sickness and Morning Sickness. The ancient Chinese sailors who used ginger to prevent seasickness were probably right. Ginger's anti-nausea action relieves motion sickness and dizziness (vertigo) better than the standard drug treatment, Dramamine, according to one study published in the British medical journal *Lancet*. In this experiment, 36 volunteers with a history of motion sickness took either 100 milligrams of Dramamine or 940 milligrams of ginger powder. Then they were seated in a computerized rocking chair programmed to trigger seasickness. People were free to stop the chair whenever they began to feel nauseated. Those taking ginger lasted 57 percent longer than those on Dramamine. In addition to motion sickness, the researchers recommended ginger capsules, ginger tea, or ginger ale for the morning sickness of pregnancy. Some doctors now recommend it for nausea associated with chemotherapy.

Digestive Aid. Ginger appears to relieve indigestion and abdominal cramping by soothing the gastrointestinal tract, making it an antispasmodic. Ginger also has anti-nausea action, and it contains some substances similar to the digestive enzymes that break down proteins.

Women's Health. Antispasmodics soothe not only the digestive tract but other smooth muscles, such as the uterus, as well. Ginger may help ease menstrual cramps.

Colds and Flu. Chinese studies show ginger helps kill influenza virus, and an Indian report shows it increases the immune system's ability to fight infection. These findings lend some support to ginger's traditional uses for colds, flu, and other infectious diseases.

Arthritis. Studies have identified anti-inflammatory substances in the herb, lending support to the traditional use of ginger for treating arthritis.

Heart Disease and Stroke. Few people in the ancient world lived long enough—or ate a diet high enough in fat— to develop heart disease or stroke, but today these diseases account for half of U.S. deaths. Ginger may help prevent them by controlling several key risk factors.

Ginger helps reduce cholesterol, according to a study published in the *New England Journal of Medicine*. It also helps lower blood pressure and prevent the internal blood clots that trigger heart attacks and some strokes.

Intriguing Possibility. One animal study shows that ginger shrinks liver tumors in experimental animals. While animal studies do not necessarily apply to humans, ginger may someday find a role in the treatment of cancer in humans.

Rx for Ginger

In food, season to taste for warm, spicy, aromatic dishes.

For motion sickness, the recommended dose is 1,500 milligrams approximately 30 minutes before travel. Commercial ginger capsules are usually most convenient, but a 12-ounce glass of ginger ale also provides the recommended amount (provided it actually contains ginger and not artificial flavor).

Use ginger tea as a digestive aid; to help treat colds and flu, nausea, morning sickness, or arthritis; or to help prevent heart disease and stroke. To make ginger tea, use 2 teaspoons of powdered or grated root per cup of boiling water. Steep 10 minutes.

Weak ginger preparations may be given to children under age 2 for colic.

The Safety Factor

Ginger's anti-nausea effect may prevent morning sickness, but traditionally the herb has a long history as a menstruation promoter. Might it cause miscarriage? In large doses it might, so pregnant women with a history of miscarriage should not use it. One study suggests that ginger's effects depend on the amount used. In the study published in *Lancet*, less than 1 gram was used to prevent nausea. To trigger menstruation, Chinese physicians recommend 20 to 28 grams.

A strong cup of ginger tea contains about 250 milligrams of the herb. A heavily spiced ginger dish contains about 500 milligrams. And an 8-ounce glass of ginger ale contains approximately 1,000 milligrams—none of which come close to the amount that promotes menstruation.

There have been no reports in the scientific literature of ginger triggering abortion or causing birth defects.

Pregnant women with no history of miscarriage should feel free to try modest amounts of ginger tea or ginger ale to treat morning sickness.

Though ginger generally relieves indigestion, some people who take it to prevent motion sickness report heartburn.

Ginger is on the Food and Drug Administration's list of herbs generally regarded as safe. For otherwise healthy adults, ginger is safe in amounts typically recommended.

Ginger should be used in medicinal amounts only in consultation with your physician. If ginger causes minor discomforts, such as heartburn, use less or stop using it. Let your doctor know if you experience any unpleasant effects or if the symptoms for which the herb is being used do not improve significantly in two weeks.

Grows in Warm Climates

Ginger is a tropical perennial that grows from a tuberous root. Each year the plant produces a round, 3-foot stem with thin, pointed, 6-inch, lance-shaped leaves and a single, large yellow and purple flower.

Ginger grows outdoors in Hawaii, Florida, southern California, New Mexico, Arizona, and Texas. It does best when well watered in partial shade in raised beds deeply cultivated with composted manure and kelp.

Ginger is propagated from young fresh roots, which contain eyes similar to those in potatoes. The ginger root sold in most supermarkets—with tough, tan skin—is neither young nor fresh, so its propagation potential is low. The best place to obtain growable ginger root is at an Asian specialty market, though some nurseries carry it. Look for gingerroot with light green skin.

Plant the roots about 3 inches deep and 12 inches apart. After 12 months, uproot the plant, harvest some roots, and replant the rest.

Ginger may also be grown indoors in deep pots with a soil mixture of loam, sand, compost, and peat moss. Indoors it needs warmth, plenty of water, and high humidity. A greenhouse environment is best.

GINKGO

What's Old Is New

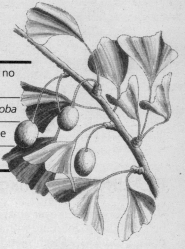

Family: Ginkgoaceae; there are no other members

Genus and species: *Ginkgo biloba*

Also known as: Maidenhair tree

Parts used: Leaves

Ginkgo is the oldest surviving tree on earth. As a healing herb, it can help the oldest surviving people. Ginkgo may prevent and help treat many conditions associated with aging: stroke, heart disease, impotence, deafness, blindness, and memory loss.

Elixir of Long Life

Ginkgo was termed "good for the heart and lungs" in China's first great herbal, the *Pen Tsao Ching* (*The Classic of Herbs*), attributed to legendary emperor/sage Shen Nung. Traditional Chinese physicians use ginkgo to treat asthma and chilblains, swelling of the hands and feet due to damp cold.

The ancient Chinese and Japanese also ate roasted ginkgo seeds as a digestive aid and to prevent drunkenness.

India's traditional Ayurvedic healers associated ginkgo

277

with long life and reportedly used it as an ingredient in soma, a longevity elixir.

Ginkgoes were introduced into Europe in 1730, and today they are popular street and park trees throughout the temperate world. But even though 18th-century horticulturists planted them throughout Europe, herbalists of that time ignored them. As a result, ginkgo's fan-shaped leaves have no history in Western herbal healing.

Today, European herbalists and mainstream physicians feel much differently. Ginkgo products are among Europe's most widely prescribed medications, with sales of $500 million a year.

HEALING with Ginkgo

Medical excitement over ginkgo comes principally from the herb's ability to interfere with the action of a substance the body produces called platelet activation factor (PAF). Discovered in 1972, PAF is involved in an enormous number of biological processes: asthma attacks, organ graft rejection, arterial blood flow, and the internal blood clots involved in heart attacks and some strokes. By inhibiting PAF, ginkgo has been shown to have enormous healing potential, particularly in conditions associated with aging.

Stroke. As people grow older, blood flow to the brain can decrease. That means less food and oxygen for brain cells. If blood flow becomes blocked, the result is a stroke, the third leading cause of death in the United States. Dozens of studies show ginkgo significantly increases blood flow to the brain and may even speed recovery from stroke.

Memory and Reaction Time. As blood flow to the brain improves, so do memory and mental functioning. In one small study involving eight women, short-term memory and reaction time improved "very significantly" after they took ginkgo.

Heart Attack. Ginkgo also improves blood flow to the heart muscle itself. And it may help prevent heart attacks by reducing the risk of the internal blood clots that trigger them.

Intermittent Claudication. When cholesterol deposits narrow the arteries in the legs, the result is intermittent claudication—pain, cramping, and weakness, particularly in the calves. Ginkgo may improve blood flow through the legs. A year-long study of 36 intermittent claudication sufferers showed ginkgo produced "significantly greater pain relief than standard treatment."

Impotence. A study published in the *Journal of Urology* showed ginkgo helps relieve impotence caused by narrowing of the arteries that supply blood to the penis. Sixty men with erection problems caused by impeded penile blood flow were given 60 milligrams of ginkgo a day. By the end of the year-long study, half the men had regained erections.

Macular Degeneration. This is deterioration of the retina, the nerve-rich area in the eye necessary for sight. Macular degeneration is the leading cause of adult blindness. In one small French study, ginkgo produced "significant improvement" in the vision of people suffering from this disease.

Cochlear Deafness. Researchers believe this form of hearing loss results from decreased blood flow to the nerves involved in hearing. One study by French researchers comparing ginkgo to standard therapy showed "significant recovery in both groups, but distinctly better improvement in the ginkgo group."

Chronic Ringing in the Ears (Tinnitus). A 13-month study of 103 chronic tinnitus sufferers done in Paris showed ginkgo "conclusively effective." Ginkgo "improved all the patients" taking the herb.

Chronic Dizziness (Vertigo). In one study, 70 people with chronic vertigo were treated for three months with either ginkgo extract or a look-alike placebo. At the conclusion of the trial, 18 percent of the the placebo-takers no longer felt dizzy, compared with 47 percent of those who took ginkgo, a highly significant difference.

Asthma. PAF causes the kind of bronchial constriction typical in asthma. Ginkgo interferes with PAF and helps prevent bronchial constriction, lending credence to the traditional Chinese use of ginkgo in treating asthma and other respiratory complaints.

Intriguing Possibilities. Preliminary reports suggest ginkgo may help prevent the rejection of transplanted organs. It may also be effective against allergies, high blood pressure, kidney problems, and Alzheimer's disease.

No wonder ginkgo is now one of the most widely prescribed drugs in Europe.

R$_x$ for Ginkgo

Ginkgo is not generally available as a bulk herb, however many herb companies offer commercial preparations. Follow package directions. Taste is not an issue because most preparations are pills.

Even if you have your own ginkgo tree, you can't just brew up some tea and expect to take advantage of the herb's healing benefits. It takes a lot of ginkgo leaves to make medicine. This is one instance in which commercial preparations are preferable.

The Safety Factor

Platelet activation factor plays a key role in blood clotting. Ginkgo's PAF-inhibiting action may cause problems for those with clotting disorders.

Some people who take extremely large amounts of the herb have reported irritability, restlessness, diarrhea, nausea, and vomiting. Recommended amounts are considered nontoxic.

For otherwise healthy nonpregnant, nonnursing adults who do not have clotting disorders, ginkgo is considered safe in amounts typically recommended.

Ginkgo should not be given to children under age 2, and except for prevention of asthma, there is no reason to give it to older children.

Ginkgo should be used in medicinal amounts only in consultation with your doctor. If ginkgo causes minor discomforts, such as nausea or diarrhea, use less or stop using it. Let your doctor know if you experience unpleasant symptoms or if the symptoms for which the herb is being used do not improve significantly in two weeks.

Males Make the Best Trees

Ginkgo is a stately, deciduous tree that reaches 100 feet with a 20-foot girth. Its flat, fan-shaped leaves have two lobes. Ginkgoes are dioecious, that is, male and female flowers appear on different trees. The females produce apricot-size, orange-yellow fruits, which contain an edible seed.

Ginkgoes are attractive street or yard trees that can be grown throughout much of the United States. Obtain a sapling from a nursery in your area. Plant only males. The fruits produced by females are messy and foul-smelling.

Plant ginkgo saplings in well-drained soil and stake them to ensure straight growth. Young trees are oddly proportioned and often look gawky, but they become stately with age. Water regularly until trees are about 20 feet tall. Then they become self-sufficient. Ginkgoes are resistant to insects and disease and grow up to 2 feet per year. In autumn, the leaves turn a beautiful gold before they fall.

GINSENG

Asia's Ultimate Tonic

Family: Araliaceae; other members include ivy

Genus and species: *Panax ginseng* (Chinese/Korean/Japanese); *Panax quinquefolius* (American); *Eleutherococcus senticosus* (Siberian)

Also known as: Man root, life root, root of immortality, Tartar root, heal-all, 'seng, 'sang

Parts used: Roots

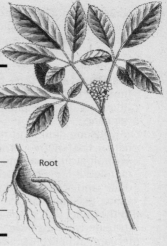

Root

Ginseng is as fascinating as it is controversial. The root of an unassuming ivylike groundcover, it has been the subject of more than 1,200 books and scientific papers, yet its effects are still hotly debated.

Advocates say it's completely safe and call it the ultimate tonic—a mild aphrodisiac that enhances memory, learning, productivity, physical stamina, and immune function, while reducing blood cholesterol and sugar (glucose) and minimizing the ravages of stress, aging, radiation, alcohol, and narcotics.

Critics say it does little, if anything, except cause a potentially hazardous "abuse syndrome."

Man Root

Ginseng is not one herb but three: Chinese or Korean or Japanese (P. *ginseng*), American (P. *quinquefolius*), and Siberian

(E. senticosus). The Siberian plant is not true ginseng, but it contains similar active chemicals, and studies show it has similar effects. As a result, all three are grouped together as "ginseng," and used interchangeably in the West.

Ginseng has a fleshy, multibranched root. If you stretch your imagination, some roots resemble the human form, with limblike branches suggesting arms and legs. The ancient Chinese called the plant "man root," *jen shen*, which became "ginseng."

Ginseng figured prominently in the first great Chinese herbal, the *Pen Tsao Ching* (*The Classic of Herbs*), compiled by the mythological emperor/sage Shen Nung. Shen Nung recommended it for "enlightening the mind and increasing wisdom," and noted that "continuous use leads to longevity." In China, ginseng's fancied resemblance to the human form led to the belief that it was a whole-body tonic, particularly for the elderly. It was widely used to treat infirmities of old age: lethargy, impotence, arthritis, senility, menopausal complaints, and loss of sexual interest. Chinese, Koreans, and Japanese still consider ginseng the best health promoter, though their calling it the "root of immortality" stretches things a bit.

More Prized Than Gold

As the popularity of ginseng spread throughout ancient Asia, demand soared and rapacious collection decimated the supply. Chinese ginseng became increasingly rare—and more valuable than gold. Unscrupulous merchants sold other roots as ginseng, and adulteration is still a problem today.

Unlike other Asian herbs that became favorites in the West (for example, ginger and cinnamon), ginseng remained a mystery in Europe until the 18th century, when missionaries informed early European botanists of its reputation as a longevity herb. Europeans scoffed at Asian claims, but those familiar with Asia—particularly the Jesuits who had many missions in China—appreciated the herb's great value there.

The Jesuits' Secret

In 1704, a French explorer returned to Paris with a sample of what turned out to be American ginseng from southern Canada. Jesuits in France alerted their brethren in Canada to its enormous value in China, and some years later, Jesuits in Montreal shipped a boatload to Canton, where other Jesuits sold it to the Chinese for what was then a king's ransom, $5 a pound.

Immediately the Jesuits began shipping to China as much ginseng as their Indian collectors could find. They made a fortune and kept the lucrative trade a secret for many years. But word eventually leaked that the celibate fathers seemed to take an unusual interest in a certain low-growing herb, which was rumored to be an aphrodisiac in far-off Cathay.

Once the word got out, ginseng was discovered growing as far south as Georgia, and it enjoyed a brief burst of popularity among American colonists interested in sexual stimulation. Most were disappointed. Virginia plantation owner William Byrd wrote in the late 17th century that ginseng "frisks the spirits," but causes none "of those naughty effects that might make men too troublesome and impertinent to their wives."

By the 1740s, few Americans were consuming ginseng, but news of its incredible value in China hit the 13 colonies like word of the California gold strike 100 years later. Shipping agents circulated handbills offering to buy the herb for the then-fabulous sum of $1 a pound. Foragers scoured the countryside, and frontier scouts, surveyors, and fur trappers collected ginseng as a sideline to their other work. Ginseng quickly became the colonies' most valuable export—more precious pound for pound than even the rarest furs.

Americans Adopt the Herb

The American Indians learned about ginseng from the Jesuits and used it to combat fatigue, stimulate appetite, and aid digestion. Some tribes mixed it into love potions.

America's 19th-century Eclectics called ginseng a stimulant

for "mental exhaustion from overwork" and prescribed it for loss of appetite, indigestion, asthma, laryngitis, bronchitis, and tuberculosis. *King's American Dispensatory* added it "invigorates the virile powers."

Contemporary herbalists echo the Chinese, recommending ginseng as a tonic stimulant that promotes vitality and longevity. They also suggest it for fever, inflammations, colds, coughs, respiratory problems, depression, menstrual difficulties, childbirth, and immune stimulation.

Wild American ginseng is no longer plentiful, but in Appalachia, collectors still forage for the herb. Wild ginseng sells to export agents for about $200 per pound. Most collectors never use the herb themselves. In the words of Georgia ginseng trader Jake Plott, "I never found it worth a damn for anything but to get money out of."

Plott's comment aptly sums up how many Western scientists feel about Asia's most revered herb. Critics dismiss its purported benefits as "folklore of the Far East" and say the studies showing benefit are seriously flawed. They also charge ginseng causes "serious side effects," including a combination of nervousness, insomnia, diarrhea, high blood pressure, and hormonal disturbances, known as "ginseng abuse syndrome."

Meanwhile, scientific literature shows ginseng is reasonably safe and beneficial for some ailments.

HEALING with Ginseng

Ginseng owes its healing value to several chemicals called ginsenosides. They are not fully understood, and their effects can be downright confusing. For example, some ginsenosides stimulate the central nervous system; others depress it. Some raise blood pressure; others reduce it. These observations need to be clarified with additional research. But researchers have learned a great deal about this herb and its many effects.

Resistance to Disease. Some advocates of ginseng call the herb an adaptogen, a technical term for what traditional herbalists call a tonic. Chief among ginseng's adaptogen advocates is Soviet researcher Israel I. Brekhman, a professor who studied ginseng for almost 30 years at the U.S.S.R. Academy of Sciences. Brekhman wrote ginseng "possesses a remarkably wide range of therapeutic activities . . . protecting the body against stress, radiation, and various chemical toxins . . . and increasing general resistance."

American scientists often view Soviet research with suspicion. But some U.S. researchers agree ginseng is an adaptogen, among them, Norman R. Farnsworth, Ph.D., research professor of Pharmacognosy at the University of Illinois School of Pharmacy, who described the herb's many effects in the journal *Economic and Medicinal Plant Research*.

The term *adaptogen* covers a broad range of effects. Various studies of Russian, Korean, and Chinese soldiers, sailors, athletes, proofreaders, factory workers, and telephone operators show the herb:

- Counteracts fatigue without caffeine and improves physical stamina. Russian, Chinese, and Korean Olympic athletes use ginseng in their training and before events, and some American athletes have begun using the herb as well.
- Counteracts the damage caused by physical and emotional stress.
- Prevents the depletion of stress-fighting hormones in the adrenal gland.
- Enhances memory.

Immune Stimulant. Ginseng appears to stimulate the immune system of both animals and humans. It revs up the white blood cells (macrophages and natural killer cells) that devour disease-causing microorganisms. Ginseng also spurs production of interferon, the body's own virus-fighting chemical, and antibodies, which fight bacterial and viral infections.

Russian researchers gave 1,500 factory workers 4 milligrams of ginseng a day. Compared with workers who did not receive the herb, the ginseng users lost significantly fewer work days due to colds, flu, tonsillitis, bronchitis, and sinus infections. Russian cosmonauts take ginseng to increase stamina and prevent illness in outer space.

American researchers have confirmed ginseng's antiviral and immune-boosting effects. In one study, ginseng eliminated chronic herpes sores, the result of herpes virus infection. After the herb treatment ended, the sores reappeared.

High Cholesterol. Ginseng reduces cholesterol, according to several American studies. It also increases good cholesterol (high-density lipoproteins, or HDLs). As good cholesterol increases, heart attack risk drops.

Heart Attack. If the arteries that supply blood to the heart have been narrowed by cholesterol deposits (atherosclerotic plaques) and blood clots form in them, the result is a heart attack. Ginseng has an anticlotting (anti-platelet) effect, which reduces the risk of these clots—and heart attack.

Diabetes. Ginseng reduces blood sugar levels, suggesting value in managing diabetes. Diabetes is a serious condition requiring professional treatment. Diabetics might try the herb in consultation with their physicians.

Liver Protection. Ginseng protects the liver from the harmful effects of drugs, alcohol, and other toxic substances. In one experiment, researchers gave what should have been fatal doses of various narcotics to experimental animals pretreated with ginseng extract. The animals survived. And in a pilot human study, ginseng improved liver function in 24 elderly people suffering from cirrhosis, liver damage from alcohol.

Radiation Therapy. Ginseng can minimize cell damage from radiation. In two studies, experimental animals were injected with various protective agents, then subjected to doses of radiation similar to those used in cancer radiation therapy. Ginseng provided the best protection against damage to healthy cells, suggesting value during cancer radiation therapy.

Cancer. Chinese researchers claim to have extended the lives of stomach cancer sufferers by as many as four years using ginseng. Soviet scientists say the herb shrinks some animal tumors.

Loss of Appetite. Asians have always considered ginseng particularly beneficial for the elderly. As people age, the senses of taste and smell deteriorate, which reduces appetite. In addition, the intestine's ability to absorb nutrients declines. As a result, some older people suffer undernourishment, which reduces their energy and alertness and increases their risk of illness. Ginseng enjoys a thousand-year-old reputation as an appetite stimulant, and one study showed it increases the ability of the intestine to absorb nutrients, thus helping prevent undernourishment.

Intriguing Possibilities. Several studies have investigated the ancient Chinese belief that ginseng is a mild sex stimulant. None involved humans, and one must be extremely careful about applying animal sex research to people. In animals, instinct controls sex. In humans, more complex social and psychological factors govern it. But, for what it's worth, Russian studies suggest ginseng treatment increases the sperm quality in bull semen. And a study published in the *American Journal of Clinical Medicine* showed that ginseng-treated experimental animals are more sexually active than animals that don't receive the herb.

A Question of Adulteration

Many ginseng studies have produced impressively beneficial results. But critics cite others that have shown no benefits whatsoever. What gives? Adulteration appears to be a big part of the answer.

Because of ginseng's rarity and enormous value, adulteration has been a problem for centuries. It still is today. It's quite possible some researchers have used "ginseng" that contained little or none of the herb. One study evaluated 54 so-called ginseng products available in U.S. health food stores. The researchers judged 60 percent "worthless" because they contained too little of the herb to have any biological effect. Twenty-five percent contained no ginseng at all.

The health food industry denounced this study, and the health food trade journal *Whole Foods* commissioned an independent test. It showed essentially the same results.

The most notorious of the nonginseng "ginsengs" was

"wild red American ginseng" or "wild desert ginseng," which appeared in health food stores during the late 1970s. Ginseng is a shade-loving, moisture-demanding plant, so "desert ginseng" is an impossibility, but many consumers fell for the fraud. The phony ginseng was actually red dock, a laxative plant. An outcry from responsible herbalists forced most "wild red ginseng" off health food store shelves by the early 1980s.

Rx for Ginseng

Even if you start with real ginseng, it may not work because it may not be mature. Ginseng roots should not be harvested until they are six years old, but sometimes younger roots are mixed in to stretch the amount, a form of adulteration which may render the herb useless.

Finally, processing can also decrease ginseng quality.

Researchers urge consumers to take "great care in selecting ginseng products." But how? Unfortunately, the only way to be absolutely certain of ginseng purity and age is to grow it yourself, which is much easier said than done. If you buy ginseng, read labels carefully. Look for products identified by species made with whole, unprocessed, six-year-old roots.

Ginseng tastes sweetish and slightly aromatic. To take advantage of ginseng's many healing benefits, use root powder, teas, capsules, or tablets, all of which are available at health food stores and through herb outlets. Recommendations range from the equivalent of about 1/2 to 1 teaspoon per day. Some sources say ginseng may be used daily. Others suggest daily use for a month, followed by a two-month layoff.

You can also make a decoction from dried, pulverized root material. Use 1/2 teaspoon per cup of water. Bring to a boil. Simmer 10 minutes. Drink up to 2 cups a day.

The Safety Factor

With controversial herbs, critics often blow any side effects out of proportion, prompting outraged proponents to counter that the herb is "completely safe." Ginseng side effects are no cause for alarm, but no drug, herbal or otherwise, should be considered completely safe.

Problems with ginseng are rare, but the medical journals contain a few dozen reports. Ginseng may cause insomnia, breast soreness, allergy symptoms, asthma attacks, increased blood pressure, and disturbances in heart rhythm (cardiac arrhythmias). People with insomnia, hay fever, and fibrocystic breasts should use it only with caution. Anyone with fever, asthma, emphysema, high blood pressure, or cardiac arrhythmia should not use it.

In addition, ginseng's anticlotting action should place it off-limits for those with clotting problems.

In Asia, ginseng is considered an herb for the elderly. It should not be given to children. Asian studies show ginseng causes no birth defects in the offspring of rats, rabbits, and lambs, but pregnant women should err on the side of caution and not use it.

Abuse of "Abuse"

Ginseng may not be completely harmless. But one study showing serious side effects—the one that came up with "ginseng abuse syndrome" (GAS)—has been found to be badly flawed.

The term was coined in a 1979 article published in the *Journal of the American Medical Association*.

The researcher studied 133 psychiatric patients who claimed to use ginseng. He said 14, or about 10 percent, developed GAS. The subjects were psychiatric patients, presumably people with problems. The researcher never bothered to identify the problems, but he freely applied his results to the general population.

The psychiatric patients *said* they used ginseng, but the researcher later admitted he made no attempt to verify that their "ginseng" was, in fact, the herb. He admitted many used "desert ginseng," which we have seen is *not* ginseng.

The subjects consumed up to 15 grams of the herb a day— many times the recommended amount. And some inhaled and injected it, methods which are unheard-of in traditional ginseng use and which strongly suggest the patients also abused illicit drugs. But the researcher never discussed his subjects' other drug use, except to mention that many used caffeine regularly throughout the two-year study.

Ginseng abuse syndrome included such symptoms as nervousness, sleeplessness, and increased blood pressure. In rare cases, ginseng may cause sleep problems or raise blood pressure, but these same symptoms are routine effects of caffeine, a drug the subjects consumed freely during the study. With results polluted by caffeine and quite possibly other drugs, it's impossible to say what caused the so-called abuse symptoms.

Another hallmark of GAS was "morning diarrhea." This may well have been caused by the nonginseng "desert ginseng," which is a laxative. Finally, the researcher charged GAS "mimics corticosteroid poisoning." Even at its worst, the purported symptoms of GAS are nothing like corticosteroid poisoning, a complex condition involving acne, unusual hair growth, fluid retention (edema), increased blood pressure and blood sugar, increased susceptibility to infection, and rounding of the face (moon face).

Nonetheless, ever since the publication of this paper, whenever medical journals or popular press reports discuss ginseng, they invariably mention "ginseng abuse syndrome" and "corticosteroid poisoning." For the record, ginseng has never been shown to cause either one.

Other Cautions

The Food and Drug Administration includes ginseng in its list of herbs generally regarded as safe. For otherwise healthy nonpregnant, nonnursing adults who do not have insomnia, hay fever, fibrocystic breasts, fever, asthma, emphysema, high blood pressure, cardiac arrhythmia, or clotting problems, ginseng is considered relatively safe in amounts typically recommended.

Ginseng should be used in medicinal amounts only in consultation with your doctor. If ginseng causes minor discomforts, such as allergy symptoms or insomnia, use less or stop using it. Let your doctor know if you experience any unpleas-

ant effects or if the symptoms for which the herb is being used do not improve significantly in two weeks.

"God and the Growers"

Ginseng is extremely difficult and expensive to grow. Prospective ginseng gardeners should heed the words of one frustrated horticulturist: "God and the growers know what they're doing, but neither one is talking."

Today, 80 percent of U.S. ginseng is grown in Marathon County, Wisconsin. Plants require shade, so growers drape nylon mesh over frames constructed along their rows. Ginseng is prone to several fungus infections, and it's a struggle to keep the young plants alive. Meanwhile, roots should be six years old at harvest, so growers must be extremely patient.

When roots are ready to be harvested, the process is painstaking. Their value in the Orient depends in part on the arrangement of their limbs. The more humanlike, the higher the price. Breaking an "arm" or "leg" off during harvesting or drying lowers the price.

Growing Your Own

Root cuttings are often diseased, so most growers start with seeds. Seeds cost $85 a pound. But seeds may also be diseased. Before planting, they must be disinfected in a solution of one part chlorine bleach and nine parts water for 10 minutes.

Plant in early autumn in well-prepared, humus-rich beds at a depth of 1/2 inch with 6-inch spacing. Ginseng grows poorly in sandy or clay soils. Maintain soil pH in the range of 5.0 to 6.0.

Be patient. Germination can take a year. Plants must be shaded, ideally under trees, but covered frames work.

Harvest roots after six years, digging carefully to prevent breaking root limbs. Dry them for one month.

GOLDENSEAL

A Potent Antibiotic

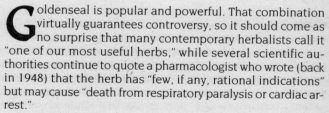

Family: Ranunculaceae; other members include buttercup, larkspur, peony

Genus and species: *Hydrastis canadensis*

Also known as: Yellow root, yellow puccoon, Indian turmeric, Indian dye, Indian paint, jaundice root, eye balm, eye root, golden root

Parts used: Rhizome and roots

Goldenseal is popular and powerful. That combination virtually guarantees controversy, so it should come as no surprise that many contemporary herbalists call it "one of our most useful herbs," while several scientific authorities continue to quote a pharmacologist who wrote (back in 1948) that the herb has "few, if any, rational indications" but may cause "death from respiratory paralysis or cardiac arrest."

On balance, there's no cause for alarm. Goldenseal may be beneficial when used carefully, though harmful effects are possible. Informed home herbalists can use it safely.

Yellow Root

The Indians of the Northeast pounded goldenseal's yellow roots (the source of most of its names) and used the yellow juice as a dye. They also used it medicinally as an eyewash (hence names "eye balm" and "eye root"), as a treatment for skin wounds, sore throat, digestive complaints, and for recovery from childbirth.

Early settlers adopted the plant but didn't use it much until the early 19th century, when Samuel Thomson, founder of Thomsonian herbal medicine, popularized it as an antiseptic. Thomson disliked the herb's Indian name, yellow root, and changed it to goldenseal.

Thomsonian medicine fell from fashion by the Civil War, but America's 19th-century Eclectics adopted goldenseal, which they called hydrastis, and greatly expanded its use. They used it externally to relieve hemorrhoids, rectal fissures, pinkeye (conjunctivitis), eczema, boils, and wounds, and internally as a digestive stimulant and treatment for colds, tonsillitis, diphtheria, uterine problems, postpartum hemorrhage, digestive ailments, and as a tonic during convalescence from any major illness.

Poor Man's Ginseng

After the Civil War, the golden herb enjoyed a golden age. It was an ingredient in many patent medicines, notably Dr. Pierce's Golden Medical Discovery, a popular tonic.

Demand soared, and goldenseal's price jumped to $1 a pound, making it almost as costly as America's most expensive healing herb, ginseng. The difference was that ginseng was collected for export to China, while goldenseal was used in the United States. Over time, goldenseal acquired some of ginseng's medicinal reputation as a panacea and longevity tonic, hence one popular name, "poor man's ginseng."

Like ginseng, goldenseal was collected to the point of near extinction. And as it became scarce, it was frequently adulterated. Today, it's farmed but still costly, and adulteration continues to be a problem.

Goldenseal was listed as an astringent and antiseptic in the U.S. *Pharmacopoeia* from 1831 to 1936, when modern antibiotics pushed it out.

Sterling Reputation for a Golden Herb

Contemporary herbalists can barely contain their enthusiasm for goldenseal. In *Back to Eden*, Jethro Kloss calls it "one of the most wonderful remedies in the entire herb kingdom. . . . A real cure-all."

Modern herbalists recommend goldenseal externally as an antiseptic to clean wounds and as treatment for eczema, ringworm, athlete's foot, itching, and conjunctivitis. They prescribe it internally for digestive upsets and colds, as a douche, and to stop excessive menstrual flow and postpartum uterine bleeding.

Most herbalists also warn goldenseal may trigger uterine contractions and "overstimulate the nervous system."

Goldenseal is also a favorite of homeopaths, who prescribe microdoses for alcoholism, asthma, indigestion, cancer, hemorrhoids, and liver ailments.

Goldenseal remains a popular folk medicine. In *Hoosier Home Remedies*, a 1985 survey of Indiana folk medicine, Varro Tyler, Ph.D., discovered the herb was used extensively as an astringent and antiseptic to treat canker sores, chapped lips, and many other external problems.

Finally, in the late 1970s, heroin addicts came to believe goldenseal tea could prevent the detection of opiates in urine specimens.

HEALING with Goldenseal

Goldenseal absolutely does not prevent the detection of opiates—or any drugs—in urine. Nor is it a cure-all.

Scientists have found that goldenseal contains two active constituents—berberine and hydrastine. Berberine, the more important, is also the active chemical in barberry. As a result, barberry and goldenseal have similar uses (and similar hazards), though goldenseal is more popular—and more expensive. Those interested in a "poor person's goldenseal" should try barberry.

Antibiotic. Goldenseal may aid in the treatment of bacterial, fungal, and protozoan infections. Berberine, which is found in goldenseal, kills many bacteria that cause diarrhea. Barberine is also effective against the protozoans that cause amoebic dysentery and giardiasis. And several reports show berberine to be effective against the cholera bacteria. In fact, in one study, Indian researchers found berberine to be more effective against cholera than the powerful antibiotic Chloromycetin. These results support goldenseal's long history as a gastrointestinal remedy, particularly for infectious diarrhea.

Immune Stimulant. In addition to killing germs, berberine may boost the immune system by revving up the white blood cells (macrophages) that devour disease-causing microorganisms.

Women's Health. In some animal studies, berberine calms the uterus, supporting its traditional use in stopping excessive menstrual flow and postpartum hemorrhage. But other studies show it stimulates uterine contractions.

Pregnant women should not use it. Women troubled by heavy menstrual flow might try it and see if it helps.

Postpartum hemorrhage is a potentially serious condition that requires prompt professional attention. If you'd like to try goldenseal in addition to standard therapy, discuss it with your physician.

Digestive Aid. Goldenseal may help soothe the intestine and stimulate bile secretion in humans, which would help digest fats.

Intriguing Possibility. Several animal studies show goldenseal helps shrink tumors, lending support to goldenseal's traditional use as a cancer treatment. In the future, there may be a role for it in cancer chemotherapy.

Rx for Goldenseal

To use goldenseal as a possible antibiotic or immune system stimulant, or to help ease menstrual flow, take it as an infusion or tincture.

For an infusion, use $1/2$ to 1 teaspoon of powdered root per cup of boiling water. Steep 10 minutes. Drink up to 2 cups a day. Goldenseal tastes bitter; add honey, sugar, or lemon, or mix with a beverage tea to improve its flavor.

In a tincture, use $1/2$ to 1 teaspoon up to twice a day.

Goldenseal should not be given to children under age 2. For older children and people over 65, start with low-strength preparations and increase strength if necessary.

The Safety Factor

The active chemicals in goldenseal have opposite effects on blood pressure. Berberine may lower it, but hydrastine may raise it. People with high blood pressure, heart disease, diabetes, glaucoma, or a history of stroke should exercise caution and not use it. If you don't know what your blood pressure is, have your physician take a reading and give you the okay before using this drug.

Beware of Bloodroot

Because of goldenseal's high cost, adulteration has been a problem for more than 100 years. One adulterant is bloodroot (*Sanguinaria canadensis*). When fresh, bloodroot is red, but when dried it turns yellow like goldenseal and tastes equally bitter. Bloodroot has powerful laxative action. In high doses, it also causes dizziness, gastrointestinal burning, intense thirst, and vomiting. If your "goldenseal" causes purging or any of these other symptoms, stop using it. It's probably bloodroot.

High doses of goldenseal may irritate the skin, mouth, and throat, and cause nausea and vomiting. Goldenseal douches may cause vaginal irritation.

The medical literature contains no reports of serious harm due to goldenseal. But hydrastine stimulates the central nervous system, and in animals, large doses have caused death from respiratory paralysis and cardiac arrest. Do *not* use more than recommended amounts of goldenseal.

Other Cautions

The Food and Drug Administration lists goldenseal as an herb of "undefined safety." For otherwise healthy nonpregnant, nonnursing adults who do not have high blood pressure, glaucoma, diabetes, or a history of heart disease or stroke, goldenseal may be used cautiously for brief periods of time in amounts typically recommended.

Goldenseal should be used in medicinal amounts only in consultation with your doctor. If goldenseal causes minor discomforts, such as stomach upset or mouth irritation, use less or stop using it. Let your doctor know if you experience unpleasant effects or if the symptoms for which the herb is being used do not improve significantly in two weeks.

Hard to Grow

Goldenseal is a small, erect perennial with a hairy, annual, purplish stem that rises from a short, knotty rhizome with yellow-brown bark and bright yellow pulp. Goldenseal has lobed leaves somewhat similar to raspberry and small, greenish white flowers, which bloom in spring and produce orange-red berries.

Goldenseal is difficult to grow. Plants may be started from seeds, but it takes five years for roots to become medicinally mature. Most authorities recommend buying two-year-old rhizomes from specialty nurseries, so you can harvest three years later.

Viable rhizomes should have a sweet, licorice-like aroma. Plant them in early fall at a depth of 1 inch with 8-inch spacing. The soil should be amended with compost, leaf mold, sand, and bonemeal. Frequently, top growth will not appear until the second summer.

Goldenseal requires moisture with good drainage and about 70 percent shade. It grows best under tree cover or shade frames.

Harvest the rhizome and roots in late fall, after frost has killed the top growth. Clean the roots and dry them until they become brittle, then powder and store them in airtight containers.

GOTU KOLA

Soothes Skin Problems

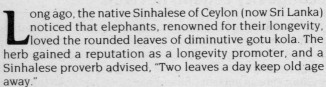

Family: Umbelliferae; other members include carrot, parsley

Genus and species: *Centella asiatica* or *Hydrocotyle asiatica*

Also known as: Sheep rot, Indian pennywort, marsh penny, water pennywort, hydrocotyle

Parts used: Leaves

Long ago, the native Sinhalese of Ceylon (now Sri Lanka) noticed that elephants, renowned for their longevity, loved the rounded leaves of diminutive gotu kola. The herb gained a reputation as a longevity promoter, and a Sinhalese proverb advised, "Two leaves a day keep old age away."

Gotu kola won't add years to your life, but it may stimulate the immune system, accelerate wound healing, help treat psoriasis, and improve circulation in the legs, which may help prevent varicose veins.

Cure for Leprosy

India's Ayurvedic herbalists first used gotu kola like ginseng to promote longevity and treat problems of aging. But over time, the herb became popular both internally and externally to treat skin diseases, including leprosy.

Philippine healers used gotu kola to treat wounds and gonorrhea. Chinese physicians used it for fever, colds, and flu.

Gotu kola got a bum rap in Europe. Several species grow there, but Europeans believed it caused foot rot in sheep (hence its once popular name, "sheep rot"), though there is no evidence this is the case.

Close relatives of gotu kola also grow in the United States, and America's 19th-century Eclectics were well aware of the herb's use as a treatment for leprosy in Asia. According to one report, "In 1852, Dr. Boileau of India, having been for many years afflicted with leprosy . . . experimented with |it| and recovered."

The Eclectics considered gotu kola safe and effective when used externally to treat skin problems. They called it a "poison" when used internally, however, asserting large doses produce "headache, dizziness, stupor, itching, and bloody passages from bowels."

Longevity Legend Revived

Gotu kola wasn't used much during the early 20th century, but after World War II it was included in an herb tea blend called Fo-Ti-Tieng, which claimed to boost longevity, reviving the ancient Sinhalese claim. The story was that one Li Ching Yun, an ancient Chinese herbalist, had used the blend regularly and lived 256 years, surviving 23 wives. The tea caught on, and gotu kola reemerged from obscurity as an herbal tonic.

Contemporary herbalists recommend gotu kola externally as a poultice for wounds. For internal use, they prescribe small doses as a tonic stimulant, and large doses as a sedative.

HEALING with Gotu Kola

Any longevity claims for gotu kola are as farfetched as the tale of Li Ching Yun. But modern science has found support for other traditional claims for this ancient herb.

Wound Healing. Gotu kola may spur wound healing. According to a study published in *Annals of Plastic Surgery*, gotu kola accelerates healing of burns and minimizes scarring. Other studies show the herb accelerates the healing of skin grafts and surgical enlargement of the vagina during childbirth (episiotomy).

Psoriasis. Supporting its traditional use for skin diseases, one small study showed that a gotu kola cream can help relieve the painful scaly red welts of psoriasis. Seven psoriasis sufferers used the cream. It healed the welts in five within two months, and only one of the five experienced any recurrence within four months after the treatment ended. Gotu kola cream is not available commercially, but you can use a compress of gotu kola infusion to help treat psoriasis.

Leprosy. Gotu kola's traditional use in treating leprosy (now called Hansen's disease) was supported by a study published in the British journal *Nature*. The bacteria that cause leprosy have a waxy coating, which protects them against attack by the immune system. Gotu kola contains a chemical (asiaticoside) that dissolves this waxy coating, allowing the immune system to destroy the bacteria.

Leg Circulation. Gotu kola also may help promote blood circulation in the lower limbs. In one study, 94 people suffering poor circulation in the legs (venous insufficiency) were given either 60 milligrams of gotu kola or a look-alike placebo. After two months, those taking the herb showed significantly improved circulation and less swelling.

Intriguing Possibilities. Poor circulation through the legs causes varicose veins. Gotu kola has not been studied specifically as a treatment for this condition, but its possible ability to improve leg circulation might help prevent and treat varicosities.

Gotu kola has a sedative effect on laboratory animals. Sedation has never been reported in humans, but some scientists claim it is possible. In animals, large doses are narcotic, causing stupor and possibly coma. Some scientists warn this reaction is also possible in humans, echoing the Eclectics, who advised against ingesting the herb. It might, however, help fight insomnia; just don't use more than recommended amounts.

Ironically, reports have also appeared claiming gotu kola causes restlessness and insomnia, which is rather odd for a purported "narcotic." Apparently these cases involved the caffeine-containing herb, kola, which was mislabeled as gotu kola. Gotu kola is not related to true kola (*Cola nitida*), the caffeine-containing nut used in cola drinks.

Rx for Gotu Kola

Use an infusion of gotu kola to help improve circulation in the legs. Or give it a try if you have insomnia. For an infusion, use $1/2$ teaspoon per cup of boiling water. Drink up to 2 cups a day. Gotu kola tastes bitter and astringent; adding sugar, honey, and lemon, or mixing it into an herbal beverage blend will improve its flavor.

To help treat wounds or psoriasis topically, try compresses made from gotu kola infusion. If results are disappointing, try a stronger infusion.

Gotu kola should not be given to children under age 2. For internal use by older children and people over 65, start with a low-strength preparation and increase strength if necessary.

The Safety Factor

The only confirmed side effect in humans is skin rash in sensitive individuals.

The chemical asiaticoside that helps against leprosy also appears to be weakly carcinogenic. A concentrated solution of the isolated chemical was applied to the skin of mice twice a week for 18 months (a long time in mouse terms), and 2.5 percent developed skin tumors. The risk to humans, if any, from occasional use of weaker, smaller doses of the whole herb remains unclear but appears minimal. Nonetheless, those with a history of cancer might reasonably decide not to use it. When in doubt, consult your physician.

Other Cautions

The Food and Drug Administration considers gotu kola an herb of "undefined safety." For otherwise healthy nonpregnant, nonnursing adults who have no history of cancer and are not taking other tranquilizers or sedatives, gotu kola is considered relatively safe in amounts typically recommended.

Gotu kola should be used in medicinal amounts only in consultation with a physician. If gotu kola causes minor discomforts, such as a rash or headache, use less or stop using it. Let your doctor know if you experience unpleasant effects or if the symptoms for which the herb is being used do not improve significantly in two weeks.

The Un-Kola

Gotu kola is not cultivated in North America, though several related species grow wild.

As a member of the Umbelliferae family, gotu kola is related to carrot, parsley, dill, and fennel, but it has neither the characteristic feathery leaves nor the umbrella arrangement (umbel) of tiny flowers. Instead, gotu kola's creeping stem grows in marshy areas and produces fan-shaped leaves about the size of an old British penny—hence its names Indian pennywort, marsh penny, and water pennywort. A cup-like clutch of inconspicuous flowers develops near the ground.

HAWTHORN

Mayflower for Heart Disease

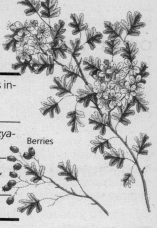

Family: Rósaceae; other members include rose, peach, almond, apple, strawberry

Genus and species: *Crataegus oxyacantha*

Also known as: Hawthorne, haw, may, mayblossom, mayflower

Parts used: Flowers, leaves, fruits

Berries

Every American schoolchild learns the Pilgrims' ship was the *Mayflower*. But few, if any, know the name refers to hawthorn, a tree known for centuries as a heart tonic and today widely used in Europe as a treatment for heart disease.

Heart disease is our leading cause of death, yet hawthorn has been virtually ignored on this side of the Atlantic. Even herb conservative Varro Tyler, Ph.D., calls hawthorn "valuable . . . a relatively harmless heart tonic which . . . yields good results."

Crown of Thorns

Hawthorn was well known in the ancient world, but not as a medicine. The Greeks and Romans linked it to hope, marriage, and fertility. Greek bridesmaids wore fragrant hawthorn blossoms, and brides carried a bough. The Romans placed hawthorn leaves in babies' cradles to ward off evil spirits.

Christianity changed hawthorn's image dramatically. Christ's crown of thorns was reputedly made of hawthorn, and as a result, it became a symbol of bad luck and death.

The hawthorn/death association was bolstered by the unpleasant aroma of some European species' flowers. These trees are pollinated by carrion-eating insects, and to attract them, their flowers emit the odor of rotting meat. A similar odor was associated with bubonic plague. (Because the disease killed so many so quickly, bodies often remained unburied for quite a while.) As a result, hawthorn was associated with plague.

Tonic for the Heart

Over the centuries, hawthorn shed its bad reputation and came to be used medicinally. Seventeenth-century English herbalist Nicholas Culpeper praised it as "a singular remedy for the stone [kidney stones], and no less effectual for dropsy [congestive heart failure]."

American pioneers also used the plant for heart problems. The 19th-century Eclectics prescribed it for the severe chest pain known as angina, and congestive heart failure (a serious heart problem with fluid buildup and shortness of breath after minor physical activity).

Modern herbals echo this advice. Most would agree with David Hoffmann's *Holistic Herbal*: "Hawthorn [is] one of the best tonic remedies for the heart. . . . It may be used safely in long-term treatment for heart weakness or failure . . . palpitations . . . angina pectoris . . . and high blood pressure."

Herbalists also suggest it for kidney stones and as a sedative for chronic insomnia.

HEALING with Hawthorn

Science appears to support what herbalists have long known. Hawthorn is a heart stimulant.

Heart Disease. Hawthorn may help the heart in several

ways: It may open (dilate) the coronary arteries, improving the heart's blood supply. It may increase the heart's pumping force. It may eliminate some types of heart-rhythm disturbances (arrhythmias). And some evidence suggests it may help limit the amount of cholesterol deposited on artery walls.

In one trial, 120 people with congestive heart failure were given either tincture of hawthorn or a look-alike placebo. The hawthorn group experienced significant improvement in heart function and reported considerably less shortness of breath.

In Germany, where herbal medicine is more mainstream than it is in the United States, three dozen hawthorn-based heart medicines are available. According to German medical herbalist Rudolph Fritz Weiss, M.D., the herb "has become one of [our] most widely used heart remedies." German physicians prescribe it to normalize heart rhythm, reduce the likelihood and severity of angina attacks, and prevent cardiac complications in elderly patients with influenza and pneumonia.

But Dr. Weiss warns hawthorn is no quick fix: "One cannot expect rapid improvement in cardiac function. [Hawthorn] has a long-term, sustained effect. . . . Hawthorn is not for cutting short angina attacks—nitroglycerine continues to be the drug of choice here. . . . [It] is safe for long-term use. With the usual therapeutic dosage, no toxic effects have been noted."

Although hawthorn is considered safe and may be effective in the treatment of angina, congestive heart failure, and cardiac arrhythmias, these are serious, potentially life-threatening conditions requiring professional medical care. Consult your physician if you'd like to use hawthorn as part of your overall treatment plan.

Rx for Hawthorn

German physicians prescribe 1 teaspoon of hawthorn tincture upon waking and before bed for periods of up to several weeks. To mask its bitter taste, mix it with sugar, honey, or lemon, or mix it into an herbal beverage blend.

For an infusion, herbalists recommend using 2 teaspoons of crushed leaves or fruits per cup of boiling water. Steep 20 minutes. Drink up to 2 cups a day.

The Safety Factor

Large amounts of hawthorn may cause sedation and/or a significant drop in blood pressure, possibly resulting in faintness.

The Food and Drug Administration lists hawthorn as an herb of "undefined safety." This heart stimulant should be used only by those diagnosed with angina, cardiac arrhythmias, or congestive heart failure—and then only in consultation with a physician. Children and pregnant and nursing women should not use hawthorn.

Flowers in May

Hawthorn is a small deciduous tree with white bark, extremely hard wood, sharp thorns, clusters of white, aromatic flowers, and brilliant red fruits, which look like small apples. It blooms from April to June depending on latitude. In Britain blossoms appear in May, hence its other names—may, mayblossom, and mayflower.

With approximately 900 North American species, hawthorn is well adapted to many environments, from urban areas to windswept hillsides.

The tree tolerates a variety of soils but prefers somewhat alkaline, rich, moist loam. Some species prefer full sun. Others grow well in partial shade. Consult a nursery for the species best suited to your area.

HOP

Beer for Better Health

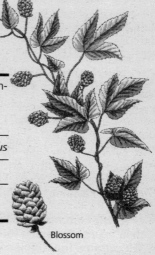

Family: Moraceae; other members include fig, mulberry; Cannabaceae; other members include hemp, marijuana

Genus and species: *Humulus lupulus*

Also known as: Humulus

Parts used: Glandular hairs of the female fruits (strobiles)

Blossom

Hop is best known as the bitter, aromatic ingredient in beer. It also has a long history in herbal healing, and some of its traditional uses have been supported by modern science.

Chinese physicians have prescribed hop for centuries as a digestive aid and treatment for leprosy, tuberculosis, and dysentery.

Ancient Greek and Roman physicians also recommended it as a digestive aid and treatment for intestinal ailments. The Roman naturalist Pliny touted the herb as a garden vegetable, the young shoots of which could be eaten in spring before they matured and grew tough and bitter. (People still eat the shoots, prepared like asparagus.)

Beer: Liquid Bread

Hop was a minor herb until about 1,000 years ago, when brewers began using it to preserve the fermented barley beverage we call beer.

Beer was an accidental offshoot of bread baking. As agriculture developed, late-prehistoric homemakers noticed that bread made from raw grain did not keep as well as bread made from sprouted grain. So before pounding their grain into flour, they soaked it in water to sprout it. If the water happened to become contaminated with yeast microorganisms from the skins of fruit, it fermented into a crude sweet beer.

Ancient beers, probably undrinkable by modern standards, were nonetheless amazingly popular. Around 2500 B.C., 40 percent of the Sumerian grain crop was used in brewing. And the world's first written legal code, Babylonia's *Code of Hammurabi*, developed in 1750 B.C., described punishments for ale houses that sold understrength or overpriced beer.

As the centuries passed, brewers added herbs to flavor their beers: marjoram, yarrow, and wormwood. Around the 9th century, the Germans began adding hop, both for its pleasantly bitter flavor and because it preserved the brew. By the 14th century, most European beers contained hop.

Outrage in England

Hop was well known in England. The vine grew wild there, and in folk medicine it was a popular appetite-stimulating digestive bitter.

But England's fermented beverage of choice was ale, a sweet, ancient-style beer without hop. Around 1500, British brewers learned of hop's preservative properties and added it, turning their sweet ales into bitter beers—and provoking national outrage.

Legions of hop haters petitioned Parliament to ban the herb as "a wicked weed that would endanger the people." Henry VIII, an ale traditionalist, agreed and banned the herb from English brewing. It remained illegal until his son, Edward VI, rescinded the ban in 1552.

But the furor refused to die. A century later, English writer John Evelyn declared, "Hop transmuted our wholesome ale into beer. This one ingredient preserves the drink indeed, but repays the pleasure in tormenting diseases and a shorter life."

Hop-Picker Fatigue

Beer brewing transformed hop from a spring vegetable into a cash crop. Hop farmers noticed the herb had two odd effects on those who harvested it. They fatigued easily and women's periods arrived early. Over time, the herb gained a reputation as a sedative and menstruation promoter.

Hop has been used ever since as a sedative, not only in tea but also in pillows. The herb's warm fragrance is supposed to induce sleep.

Seventeenth-century English herbalist Nicholas Culpeper recommended hop "in opening obstructions of the liver and spleen . . . cleansing the blood . . . helping cure the French disease [syphilis], and bringing down women's courses [menstruation]." Culpeper also added his two pence to the lingering beer/ale controversy, writing that hop's medicinal uses made "beer . . . better than ale."

From Sedative to Patent Medicine

In North America, the Indians used native American hop as a sedative and a digestive aid.

America's 19th-century Eclectics considered hop a digestive aid and treatment for the "morbid excitement of delerium tremens." But they were unimpressed with its reputation as a sedative, warning it "often failed."

Hop was listed as a sedative in the U.S. *Pharmacopoeia* from 1831 to 1916. Throughout the 19th century, it was an ingredient in many patent medicines, including Hop Bitters, a popular herb tonic in a 30-percent alcohol base. Its advertising slogan typified patent medicine claims in the era before the Food and Drug Administration (FDA): "Take Hop Bitters three times a day, and you will have no doctor bills to pay."

During the 1950s, jazz musicians who smoked marijuana were called "hopheads," and marijuana caused users to feel "hopped up." Hop is botanically related to marijuana, but smoking the herb does not produce intoxication.

Contemporary herbalists recommend hop primarily as a sedative, tranquilizer, and digestive aid.

HEALING with Hop

Those old brewers may have known what they were doing. Hop contains two chemicals (humulone and lupulone) that can kill bacteria that cause spoiling.

Infection Prevention. The bacteria fighters in hop also may help prevent infection. Hop is not a major herbal antibiotic, but for garden first aid, press some crushed flower tops into cuts and scrapes on the way to washing and bandaging them.

One study shows hop effective against tuberculosis bacteria, lending some credence to one of its traditional Chinese uses.

Sedative. For decades, scientists scoffed at hop's long-time use as a sedative. Then in 1983, a sedative chemical (2-methyl–3-butene–2-ol) was discovered in the plant. This chemical is present in only trace amounts in the fresh leaves, but as the herb dries and ages, its concentration increases. If you use hop as a possible sedative, use dried, aged herb.

Digestive Aid. Hop may relax the smooth muscle lining of the digestive tract, according to French researchers, supporting its traditional use as an antispasmodic digestive herb.

Women's Health. German researchers claim hop contains chemicals similar to the female sex hormone estrogen, which may help to explain some of the menstrual changes in women hop pickers. Other studies dispute this finding. Currently, the issue remains unresolved.

Rx for Hop

For possible infection prevention and as a digestive aid, use the freshest hop you can find. For insomnia, use dried, aged herb.

To make an infusion, use 2 teaspoons of herb per cup of boiling water. Steep 5 minutes. Hop tastes warm and pleasantly bitter.

Hop should not be given to children under age 2. For older children and people over 65, start with low-strength preparations and increase strength if necessary.

The Safety Factor

Many hop pickers develop a rash called hop dermatitis. Otherwise, there are no reports of harm from this herb.

In case the Germans are right about hop containing chemicals similar to the female sex hormone estrogen, pregnant women should not use it. Women with estrogen-dependent breast cancer should also avoid it.

The FDA includes hop on its list of herbs generally regarded as safe. For otherwise healthy nonpregnant, nonnursing adults who are not taking other sedatives, hop is considered safe in amounts typically recommended.

Hop should be used in medicinal amounts only in consultation with your doctor. If hop causes minor discomforts, such as stomach upset or diarrhea, use less or stop using it. Let your doctor know if you experience unpleasant symptoms or if the symptoms for which the herb is being used do not improve significantly in two weeks.

The Vine Climbs

Hop is a resinous, hairy, climbing, perennial vine resembling grape. Grown commercially in Bavaria, Germany, and in the

Pacific Northwest in pole-studded fields called hop yards, mature vines often reach 25 feet.

Hop can be grown from seeds, but most growers use root cuttings taken in spring or fall. Plant cuttings in hills, three roots per hill, with hills 18 inches apart.

Hop needs deeply cultivated, rich, moist soil, and full sun. Water frequently.

Harvest the female flowers in fall when they feel firm, turn amber-colored, and are covered with yellow dust. Dry them immediately in an oven no hotter than 150°F.

HOREHOUND

For Cough, Colds, and Flu

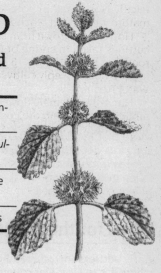

Family: Labiatae; other members include mint

Genus and species: *Marrubium vulgare*

Also known as: Hoarhound, white horehound, marrubium

Parts used: Leaves and flower tops

Horehound has been a popular herbal expectorant and cough remedy for almost 2,000 years. Even herb-medicine skeptics grant its safety and effectiveness. Then out of the blue in 1989, the Food and Drug Administration (FDA) banned it from over-the-counter cough remedies, claiming it was ineffective. The action left herbalists shaking their heads. Worse yet, the FDA decreed another expectorant "effective," over the objections of many scientists.

Roman Poison Antidote and More

Horehound was first used medicinally in ancient Rome as an ingredient in the multi-ingredient (and ineffective) poison antidotes known as *theriaca*. Medieval Europeans generalized from this use and came up with the belief that the herb provided protection from witches' spells.

315

The Roman physician Galen was the first to recommend horehound for coughs and respiratory problems, and it's been used as an expectorant ever since.

German abbess/herbalist Hildegard of Bingen considered it one of the best herbs for colds.

England's John Gerard wrote: "Syrup made of the greene fresh leaves and sugar is a most singular remedie against cough and wheezings of the lungs."

Seventeenth-century English herbalist Nicholas Culpeper wrote that in addition to curing "those that have taken poison . . . a decoction of the dried herb taken with honey is a remedy for those that are short-winded, have a cough, or are fallen into consumption. . . . It helpeth to expectorate tough phlegm from the chest."

Good for the Lungs

Early settlers introduced horehound into North America, where it was a popular cough, cold, and tuberculosis remedy. Folk herbalists also considered it a laxative, menstruation promoter, and treatment for hepatitis, malaria, intestinal worms, and menstrual problems.

America's 19th-century Eclectic physicians prescribed it for coughs, colds, asthma, intestinal worms, and menstrual complaints.

Most contemporary herbalists recommend horehound only for minor respiratory problems: coughs, colds, and bronchitis.

HEALING with Horehound

The FDA order removing horehound from cough and cold remedies may say more about the watchdog agency's shortcomings than it does about the herb's.

Expectorant. Horehound contains a chemical (marrubiin), which Russian and German studies show has phlegm-loosening (expectorant) properties. In Europe, the herb has been used for decades in a large number of cough syrups and lozenges. It has been widely used in the United States as well. Even herb conservative Varro Tyler, Ph.D., calls it "an effective expectorant."

The FDA horehound ban followed the recommendation of an agency advisory panel, which decreed only one expectorant, guaifenesin, safe and effective. Ironically, many lung experts consider guaifenesin *ineffective*.

The FDA order covers only horehound preparations marketed as cough remedies. The herb is still available in bulk and in some sore-throat products. As this book goes to press, herbalists say they plan to challenge the FDA ruling.

Intriguing Possibilities. Animal studies performed in Europe show horehound opens (dilates) blood vessels, which suggests possible value in treating high blood pressure.

Other animal studies show that in small amounts, horehound helps normalize irregular heart rhythm (arrhythmias), but in large amounts can *cause* them.

Rx for Horehound

For a cough-remedy infusion, use ½ to 1 teaspoon of dried leaves per cup of boiling water. Steep for 10 minutes. Drink up to 3 cups a day. To offset its bitter taste, add sugar or honey.

In a tincture, take ¼ to ½ teaspoon up to three times a day.

Horehound should not be given to children under age 2. For older children and people over 65, start with low-strength preparations and increase strength if necessary.

The Safety Factor

There have been no reports of adverse reactions to horehound in humans. But because horehound in large doses may cause cardiac arrhythmias, those with heart disease should avoid it.

Horehound's traditional use as a menstruation promoter has not been confirmed scientifically, but it would be prudent for pregnant women to exercise caution.

For otherwise healthy nonpregnant, nonnursing adults who do not have heart disease, horehound is considered relatively safe in amounts typically recommended. Horehound should be used in medicinal amounts only in consultation with a physician. If horehound causes minor discomforts, such as stomach upset or diarrhea, use less or stop using it. Let your doctor know if you experience unpleasant symptoms or if a cough does not improve significantly in two weeks. If a cough brings up brown, black, or bloody phlegm, consult a physician immediately.

A Furry Pest of a Plant

Horehound is a spreading, pleasantly aromatic, perennial with square annual stems that reach about 18 inches. The leaves are rounded, wrinkled, and deeply veined with tiny white flowers that develop at the stem/leaf stalk junctions. The entire plant is covered with soft hairs, giving it a woolly appearance and a grayish-white cast.

A self-seeder, horehound grows so easily that it may become a pest. It needs little water, tolerates poor soil, and does best in full sun but tolerates partial shade.

Plant seeds just under the surface in either spring or fall. Thin seedlings to 9-inch spacing.

Horehound does not bloom until its second year, but you can harvest leaves and top growth after one growing season.

In the soil, the herb exudes a musky odor some people dislike, but as the plant dries, the odor disappears.

HORSETAIL

An Herbal Gold Mine

Family: Equisetaceae; the family is extinct except for horsetail

Genus and species: *Equisetum arvense*

Also known as: Equisetum, scouring rush, pewterwort, shave grass, corncob plant, bottle brush

Parts used: Stems

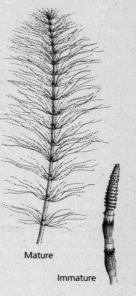

Mature

Immature

A ll that's gold does not necessarily glitter. Take horsetail. This bamboolike marsh dweller is capable of absorbing gold dissolved in water. What makes that of interest to herbalists is that doctors often prescribe preparations containing gold for rheumatoid arthritis, and horsetail has a long history as an herbal remedy for joint pain.

Scouring Rush

Centuries before anyone realized horsetail contains gold, the ancients discovered its value as an abrasive cleanser. As the centuries passed, it was used to scour pots, polish pewter, and sand or "shave" wood, hence its popular names—scouring rush, shave grass, and pewterwort (*wort* is Old English for *plant*).

During ancient famines, Romans ate horsetail shoots, which look like asparagus but are neither as tasty nor as nutritious. (Backpacking guides still recommend the tough, stringy shoots for wilderness foragers.)

Ancient Chinese physicians used this herb to treat wounds, hemorrhoids, arthritis, and dysentery.

The Roman physician Galen claimed horsetail healed severed tendons and ligaments and helped stop nosebleeds. Over the centuries, the herb gained a reputation as a wound healer.

Seventeenth-century English herbalist Nicholas Culpeper called horsetail "very powerful to stop bleeding . . . [and] heal ulcers . . . the juice or decoction being drunk . . . or applied outwardly. . . . It solders together wounds and cures all ruptures."

Used for Urinary Problems

As time passed, horsetail shed its reputation as a wound healer and gained one as a diuretic to treat water retention and as a urinary remedy. It was used to treat painful urination, gonorrhea, kidney infections, urinary tract infections, and dropsy (congestive heart failure).

America's 19th-century Eclectics prescribed horsetail as a diuretic and urinary antiseptic for incontinence, gonorrhea, kidney stones, kidney infections, urinary complaints, and congestive heart failure.

Homeopaths prescribe microdoses of the herb for urinary problems: bladder infections, bed-wetting, incontinence, and urethritis.

Contemporary herbalists recommend it externally for wounds and internally for urinary and prostate problems.

HEALING with Horsetail

Horsetail is not a major medicinal herb, but if California's Gold Rush '49ers were alive today, they'd say, "There's gold in them thar herbs!"

Arthritis. Horsetail absorbs gold dissolved in water better than most plants, as much as 4 ounces per ton of fresh stalks. Of course, the amount of gold in a cup of horsetail tea is quite small, but small amounts of gold are used to treat rheumatoid arthritis, and the Chinese used horsetail for this disease. If you'd like to include horsetail as part of an overall rheumatoid arthritis treatment plan, discuss it with your physician.

Diuretic. Horsetail contains a weak diuretic chemical (equisetonin), lending support to its traditional use as a urinary stimulant.

Dead-End File. Horsetail contains nicotine, and some herbalists suggest it as a nicotine substitute for smokers attempting to quit. However, compared to the amount in cigarettes, horsetail's nicotine content is minute, only about 0.00004 percent, and is unlikely to satisfy a smoker's craving. Prescription nicotine gum (Nicorette) would be a better alternative.

Rx for Horsetail

To help treat water retention or rheumatoid arthritis (in consultation with your physician), use either an infusion or tincture. For an infusion, use 1 to 2 teaspoons of dried herb per cup of water. Steep 10 minutes. Drink up to 2 cups a day. Horsetail has little taste.

In a tincture, use 1/2 to 1 teaspoon up to twice a day.

Horsetail should not be given to children under age 2. For older children and people over 65, start with low-strength preparations and increase strength if necessary.

The Safety Factor

Horsetail is relatively high in selenium. Too much selenium may cause birth defects. In marshes downstream from heavily fertilized agricultural areas, horsetail may have hazardously high selenium levels. Pregnant women should not use this herb.

Horsetail contains a chemical (equisetine) that in large

amounts is a nerve poison. Animals fed the herb have suffered fever, weight loss, muscle weakness, and abnormal pulse rate. Animal fatalities have also been reported. Children have reportedly suffered nonfatal reactions after using the hollow stems as toy blowguns and ingesting the juice. Don't let children play with this herb.

Other Cautions

Because of the problems it has caused in animals, the Food and Drug Administration lists horsetail as an herb of "undefined safety." For otherwise healthy nonpregnant, nonnursing adults who are not taking other diuretics, horsetail is considered relatively safe when used cautiously for brief periods in amounts typically recommended.

Horsetail should be used in medicinal amounts only in consultation with your doctor. If horsetail causes minor discomforts, such as stomach upset or diarrhea, use less or stop using it. Let your doctor know if you experience any unpleasant effects or if the symptoms for which the herb is being used do not improve significantly in two weeks.

Giant of the Marshes

Horsetail is the sole descendant of the giant fernlike plants that covered the earth some 200 million years ago. The herb's creeping rhizome sends up hollow, jointed, virtually leafless, bamboolike stalks that reach 6 feet. At the ends of the stalks, spore-bearing structures (catkins) develop which resemble horse tails, corncobs, or bottle brushes, hence some of the herb's names.

Horsetails may be purchased from specialty nurseries, or root cuttings may be taken from wild plants in the spring when the spearlike stems have reached a few inches.

Set plants or cuttings just under the surface of marshy soil. Keep it wet. If you do not want the plant to spread, contain it by embedding sheet metal in the soil to a depth of 18 inches.

Harvest the stalks in the fall.

Make sure children do not suck on the hollow stems.

HYSSOP

The Biblical Antiseptic

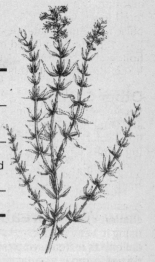

Family: Labiatae; other members include mint

Genus and species: *Hyssopus officinalis*

Also known as: No other names, however, many other plants are called hyssop

Parts used: Leaves and flowers

The Book of Psalms (51:9) says, "Purge me with hyssop and I shall be clean." But the biblical cleanser does more than clean. It may work as an antiseptic for infections like cold sores and genital herpes.

Temple Cleaner

Jewish priests used strong-smelling hyssop 2,500 years ago to clean the temple in Jerusalem and other places of worship. The Greeks adopted it, and the physician Dioscorides prescribed the herb in tea for cough, wheezing, and shortness of breath, in plasters and chest rubs, and as an aromatic nasal and chest decongestant.

The German abbess/herbalist Hildegard of Bingen wrote hyssop "cleanses the lungs." She also recommended a meal of chicken cooked in hyssop and wine as a treatment for "sadness" (depression).

In 17th-century Europe, hyssop was a popular air freshener or "strewing herb." Crushed leaves and flower tops were scattered around homes to mask odors at a time when people rarely bathed and when farm animals often shared human living quarters.

When bathing became popular and strewing ceased, hyssop was placed in scent baskets in sickrooms.

Seventeenth-century English herbalist Nicholas Culpeper echoed Dioscorides' endorsement of hyssop for chest ailments: "It expelleth tough phlegm and is effectual for all griefs of the chest and lungs." He also claimed: "It killeth worms in the belly. . . . Boiled with figs it makes an excellent gargle for quinsey [tonsillitis] . . . Boiled in wine, it is good to wash inflammations . . . the head being anointed with the oil, it killeth lice."

New World Treatments

Colonists introduced hyssop into North America and continued using it to treat chest congestions. Hyssop also developed a reputation as a menstruation promoter and as a means to induce abortions. (It won't do either.)

But as time passed, hyssop's popularity waned. America's 19th-century Eclectics prescribed it externally to relieve the pain of bruises, and internally as a gargle for sore throat and tonsillitis and as a treatment for asthma and coughing.

Contemporary herbalists recommend hyssop compresses and poultices for bruises, burns, and wounds, and an infusion for colds, coughs, bronchitis, flatulence, indigestion, menstruation promotion, and even epileptic seizures. Some herbalists point to the fact that the microorganism that produces penicillin (*Penicillium*) grows on hyssop leaves as proof of its effectiveness for wounds and chest infections.

HEALING with Hyssop

The biblical cleanser won't whiten and brighten your bathroom bowl as modern cleansers do, but the herb's main traditional uses have some scientific support.

Herpes. Hyssop inhibits the growth of herpes simplex virus, which causes genital herpes and cold sores. Try the infusion in a compress if you have this chronic, recurring infection.

Cough. Hyssop oil contains several soothing camphorlike constituents and one expectorant chemical (marrubiin), which loosens phlegm so it can be coughed up more easily. Scientific sources agree it's a "reasonably effective" treatment for the cough and respiratory irritation of colds and flu.

Dead-End File. *Penicillium* does indeed grow on hyssop. It also grows just about everywhere else on earth. The assertion that hyssop heals because it carries penicillin is nonsense.

Rx for Hyssop

To make a compress, use 1 ounce of dried herb per pint of boiling water. Steep 15 minutes and cool. Soak a clean cloth in the infusion and apply to cold sores and genital herpes as needed.

For an infusion, use 2 teaspoons of herb per cup of boiling water. Steep 10 minutes. Drink up to 3 cups a day to treat cough. Hyssop has a strong, camphorlike smell and tastes bitter. Add sugar, honey, or lemon, or mix it with an herbal beverage blend to improve flavor.

If you prefer a tincture, use 1 teaspoon up to three times a day.

Hyssop should not be given to children under age 2. For older children and people over 65, start with low-strength preparations and increase strength if necessary.

The Safety Factor

Hyssop has not been shown to stimulate the uterus, but its traditional use to stimulate abortion should discourage pregnant women from using it. No reports of harm from hyssop appear in world medical literature.

Just make sure the "hyssop" you use is H. *officinalis*. Several other North American plants are also called hyssop: hedge hyssop (*Gratiola officinalis*), the giant hyssops (several species of the genus *Agastache*), and the water hyssops (several species of *Bacopa*). These plants should not be ingested.

Other Cautions

Hyssop is included in the Food and Drug Administration's list of herbs generally regarded as safe. For otherwise healthy nonpregnant, nonnursing adults, hyssop is considered safe in amounts typically recommended.

Hyssop should be used in medicinal amounts only in consultation with your doctor. If hyssop causes minor discomforts, such as stomach upset or diarrhea, use less or stop using it. Let your doctor know if you experience any unpleasant effects or if the symptoms for which the herb is being used do not improve significantly in two weeks.

Magnet for Bees

If you want bees in your garden, plant this pretty, hardy, shrubby perennial. Hyssop also has a reputation for enhancing the flavor of grapes and increasing the yield of cabbages planted nearby.

Hyssop has small, lance-shaped leaves, and the mints' characteristic square stems. The plant reaches 2 feet and has a medicinal odor, which becomes more mintlike when the leaves are crushed. Dense clusters of blue or violet flowers form on 6-inch spikes atop the stems in summer and early fall.

Hyssop enjoys dry, sunny locations and tolerates most soils. In partial shade, it tends to become leggy. Hyssop may be propagated from seeds, cuttings, or root divisions. Seeds should be sown 1/4 inch deep after danger of frost has passed. Cuttings and divisions may be rooted either indoors or outdoors in a cool, shady place.

Thin established plants to 12-inch spacing. Add compost

each spring. Water seedlings every few days. Mature plants prefer a drier environment and require little care.

Once the plant reaches about 18 inches and exudes its characteristic aroma, cut back the tops to stimulate leaf growth. Leaves may be harvested at any time. Cut back the entire plant to 4 inches above ground just before it flowers. Dry and store in airtight containers.

JUNIPER

The Gin-Flavored Healer

Family: Cupressaceae; other members include cypress

Genus and species: *Juniperus communis*

Also known as: Genvrier, geneva

Parts used: "Berries," actually miniature female cones

If you've ever had a martini, you know juniper. Aromatic juniper berries are the source of gin. Juniper also increases urine production—making this herb a possible treatment for premenstrual syndrome, high blood pressure, and congestive heart failure.

French Fumigant

During the Middle Ages, Europeans believed planting a juniper beside the front door kept witches out. Unfortunately, the tree did not provide complete protection. A witch could still enter if she correctly guessed the number of its needles.

As time passed, juniper's protective reputation evolved into the belief that its smoke prevented leprosy and bubonic plague. As recently as World War II, French nurses burned juniper in hospital rooms to fumigate them.

By the 17th century, juniper was a popular diuretic, used to increase urine production. English herbalist Nicholas Culpeper wrote the herb "provokes urine exceedingly. . . . [Juniper] is so powerful a remedy against dropsy [congestive heart failure], it cures the disease." In addition, Culpeper prescribed juniper for "cough, shortness of breath, consumption [tuberculosis] . . . to provoke terms [menstruation] . . . and give safe and speedy delivery to women with child."

Zuni Childbirth Herb

American Indians independently discovered juniper's childbirth-assisting properties. When the Spanish explorer Coronado entered what is now New Mexico in 1540 looking for the mythical, gold-encrusted Seven Cities of Cíbola, he found Zuni women using juniper berries to promote uterine recovery after childbirth. They also used it to treat wound infections and arthritis.

America's 19th-century Eclectics dismissed the use of juniper in childbirth but endorsed it strongly for congestive heart failure. The Eclectics also prescribed juniper externally for eczema and psoriasis, and internally to treat gonorrhea, bladder and kidney infections, and other genitourinary problems.

Contemporary herbalists recommend juniper externally as an antiseptic, and internally for bladder infections, arthritis, intestinal cramps, and gout. One suggests it as a urinary deodorant in cases of chronic incontinence because the herb gives urine the fragrance of violets. Another claims juniper "destroys all fungi."

In Dutch

But medicinal claims for juniper take a backseat to its use in gin, invented by the Dutch during the 17th century. Our word *gin* comes from the Dutch word for juniper, *geniver*. The English took to gin so enthusiastically that references to its native land still pepper the English language. Drink too much gin, and you're likely to get in trouble or "in Dutch."

HEALING with Juniper

Juniper's aromatic oil contains a diuretic chemical (terpinen-4-ol), which increases the fluid-filtering rate of the kidneys, supporting its traditional use as a diuretic. In fact, it's an ingredient in the over-the-counter diuretic, Odrinil.

High Blood Pressure. Physicians often prescribe diuretics to treat high blood pressure. High blood pressure is a serious condition requiring professional care. If you'd like to use juniper as part of your treatment plan, discuss it with your physician.

Diuretics deplete the body of potassium, an essential mineral. If you use juniper, eat foods high in potassium, such as bananas and fresh vegetables.

Congestive Heart Failure. Culpeper exaggerated when he said juniper "cured" this condition. But as a diuretic, the herb can be a part of an overall treatment plan. Heart failure is a serious condition requiring professional care. If you'd like to use it, discuss it with your physician.

Women's Health. In animal studies, juniper stimulates uterine contractions. Pregnant women should not use it (except at term under the supervision of a physician, when it might help stimulate labor). Other women might try it to help begin their periods.

Since diuretics help relieve the bloated feeling caused by premenstrual fluid retention, women bothered by premenstrual syndrome might try juniper during the uncomfortable days right before their periods.

Arthritis. Juniper may have anti-inflammatory properties, suggesting it may have value in treating arthritis—one of its age-old Indian uses. In Germany, where herbal medicine is considerably more mainstream than it is in the United States, physicians prescribe juniper preparations for arthritis and gout.

Dead-End File. Juniper does not "destroy all fungi," and it has never been shown effective for gonorrhea or bladder or kidney infections.

Rx for Juniper

If you want to use it as a diuretic, or try to treat the inflammation associated with arthritis, or attempt to bring on your period, take juniper as an infusion. For an infusion, use 1 teaspoon of bruised berries per cup of boiling water. Steep 10 to 20 minutes. Drink up to 2 cups a day for no more than 6 weeks. Juniper has a strong, pleasantly aromatic taste.

Juniper should not be given to children under age 2. For older children and people over 65, start with low-strength preparations and increase strength if necessary.

The Safety Factor

High doses of juniper cause kidney irritation, and possibly kidney damage. The herb should not be used by anyone with a kidney infection or a history of kidney impairment. Even low doses taken over long periods may cause problems. "The rule," writes German medical herbalist Rudolph Fritz Weiss, M.D., "is never take juniper for longer than six weeks."

Overdose symptoms include diarrhea, intestinal pain, kidney pain, protein in the urine (albuminuria), blood in the urine (hematuria), purplish urine, rapid heartbeat, and elevated blood pressure.

If juniper causes any overdose symptoms, stop using it.

Up to one-third of hay fever sufferers develop allergy symptoms from exposure to juniper, according to a study in *Clinical Allergy*. If you have hay fever you might want to avoid this herb.

Other Cautions

Oddly enough, given its potential kidney toxicity, the Food and Drug Administration includes juniper in its list of herbs generally regarded as safe. For otherwise healthy nonpregnant, nonnursing adults who do not have kidney disease and are not taking other diuretics, juniper is considered relatively safe when used cautiously for short periods of time in amounts typically recommended.

Juniper should be used in medicinal amounts only in consultation with your doctor. Let your doctor know if you experience any unpleasant effects or if the symptoms for which the herb is being used do not improve significantly in two weeks.

Many elderly people suffer kidney impairment. Those over 65 should consult a physician about their kidney function before taking this herb.

Plant Both Genders for Berries

The genus *Juniperus* contains more than 70 species of aromatic evergreens. Most are small trees, but some grow to 40 feet. The species most widely used in herbal healing, common juniper (*J. communis*) reaches 6 to 20 feet, depending on locale. Its close, tangled, spreading branches are covered with reddish brown bark, sticky gum, and pointed, ½-inch needles. Males produce yellow flowers and females green flowers. The females also produce scaly, green, ¼-inch, aromatic cones ("berries"), which turn blue-black during their two-year maturation.

If you want berries, be sure to plant both male and female junipers, or the females will not fruit. Junipers usually prefer sandy soil and full sun, but they adapt to many soil and climate conditions. Consult a nursery for advice that is specific to your locale.

Females produce immature (green) and mature (blue-black) berries simultaneously. Harvest only the mature berries in fall. Dry them in the sun. When dry, they turn a dull black. Store them in airtight containers to preserve their volatile oil.

KELP

Protector from the Sea

Family: Fucaceae; other members include other seaweeds

Genus and species: *Fucus versiculosus* and species of three other genuses: *Laminaria, Macrocystis,* and *Nereocystis*

Also known as: Bladderwrack, seawrack, fucus, bladder fucus, cutweed, and sea vegetables; in Japan, wakame, arame, kombu, and hijiki

Parts used: Stemlike and leaflike parts

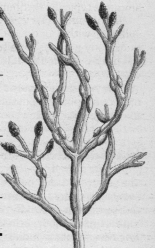

Kelp, as a source of iodine, used to be the treatment of choice for goiter—a thyroid enlargement caused by iodine deficiency. A few modern herbals still recommend kelp for the thyroid. But today kelp is more known as a protector from radiation, heart disease, and toxic heavy metals.

Fisherman's Friend

Kelp is a type of seaweed, specifically long-frond brown algae, which grows to lengths of 200 feet off Japan, Europe, and North America.

Ancient seafarers were well acquainted with the kelp beds off England and France. Early fishermen burned the plant for fuel and wrapped, baked, and ate fish in it. Unlike the Japanese, who eat a great deal of seaweed, Europeans never

333

developed much taste for kelp. But 18th-century physicians noticed that people who lived along the Atlantic coast rarely developed goiters—the large growths in the neck that were later shown to be enlarged thyroid glands.

Iodine: The Weight-Loss Connection

In 1750 a British physician introduced a cure for goiter—charred kelp in a vegetable-oil base. It worked, but no one knew why until 1812, when chemists identified iodine in the plant and physicians learned goiters were caused by iodine deficiency.

For several decades, Europeans and North Americans harvested kelp for its iodine. The fronds were cut off exposed rocks at low tide, hence one popular name, cut weed. Eventually other iodine sources replaced kelp, and the harvesting ceased.

During the 1860s, British and French physicians observed that people taking iodine for other reasons seemed to lose weight more easily. The iodine stimulated their thyroid, which boosted their metabolism, and they burned calories faster. Kelp gained a reputation as a treatment for obesity, which it retains to this day.

America's 19th-century Eclectics had no use for kelp, but they prized its iodine. They used iodine as an antiseptic for treating wounds and prescribed tincture of iodine internally for tuberculosis, liver and spleen disorders, syphilis, vaginal discharge, menstrual cramps, menstruation promotion, ovarian tumors, and enlargment of the testicles and uterus.

The Eclectics were also well aware that iodine overdose caused poisoning (iodism) involving fever, vomiting, thirst, diarrhea, abdominal pain, heart rhythm disturbances (arrhythmias), and "violent priapism" (painful, persistent penile erection unrelated to sexual desire).

Only a few contemporary herbalists still mention kelp for goiter, other thyroid disorders, arthritis, and obesity.

HEALING with Kelp

Kelp is definitely high in iodine. Back in the days before iodized salt, when iodine deficiency was a real problem, kelp was a real blessing. But today, iodine deficiency is virtually unheard-of in developed countries. To function normally, the body needs only a minute amount of iodine (150 micrograms a day)—an amount more than supplied by iodized salt. Additional iodine has no significant effect—until you consume enough to cause iodism, which is almost impossible just from eating kelp.

Kelp is a healing herb today because it contains another chemical (sodium alginate, also known simply as alginate), which is beneficial for health problems unique to the 20th century: radiation exposure, heavy metal toxicity, and heart disease.

Radiation Protection. The sodium alginate in kelp helps prevent absorption of radioactive strontium 90, a by-product of nuclear explosions and nuclear power and weapons facilities. Strontium 90, one of many toxic heavy metals, accumulates in bone tissue and has been linked to several cancers: leukemia, bone cancer, and Hodgkin's disease. Aboveground nuclear testing released a great deal of strontium 90. Nuclear accidents, including those at Three Mile Island and Chernobyl, have also released large quantities. In fact, so much strontium 90 has been released into the atmosphere, the bone tissue of every person on earth probably contains detectable levels.

Many animal studies show alginate supplements reduce strontium–90 absorption by as much as 83 percent. The herb's anti-strontium effect extends to human children and adults, according to a report in the *International Journal of Radiation Biology*.

The U.S. Atomic Energy Commission (now the Nuclear Regulatory Commission) guidelines advocate 3 ounces of kelp a week or 2 tablespoons of alginate supplement a day to prevent strontium–90 absorption.

However, sodium alginate mainly prevents the absorption

of *newly ingested* heavy metals. It works only in the gastrointestinal tract. It has little effect on past exposures. It does not significantly eliminate strontium and other pollutants already deposited in bone and other tissues. But since emissions from nuclear facilities continue to expose us to strontium 90 and other heavy metals, kelp or alginate supplementation is a good idea, especially for anyone who works in a nuclear facility, lives near one, or is occupationally exposed to heavy metals.

Toxic Heavy Metals. Strontium 90 is just one of many toxic heavy metals. Studies at McGill University in Montreal show that kelp also protects the body from several others: barium, cadmium, plutonium, and cesium.

Heart Disease. Some animal studies show kelp may help reduce cholesterol and blood pressure. On the other hand, kelp is also high in sodium, which may raise some people's blood pressure. Salt-sensitive individuals with high blood pressure should not consume large amounts of kelp. Others may include the herb in a comprehensive heart-disease prevention program.

Infection Prevention. Kelp is not an herbal antibiotic, but it does interfere with the growth of some bacteria and fungi. Cuts exposed to seawater are often slow to heal and prone to infection. Kelp might be useful as an emergency bandage for boating, fishing, surfing, and diving injuries.

Dead-End File. Kelp has never been shown to treat arthritis, help the liver or spleen, or treat any sexual infections or reproductive problems.

If thyroid function is normal, kelp does not promote weight loss.

Rx for Kelp

To most people, kelp tastes unpleasant. To take advantage of the protection from environmental pollution that kelp offers, tablets are the way to go. They're available where supplements are sold. Follow package directions.

If you decide to try an infusion, use 2 to 3 teaspoons of

dried powdered frond per cup of boiling water. Steep 10 minutes. Drink up to 3 cups a day.

Low-strength kelp preparations may be given cautiously to children under age 2. For older children and people over 65, start with low-strength preparations and increase strength if necessary.

The Safety Factor

If you're really adventurous, you might try some kelp recipes from a Japanese cookbook or else develop a taste for sushi, which makes considerable use of kelp.

The Food and Drug Administration includes kelp in its list of herbs generally regarded as safe. For otherwise healthy nonpregnant, nonnursing adults who do not have thyroid disorders or high blood pressure, kelp is considered safe in amounts typically recommended.

Kelp should be used in medicinal amounts only in consultation with your doctor. If kelp causes minor discomforts, such as stomach upset or diarrhea, use less or stop using it.

Let your doctor know if you experience any unpleasant symptoms or if the symptoms for which the herb is being used do not improve significantly in two weeks.

Don't Collect It, Buy It

Kelp grows in the cold water off the Atlantic and Pacific coasts of North America. It has a strong, foul odor when fresh, but baking deodorizes it. Authorities discourage using kelp collected close to shore because it may be contaminated by industrial pollutants. If you use kelp, buy it from commercial sources.

KOLA

Soda Pop Versus Asthma

Family: Sterculiaceae; other members include cocoa

Genus and species: *Cola nitida, C. vera, C. acuminata*

Also known as: Cola

Parts used: Seed leaves (cotyledons) known as nuts

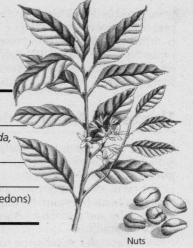

Nuts

Cola drinks account for a whopping 70 percent of the enormous U.S. soft drink market. Americans might drink even more if they knew the tropical nut that helps flavor them may help manage asthma.

Fabulous Virtues

West Africans have used kola since prehistoric times. They chewed the seeds for their stimulant effect and used them to treat fevers.

West African slaves introduced the kola tree into Brazil and the Caribbean. Kola became a favorite Caribbean diuretic to treat water retention, a digestive aid, and a folk remedy for diarrhea, fatigue, and heart problems. Over time, kola's stimulant properties led to the belief that it was an aphrodisiac.

Kola arrived in the United States after the Civil War. The 19th-century Eclectics noted that Caribbeans ascribed "innumerable fabulous virtues" to it. The Eclectics correctly identified the stimulants in kola as the same ones in cocoa. They prescribed kola to "overcome mental depression" and prepare for "severe physical and mental exertion." They also recommended it to relieve diarrhea, pneumonia, typhoid fever, migraine headaches, seasickness, morning sickness, and "attempts to break the tobacco habit."

Things Go Better with . . .

Because it was used medicinally, 19th-century pharmacists stocked kola. Legend has it that on May 8, 1886, Atlanta pharmacist John Styth Pemberton mixed some sugar with extracts of kola and coca (the source of cocaine) in a three-legged brass pot in his backyard. He added carbonated water to his sweet syrup and created a refreshing drink his bookkeeper dubbed Coca-Cola.

Two years later, Pemberton sold all rights to his beverage to Atlanta businessman Asa Candler for $2,300. Candler was an imaginative marketer, and by 1895, Coke had become America's first national soft drink. Today, Coca-Cola is the best-known product in the world. People request it 250 million times a day in 80 languages in 135 countries. Since its development, Coca-Cola's formula has been a closely guarded secret. The formula has evolved over the years. When the United States outlawed cocaine, the drug was removed from Coke. Today Coca-Cola is known to contain decocainized coca leaf extract and a small amount of kola.

Modern herbalists recommend kola for its "marked stimulating effect on human consciousness," according to David Hoffmann's *Holistic Herbal*, and as a treatment for diarrhea, depression, nervous debility, migraine headache, and loss of appetite.

HEALING with Kola

Some herbals claim kola contains more caffeine than coffee. Not so. A 6-ounce cup of brewed coffee contains about 100 milligrams of caffeine. A cup of instant coffee contains 65 milligrams, and a 12-ounce can of a cola soft drink contains about 50. However, most of this caffeine comes not from the kola nut but from added caffeine.

Asthma. Caffeine and kola both open (dilate) the bronchial passages. An article in the *Journal of the American Medical Association* recommended cola drinks to help manage childhood asthma because kids like them better than standard asthma medication. (For more on the benefits of caffeine, see "Coffee" on page 182.)

Rₓ for Kola

Cola beverages are the most convenient way to enjoy small amounts of this pleasant-tasting herb. Enjoy them as a possible aid for asthma or for a quick pick-me-up.

If you prefer to make a decoction, place 1 to 2 teaspoons of powdered nuts in a cup of water. Bring to a boil and simmer 10 minutes. Drink up to 3 cups a day.

Small amounts of kola may be given cautiously to children under age 2.

The Safety Factor

Because kola contains caffeine, it should be avoided by pregnant women or those with insomnia, diabetes, anxiety problems, digestive disorders, chronic high blood pressure, high cholesterol, heart disease, or a history of stroke. (For details, see "Coffee.")

Kola is included on the Food and Drug Administration's (FDA) list of herbs generally regarded as safe. However, a recent FDA panel recommended removing caffeine from the "safe" list. If this happens, kola might also be removed.

For otherwise healthy nonpregnant, nonnursing adults who have no history of the conditions listed above and who are not taking other medications containing caffeine, kola is considered safe in amounts typically recommended.

Kola should be used in medicinal amounts only in consultation with your doctor. If kola causes minor discomforts, such as insomnia, irritability, or stomach upset, use less or stop using it. Let your doctor know if you experience any unpleasant symptoms or the symptoms for which the herb is being used do not improve significantly in two weeks.

Prefers a Warm Climate

Kola is a 40-foot tree that grows in West Africa, the Caribbean, Brazil, Sri Lanka, and Indonesia. Kolas have beautiful yellow flowers with purple spots and produce chocolate-colored seed pods in spring and fall. In most plants, the "nut" refers to the whole seed, but the kola nut is only part of the seed, specifically the embryonic leaves (cotyledons) inside the seed coat. They are dried and powdered.

LICORICE

Beneficial—and Controversial

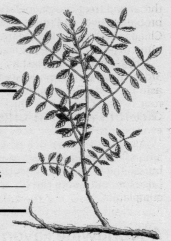

Family: Leguminosae; other members include beans, peas

Genus and species: *Glycyrrhiza glabra*

Also known as: No other names

Parts used: Rhizome and roots

Licorice is one of the most beneficial—and controversial—healing herbs. Advocates claim it has been used safely around the world for thousands of years to treat cough, colds, rashes, arthritis, ulcers, hepatitis, cirrhosis, and infections. Critics concede the herb's effectiveness but insist its "potentially life-threatening side effects" make it too dangerous to use.

The licorice extracts used in candies have, in some cases, caused some harm when used in large amounts. But for otherwise healthy adults who use licorice in moderation, this healer's benefits greatly outweigh its risks.

Sweet Root by Another Name

Licorice appears prominently in the first great Chinese herbal, the *Pen Tsao Ching* (*Classic of Herbs*), written more than 5,000 years ago according to legend.

Ever since, licorice has been one of China's most popular healing herbs. Chinese physicians prescribe it to soothe the

342

throat and treat cough, malaria, food poisoning, respiratory problems, liver and uterine complaints, and some cancers. Chinese herbalists also use the herb's sweetness to mask the bitter taste of other herbal medicines.

The herb has a long history in the West, as well. During the 3rd century B.C., Hippocrates extolled licorice for cough, asthma, and other respiratory complaints. He called it sweet root, in Greek, *glukos riza*, which evolved into the herb's genus, *Glycyrrhiza*. The Romans changed *Glycyrrhiza* to *Liquiritia*, which evolved into licorice.

Amid the treasures of King Tut's tomb, archeologists found a bundle of licorice sticks. More than 1,300 years after Tut's burial, the Greek physician Dioscorides prescribed licorice juice for colds, sore throat, and chest and gastrointestinal complaints.

A Worldwide Favorite

German abbess/herbalist Hildegard of Bingen prescribed licorice for stomach and heart problems. It was mentioned frequently in 14th- and 15th-century German and Italian herbals as a cough and respiratory remedy.

Seventeenth-century English herbalist Nicholas Culpeper called licorice "a fine medicine . . . for those that have dry cough or hoarseness, wheezing or shortness of breath, phthisis [tuberculosis], heat of urine [burning], and griefs of the breast and lungs."

North American colonists found the Indians drinking a tea brewed from American licorice as a cough remedy, laxative, earache treatment, and mask for the bitter flavor of other herbs.

America's 19th-century Eclectics prescribed licorice for urinary problems, cough, colds, and other "bronchial and pectoral [chest] affections."

Among American folk herbalists, licorice was considered a treatment for menstrual discomforts. It was included in Lydia E. Pinkham's Vegetable Compound, the popular 19th-century patent medicine for menstrual complaints, and it remains an ingredient in the product's current formulation.

Licorice has also been used to treat a variety of cancers in many cultures.

Contemporary herbalists recommend licorice for its soothing effects on the respiratory, genitourinary, and gastrointestinal tracts, especially as a treatment for ulcers. Herbalists continue to recommend licorice to mask the bitter taste of other healing herbs. A few mention the herb's hormonelike action and recommend it in the treatment of Addison's disease, a disease in which the adrenal gland produces abnormally low amounts of certain of its hormones.

HEALING with Licorice

True to its Greek name, sweet root, licorice is 50 times sweeter than sugar. Licorice contains a remarkable chemical (glycyrrhetinic acid, or GA) with a broad range of benefits. But a bitter battle has erupted over the sweet root's hazards.

Cough Remedy. Several studies support licorice's ancient use as a cough remedy. GA has some cough-suppressant properties. In Europe, it's used extensively in cough formulas.

Ulcers. Back in 1946, a Dutch pharmacist noticed that licorice candies and cough remedies were unusually popular with customers who had gastrointestinal ulcers. They told him licorice provided better, longer-lasting relief than other ulcer medicines. Intrigued, the phamacist published a report in a Dutch medical journal.

Soon studies published in *Lancet* and the *Journal of the American Medical Association* showed concentrated GA extracted from licorice heals ulcers in both animals and people. Unfortunately, it also causes swelling of the ankles—a classic sign of water retention. Water retention is potentially serious. It can lead to elevated blood pressure, which can be dangerous for pregnant and nursing women and anyone with diabetes, glaucoma, high blood pressure, heart disease, or a history of stroke.

By the late 1970s, mainstream medicine had an amazingly effective ulcer drug, cimetidine (Tagamet), currently one of the world's most widely prescribed medications. How does GA stack up against Tagamet? Several studies compared the two. Tagamet was more effective for stomach ulcers, but the two were equally effective for small intestinal (duodenal) ulcers, with the licorice extract actually providing better protection against relapses. But GA water retention continued to be a problem.

As time passed, researchers learned why GA caused water retention. The chemical acts like the adrenal hormone aldosterone, which is involved in salt and water metabolism. Large amounts can cause a potentially serious condition (pseudoaldosteronism), symptoms of which include headache, lethargy, water retention, elevated blood pressure, and possibly heart failure.

Fortunately, scientists discovered they could retain licorice's ulcer-healing benefits but eliminate its hormonal side effects by removing 97 percent of its GA, creating a new herbal medicine, DGL (deglycyrrhizinated licorice).

As European and British journals published studies demonstrating DGL's anti-ulcer effectiveness without serious side effects, American researchers, who had dismissed GA as too hazardous, took a second look. But during the late 1970s several studies using improperly prepared DGL delivered results that made the medicine appear to be totally ineffective against ulcers. These unfortunate results crushed interest in the United States. It turned out the ineffective DGL preparations released very little medicine (poor bioavailability).

Today, DGL holds little interest for most U.S. ulcer researchers, but European researchers continue to publish impressive results. A 12-week study of 874 duodenal-ulcer sufferers published in the *Irish Medical Journal* showed DGL healed their ulcers faster than Tagamet with no hormonal side effects.

If future studies corroborate these results, American physicians may one day use DGL to treat duodenal ulcers. In the meantime, ulcer sufferers interested in incorporating licorice into their treatment plans should discuss the herb with their physicians.

Arthritis. Licorice also has anti-inflammatory and antiarthritic properties. One study showed GA could be applied like hydrocortisone creams to treat skin inflammations, such as eczema. These findings led to studies showing licorice taken internally also has anti-inflammatory, specifically antiarthritic, effects. Arthritis sufferers interested in licorice should discuss the herb with their physicians.

Herpes. Licorice stimulates cell production of interferon, the body's own antiviral compound, according to a study published in *Microbiology and Immunology*. Not surprisingly, other studies show it fights *Herpes simplex* virus, the cause of genital herpes and cold sores. Sprinkling some powdered licorice root on clean sores may help heal herpes.

Infection. Many laboratory studies show licorice also fights disease-causing bacteria (*Staphylococci* and *Streptococci*) and the fungus responsible for vaginal yeast infections (*Candida albicans*). Sprinkling some powdered licorice root on clean wounds may help prevent infection.

Hepatitis, Cirrhosis. Chinese physicians have used licorice for centuries to treat liver problems. Asian studies show the herb helps control hepatitis and improve liver function in people with cirrhosis. Hepatitis and cirrhosis are serious conditions requiring professional care. If you'd like to try licorice for liver disease, discuss it with your physician.

Intriguing Possibility. Immune stimulation may help explain licorice's antitumor activity against cancerous melanomas in experimental animals. It's too early to call the herb a treatment for these tumors, but in the future it might become one.

R$_x$ for Licorice

To help prevent wound infection, sprinkle powdered licorice on minor wounds after washing them with soap and water. It can also be used in this way on herpes sores, but check with your physician before doing so.

To help soothe a sore throat, add a pinch of sweet-tasting licorice to any herbal beverage tea.

If you want to take advantage of licorice's more powerful healing action—against liver disease, ulcers, or arthritis—discuss the herb with your physician. To make a possible infection-fighting decoction, gently boil ½ teaspoon of powdered herb per cup of water for 10 minutes. Drink up to 2 cups a day.

In a tincture, use ½ to 1 teaspoon up to twice a day.

Licorice should not be given to children under age 2. For older children and people over 65, start with low-strength preparations and increase strength if necessary.

The Safety Factor

U.S. medical journals have been slow to pick up on licorice's successes, but they've jumped all over its potential for causing pseudoaldosteronism. The problem is real, and some people should not use licorice. But in moderation, most people can use it safely.

There have been no reports of licorice sticks or the powdered herb causing problems. The problems—about 25 reports in the world medical literature—have been caused by the highly concentrated licorice extracts used in some candies, laxatives, and tobacco products. And most have resulted from overindulgence in licorice candies.

Remember, though, that most U.S. "licorice" contains anise, not licorice. Real licorice is available, however, in specialty shops. The *Journal of the American Medical Association* recounted the case of a man who ate 2 to 4 ounces of real licorice candies a day for seven years. He developed weakness and hormone disturbances requiring hospitalization. Another overdose victim ate more than a pound of licorice candy a day for nine days. He, too, required hospital treatment.

Licorice-Laced Products

One woman suffered weakness after taking 4 tablespoons of Lydia Pinkham's Vegetable Compound a day for three months. (As a menstrual remedy, it should be taken only a few days a month.) According to a report in the *New England Journal of Medicine*, she recovered two weeks after she stopped using the compound.

Licorice-laced chewing tobacco can also cause problems. One man chewed a dozen 3-ounce bags a day and swallowed his saliva instead of spitting it out. He developed weakness and had to be hospitalized. Of course, his symptoms could have been caused by substances in the chewing tobacco other than licorice—nicotine, for example.

These cases raise important points: Pregnant and nursing women, and anyone with a history of diabetes, glaucoma, high blood pressure, stroke, or heart disease should be cautious regarding consumption of licorice. In these people it might raise their blood pressure and cause potentially serious problems.

On the other hand, the vast majority of overdose reports have involved huge doses of highly concentrated licorice extracts—not the whole herb. Otherwise healthy people may use the herb cautiously, but should familiarize themselves with overdose symptoms: headache, facial puffiness, ankle swelling, weakness, and lethargy.

Other Cautions

Despite its well-publicized potential hazards, licorice is included in the Food and Drug Administration's list of herbs generally regarded as safe. For otherwise healthy nonpregnant, nonnursing adults who do not have diabetes, glaucoma, high blood pressure, or a history of heart disease or stroke and are not taking digitalis-like medications, licorice is considered relatively safe when used cautiously in amounts typically recommended for brief periods.

Licorice should be used in medicinal amounts only in consultation with your doctor. If licorice causes minor discomforts, such as stomach upset or diarrhea, use less or stop using it. Let your doctor know if you experience unpleasant effects or if the symptoms for which the herb is being used do not improve significantly in two weeks.

Beautiful Candy Plant

Licorice is an erect, hardy perennial that reaches 3 to 7 feet. Small, alternate, inch-long leaflets and $\frac{1}{2}$-inch purple mid-summer flowers give the plant a graceful beauty. Mature plants have a long taproot that sends out creeping horizontal rhizomes (stolons), the source of other shoots and more branching roots, creating a tangled mass of underground growth. Licorice roots have brown bark, and sweet, juicy, yellow pulp.

Hard freezes kill licorice. It grows best in warm, sunny climates, or in greenhouses in pots 48 inches deep. Greenhouse licorice often requires artificial light.

Licorice is usually propagated from root cuttings containing eyes. Plant them vertically about an inch below the surface, with 18-inch spacing. Beds should be rich, well dug, well manured, well drained—and contained. Once established, this herb can become extremely invasive. Contain it.

Licorice requires little care other than weeding. Expect slow growth the first year or two. Harvest rhizomes and roots during the fall of the third or fourth year. The year you plan to harvest, pinch the flowers back. Flowering drains some of the roots' sweep sap. Thick roots should be split to dry. Shade-dry roots for six months.

MARJORAM

Spicy Stomach Settler

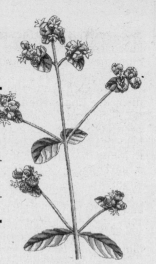

Family: Labiatae; other members include mints

Genus and species: *Origanum majorana* and other *Origanum* species

Also known as: Knotted marjoram, oregano

Parts used: Leaves and flower tops

Marjoram is usually considered a culinary spice, not a healing herb. This is unfortunate, because science has supported its value as a digestive aid and discovered it may help treat herpes.

The ancient Greeks believed marjoram was first cultivated by Aphrodite, goddess of love, whose touch produced its fragrant aroma. Greek couples wore marjoram wreaths at their weddings. The Greeks also believed that if a girl placed marjoram in her bed, Aphrodite would visit her dreams and reveal the identity of her future spouse. Today in parts of Europe, girls who want sweet marriages place marjoram sprigs in their hope chests. (For fresher-smelling sheets, hang a few sprigs in your linen closet.)

Roman Digestive Aid

Early Greek physicians used marjoram as an antidote for snakebite and a treatment for muscle and joint pains. But the herb did not become widely used in healing until the Romans discovered it settled the stomach. Roman herbalists also believed it could heal bruises, alleviate menstrual cramps, promote menstruation, and treat pinkeye (conjunctivitis) and other eye problems.

By the 17th century, marjoram was widely used in herbal medicine. English herbalist Nicholas Culpeper called it "an excellent remedy for the brain . . . and stomach. . . . The decoction thereof . . . draweth forth much phlegm . . . [and] helpeth all diseases of the chest. The oil thereof is comfortable to joints that are stiff. It helpeth griefs of the womb [menstrual cramps] . . . [and] provoketh women's courses [menstruation]."

Early colonists introduced marjoram into North America and used it as both a kitchen and medicinal herb. America's 19th-century Eclectics recommended it as a tonic stimulant and menstruation promoter. Folk healers also used marjoram to treat infant colic, arthritis, and some cancers.

Contemporary herbalists recommend marjoram as a digestive aid, tranquilizer, and cough remedy. Some say it helps relieve menstrual cramps without promoting menstruation. Others say it encourages menstruation. Various herbalists recommend marjoram tea for headaches, before bed to prevent insomnia, and before travel to prevent motion sickness.

Marjoram or Oregano?

Cookbooks often suggest replacing oregano with marjoram for sweeter, spicier sauces. But the fact is, the oregano on your spice rack *might be* marjoram. All marjoram species are also called oregano. But only a few of the 50 plants called oregano are ever called marjoram. Many palates cannot tell the difference between the two (see "Oregano" on page 399).

HEALING with Marjoram

The Romans were probably right about marjoram soothing the stomach.

Digestive Aid. Marjoram appears to soothe the digestive tract (making it an antispasmodic). Marjoram's stomach-settling activity may also explain its use in preventing motion sickness, which typically involves gastrointestinal symptoms.

Women's Health. Antispasmodics soothe not only the smooth muscle lining of the digestive tract but other smooth muscles, such as the uterus, as well. This possibly accounts for the herb's use in the treatment of menstrual cramps.

In recommended medicinal amounts, marjoram is unlikely to stimulate menstruation, even though it has a reputation for doing so and has been used this way for centuries. Pregnant women should not use more than culinary amounts. Other women might try it to trigger menstruation. It might be helpful on rare occasions.

Herpes. Test-tube studies show marjoram inhibits the growth of *Herpes simplex*, the virus that causes genital herpes and cold sores. If you have recurrent herpes, try sprinkling some powdered herb or using a few drops of tincture on cold sores or genital herpes. It may be of some help, although there is no evidence that it has any clinical effect against herpes at this time.

Dead-End File. Marjoram has never been shown to relieve joint stiffness.

Rx for Marjoram

Take marjoram as an infusion or tincture to take advantage of its stomach-soothing potential or to try to bring on menstruation. For a sweet, pleasantly spicy infusion, use 1 to 2 teaspoons of dried leaves and flower tops per cup of boiling water. Steep 10 minutes. Drink up to 3 cups a day.

In a tincture, use 1/2 to 1 teaspoon up to three times a day.

Sprinkle some dried powdered herb on cold sores or genital herpes sores.

Low-strength marjoram preparations may be given cautiously to children under age 2 for colic. For older children and people over 65, start with low-strength preparations and increase strength if necessary.

The Safety Factor

The medical literature contains no reports of harm from marjoram.

Marjoram is included in the Food and Drug Administration's list of herbs generally regarded as safe. For otherwise healthy nonpregnant, nonnursing adults, marjoram is considered safe in amounts typically recommended.

Marjoram should be used in medicinal amounts only in consultation with your doctor. If marjoram causes minor discomforts, such as stomach upset or diarrhea, use less or stop using it. Let your doctor know if you experience unpleasant effects or if the symptoms for which the herb is being used do not improve significantly in two weeks.

A Spicy Favorite

In its native Spain, Portugal, and North Africa, O. *majorana* is a perennial. But it's grown as an annual in North America.

Marjoram is a hairy plant with square purplish stems. The leaves are small and oval. Its white, pink, or lavender flowers bloom in late summer and cluster close together in knots, hence the name knotted marjoram.

Once marjoram's tiny, slow-germinating seeds sprout, the plant grows easily. For best results, germinate it indoors, then transplant it outdoors after danger of frost has passed. Arrange seedlings in groups of three spaced every 8 inches. Five clumps (15 plants) satisfy most families' cooking needs.

Marjoram grows best under full sun in rich, well-drained soil. Weed frequently until the plants have become established. Pinch the flower buds back to increase bushiness and leaf yield.

Harvest leaves anytime after flower buds form. In autumn harvest the entire plant to 1 inch aboveground. Marjoram dries easily. Store it in airtight containers.

MARSH MALLOW

Confection with Healing Roots

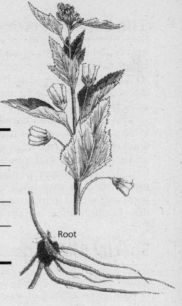

Family: Malvaceae; other members include cotton, hollyhock, hibiscus

Genus and species: *Althaea officinalis*

Also known as: Althea, cheeses

Parts used: Roots; sometimes leaves and flowers

Root

Yes, this plant inspired the pillowy white confection we toast over camp fires. But today's marshmallows contain none of their namesake herb and bear no resemblance to the marsh mallow sweets of old. It's a shame so few people know this herb as anything other than a candy, because marsh mallow has been widely used in healing for 2,500 years.

Food for Famines

Marsh mallow was a food before it was a medicine. The Book of Job (30:4) mentions a plant (translated as mallow or broom) that was eaten during famines. And during the Middle Ages when crops failed, people boiled marsh mallow roots, then fried them with onions in butter. Backpacking guides suggest the plant for wilderness foragers today.

The plant's history as a healer goes back to Hippocrates, who prescribed a decoction of marsh mallow roots to treat bruises and blood loss from wounds. Four hundred years later, the Greek physician Dioscorides recommended marsh mallow root poultices for insect bites and stings and prescribed the decoction for toothache and vomiting and as an antidote to poisons.

The Romans loved marsh mallow. The Roman naturalist Pliny wrote, "Whosoever shall take a spoonful of the mallows shall that day be free from all diseases."

Tenth-century Arab physicians used mallow leaf poultices to treat inflammations, and early European folk healers used marsh mallow root both internally and externally for its soothing action in treating toothache, sore throat, digestive upsets, and urinary irritation.

Special Blessings

Marsh mallow was a special favorite of 17th-century English herbalist Nicholas Culpeper: "You may remember that not long since, there was a raging disease called the bloody flux . . . the college of physicians not knowing what to make of it. My son was taken with [it] and . . . the only thing I gave him was mallows bruised and boiled in milk and drunk. In two days (the blessing of God be upon it) it cured him. And I here, to show my thankfulness to God in communicating it to his creatures, leave it to posterity."

Culpeper recommended marsh mallow roots, leaves, and seeds for their soothing action in "agues [fever] . . . torments of the belly . . . pleurisy, phthisis [tuberculosis], and other diseases of the chest . . . coughs, hoarseness . . . shortness of breath, wheezing, cramps . . . and swellings in women's breasts. . . . and other offensive humors."

The colonists introduced marsh mallow into North America, and by the mid-19th century, it was included in the U.S. *Pharmacopoeia*. The Eclectics prescribed it externally for "wounds, bruises, burns, scalds, and swellings of every kind." Internally, they recommended the root decoction for colds, hoarseness, diarrhea, gonorrhea, gastrointestinal problems, and "nearly every affection of the kidney and bladder."

Contemporary herbalists generally limit their marsh mallow recommendations to respiratory and gastrointestinal irritation. Some tout it for urinary complaints.

Thank the French for the spongy confection that bears this herb's name. They first candied marsh mallow roots centuries ago. They peeled the root bark, exposing the white pulp, and boiled it to soften it and release its sweetness. Then they added sugar. The result: sweet, white, somewhat spongy sticks, which over time evolved into today's camp fire treat.

HEALING with Marsh Mallow

The spongy material in marsh mallow roots is called mucilage. When it comes in contact with water, it swells and forms a gel.

Cuts and Wounds. Externally, marsh mallow gel may help soothe cuts, scrapes, wounds, and burns.

Respiratory Woes. Taken internally, it may help relieve upset stomach and the respiratory rawness associated with sore throat, cough, colds, flu, and bronchitis.

Immune System. In one recent experiment, marsh mallow enhanced white blood cells' ability to devour disease microbes (phagocytosis), suggesting that its traditional use in wound treatment and gastrointestinal infections may have been therapeutic as well as soothing.

Intriguing Possibility. One animal study indicated the root reduces blood sugar (glucose), suggesting possible value in managing diabetes.

Rx for Marsh Mallow

Enjoy a sweet decoction to take advantage of marsh mallow's soothing potential and possible infection-fighting abilities.

To make a decoction, gently boil $\frac{1}{2}$ to 1 teaspoon of chopped or crushed root per cup of water for 10 to 15 minutes. Drink up to 3 cups a day.

To prepare marsh mallow for external use, chop the root very fine and add enough water to make a gooey gel. Apply the gel directly to superficial wounds or sunburn. If you have a serious wound or sunburn, see your physician to obtain advice regarding treatment.

Low-strength marsh mallow decoctions may be given cautiously to children under age 2.

The Safety Factor

The medical literature contains no reports of any harm from marsh mallow.

For otherwise healthy nonpregnant, nonnursing adults, marsh mallow is considered safe in amounts typically recommended.

Marsh mallow should be used in medicinal amounts only in consultation with your doctor. If marsh mallow causes minor discomforts, such as stomach upset or diarrhea, use less or stop using it. Let your doctor know if you experience unpleasant effects or if the symptoms for which the herb is being used do not improve significantly in two weeks.

Found in Bogs

Marsh mallow grows, not surprisingly, in marshes, bogs, damp meadows, and along streambanks. The plant is a downy, erect, 5-foot perennial with a long taproot. The stems, which die back each autumn, are hairy and branching. The roundish, gray-green leaves, 1 to 3 inches long, are lobed, toothed, and covered with velvety hairs. The flowers, pink or white, bloom in summer. They are up to 2 inches across and give rise to round fruits called "cheeses," one of the herb's names.

In moist soil under full sun, marsh mallow is a hardy plant

that grows easily from seeds, cuttings, or root divisions. Seeds should be planted in spring, root divisions in autumn. Thin them to a 2-foot spacing.

Do not harvest roots from plants less than two years old. In autumn, when the top growth has died back, dig out mature roots and remove the lateral rootlets. Wash, peel, and dry them whole or in slices.

MATÉ

The High-C Stimulant

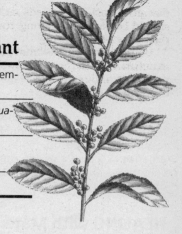

Family: Aquifoliaceae; other members include holly

Genus and species: *Ilex paraguayensis* or *I. paraguariensis*

Also known as: Yerba maté, Paraguay tea, Jesuit tea

Parts used: Leaves

More than 300 years ago, Jesuit missionaries noticed that South American Indians ate a virtually all-meat diet yet did not develop "sailor's sickness" (scurvy), which decimated European mariners who ate a similar diet at sea. The Jesuits decided the Indians must be protected by the tea they drank out of cups made from calabash gourds. They named it *maté*, from the Spanish for "gourd," and began cultivating the hollylike shrub and drinking the bitter tea made from its leathery leaves.

Maté (pronounced MAH-*tay*), also called yerba maté or Paraguay tea, was introduced into the United States in the 1970s as a noncaffeine coffee substitute. That claim was in error. Maté contains caffeine. It also contains vitamin C, making it more nutritious than other caffeine-containing herbs (coffee, tea, kola, and cocoa).

Jesuit Tea

The Jesuits introduced maté to European colonists, and today it is one of South America's favorite stimulants. In Argentina,

Paraguay, and Uruguay, it's considerably more popular than either coffee or tea. More than 200 brands of maté are currently marketed in Argentina alone. Argentinians consume 11 pounds per capita of maté annually. In Uruguay, the figure is 22 pounds. South American breads often have maté added, and the herb is a key ingredient in a popular South American soft drink.

South Americans consider maté not only a pleasant stimulant but also an appetite suppressant and a diuretic that treats water retention. Although there has been no scientific research to back it up, maté has long been used in South America as a digestive aid. Argentinian cowboys (gauchos) sometimes live on just meat and maté like the Indians of old.

HEALING with Maté

A 6-ounce cup of maté contains about 50 milligrams of caffeine, about as much as a cup of tea or a can of cola soda. Instant coffee contains a little more caffeine (65 milligrams per cup). Brewed coffee contains two to three times as much (100 to 150 milligrams per cup). (For details on caffeine's benefits, see "Coffee" on page 182.)

Because maté contains only one-third to one-half as much caffeine as a comparable-size cup of brewed coffee, its effects would be only a fraction as intense.

Colds and Flu. Some experts recommend vitamin C for colds. The herb is fairly high in vitamin C and is, in fact, the most nutritious stimulating beverage. (The Jesuits were right about maté preventing scurvy.) Drinking maté when you have a cold will provide one additional source of vitamin C.

Premenstrual Syndrome. Diuretics help relieve the bloated feeling caused by premenstrual fluid retention. Women bothered by PMS might try maté during the uncomfortable days just before their periods.

Rx for Maté

For a pleasantly bitter infusion, use 1 teaspoon of dried herb per cup of boiling water. Steep 10 minutes. Drink up to 3 cups a day. Some people object to maté's odor, although others learn to enjoy it. Add honey and lemon if you need to.

Maté should not be given to children under age 2. For older children and people over 65, start with low-strength preparations and increase strength if necessary.

The Safety Factor

Caffeine is classically addictive and large amounts may cause significant harm (see "Coffee"). However, because of maté's lower caffeine content, cup for cup, it should cause fewer problems.

Maté contains tannins, which have both pro- and anti-cancer action. A Uruguayan study published in the *Journal of the National Cancer Institute* showed heavy maté users have an increased risk of esophageal cancer. The *average* Uruguayan consumes 22 pounds of this herb a year, so God knows how much *heavy* Uruguayan users consume. This finding appears to have no real significance to Americans who drink an occasional cup of maté tea. Those with esophageal cancer should not use it, however.

Other Cautions

For otherwise healthy nonpregnant, nonnursing adults who are not taking other substances or medications containing caffeine, maté is considered relatively safe in amounts typically recommended.

Maté should be used in medicinal amounts only in consultation with your doctor. If maté causes minor discomforts, such as stomach upset or diarrhea, use less or stop using it. Let your doctor know if you experience unpleasant effects or if the symptoms for which the herb is being used do not improve significantly in two weeks.

South American Native

Maté is not cultivated in the United States. In South America, it grows wild near streams, but it is also extensively cultivated, especially in Argentina. Maté is a perennial shrub with spineless, oval, toothed, leathery leaves. Its fruits (berries) are red, black, or yellow, and about the size of black peppercorns.

MEADOWSWEET

Herbal Aspirin

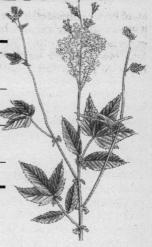

Family: Rosaceae; other members include rose, almond, apple, raspberry, cherry

Genus and species: *Filipendula ulmaria*, formerly *Spiraea ulmaria*

Also known as: Spiraea, bridewort, queen-of-the-meadow

Parts used: Leaves and flower tops

It's a rare medicine cabinet that doesn't contain aspirin, but it's even rarer to find anyone who knows we owe the word "aspirin" to the beautiful, aromatic meadowsweet.

Original Air Freshener

During the Middle Ages, meadowsweet's delicate almond fragrance made it a popular air freshener, or "strewing herb." It was scattered around homes at a time when people rarely bathed and when farm animals often shared human living quarters. Later, this herb's sweet aroma and lovely blossoms earned it a place in bridal bouquets, hence the name bridewort. Later herbalists recommended meadowsweet to treat fevers, arthritis, "falling sickness" (epilepsy), and respiratory ailments.

Colonists introduced the plant into North America, and the 19th-century Eclectics considered it "an excellent astringent . . . in diarrhea. [It] is less offensive to the stomach than other agents of its kind." They also prescribed it for menstrual cramps and vaginal discharges.

From Salicin to Aspirin

In 1839, a German chemist discovered meadowsweet flower buds contained salicin, the same chemical isolated from white willow bark 11 years earlier. Salicin has powerful pain-relieving (analgesic), fever-reducing, and anti-inflammatory properties. Unfortunately, salicin (and its close chemical relatives, notably salicylic acid) also causes potentially hazardous side effects: stomach upset, nausea, diarrhea, stomach bleeding, ringing in the ears (tinnitus), and at high doses even respiratory paralysis and death.

Chemists began tinkering with salicylic acid, hoping to preserve its benefits while minimizing its hazards. In 1853, German chemists working with an extract of meadowsweet synthesized acetylsalicylic acid. The new drug still had salicylic acid's side effects but was much more potent. To name the new drug, they took the *a* from *acetyl*—the chemical they added to the extract—and *spirin* from meadowsweet's Latin name, *Spiraea*, and came up with aspirin. News of aspirin's development was published in an obscure German medical journal and forgotten for almost 50 years.

Bayer Does It Better

Then in the late 1890s, a German chemist, Felix Hoffman, became upset that his father's rheumatoid arthritis medication brought him so little relief. Hoffman worked at the Fredrich Bayer pharmaceutical company, and he began combing the journals for leads to a better arthritis treatment. He came upon the old reports of aspirin and prepared the drug. His father improved significantly after taking it. At first, Bayer officials were not interested in Hoffman's arthritis remedy, but eventually they saw its potential, and in 1899 they introduced acetylsalicylic acid in Europe and North America under the brand name *Aspirin*.

Aspirin quickly became the household drug of choice for a broad range of everyday medical needs. But in one of the earliest U.S. trademark-protection battles, Bayer lost its trademark to *aspirin*. The court ruled the word had passed into general usage.

Contemporary herbalists recommend meadowsweet for colds and flu, nausea, heartburn and other digestive upsets, muscle aches, dropsy (congestive heart failure), and childhood diarrhea.

HEALING with Meadowsweet

Meadowsweet gave us aspirin, but don't expect the herb to do everything aspirin does.

Pain Relief. Meadowsweet does not pack aspirin's pain-relieving, fever-reducing, and anti-inflammatory punch. The herb is low in salicylate, and even strong infusions may not reduce fever or relieve pain. Tinctures provide more salicylate and greater pain relief.

On the other hand, meadowsweet is less likely to cause aspirin's major side effect, stomach upset. In fact, recent European studies show the herb actually *protects* experimental animals from aspirin-induced stomach ulcers, a finding that supports the Eclectic observation that meadowsweet is gentle to the stomach.

If you'd rather take an herbal preparation than a pill, try meadowsweet for headache, arthritis, menstrual cramps, low-grade fever, and other pains and inflammations, especially if aspirin upsets your stomach. It might help.

Diarrhea. A European study showed meadowsweet effective against one of the bacteria that cause diarrhea (*Shigella dysenteriae*), lending some credence to its traditional use for this condition.

Intriguing Possibilities. Aspirin helps prevent the internal blood clots that trigger heart attack. Meadowsweet's effect on heart disease, if any, has not been researched, but it seems reasonable to presume the herb may have a similar effect.

One study showed salicin reduces blood sugar (glucose) levels, suggesting possible value in the management of diabetes.

Rₓ for Meadowsweet

For a pleasantly astringent infusion, use 1 to 2 teaspoons of dried herb per cup of boiling water. Steep 10 minutes. Drink up to 3 cups a day.

In a tincture, take ½ to 1 teaspoon up to three times a day.

Meadowsweet should not be given to children under age 2 or children under 16 suffering fevers from colds, flu, or chicken pox. For other children and people over 65, start with low-strength preparations and increase strength if necessary.

The Safety Factor

Recent European animal studies suggest meadowsweet may stimulate uterine contractions. The herb has no history of use as a menstruation promoter, but aspirin has been associated with an increased risk of birth defects, so pregnant women should not use it.

In children under 16 suffering fevers from colds, flu, or chicken pox, aspirin is associated with Reye's syndrome, a rare but potentially fatal condition. Meadowsweet has never been associated with Reye's syndrome, but because it's related to aspirin, parents should not give it to children with fevers caused by those illnesses.

Other Cautions

The Food and Drug Administration lists meadowsweet as an herb of "undefined safety." For otherwise healthy nonpregnant, nonnursing adults who do not have ulcers or gastritis and are not taking other medications containing aspirin or salicylates, meadowsweet is considered safe in amounts typically recommended.

If meadowsweet causes minor discomforts, such as stomach upset or ringing in the ears, use less or stop using it. Let your doctor know if you experience any unpleasant effects or if the symptoms for which the herb is being used do not improve significantly in two weeks.

Queen-of-the-Meadow

Meadowsweet is a perennial with stems that reach 2 to 6 feet. It has elm-like leaves and large drooping clusters of small coiled white or pink flowers, which bloom throughout summer and have a fragrant, sweet almond aroma. It stands taller and has more striking flowers than most other meadow plants, hence its name queen-of-the-meadow.

Meadowsweet grows wild from Newfoundland to Ohio in marshes, along streambanks, and in moist forests and meadows. It is best propagated from cuttings of its creeping, perennial, underground stem (rhizome). Meadowsweet does best in rich, moist, well-drained soil under partial shade. Harvest the leaves and flower tops when the plant is in bloom.

MINTS

Marvelous Menthol

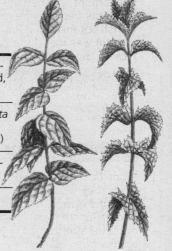

Family: Labiatae; other members include balm, basil, catnip, horehound, marjoram, pennyroyal

Genus and species: *Mentha piperita* (peppermint); *M. spicata, M. viridis, M. aquatica, M. cardiaca* (spearmint)

Also known as: Hundreds of different kinds of mint

Parts used: Leaves and flower tops

Spearmint   Black peppermint

Have you ever had an after-dinner mint? These familiar candies evolved from the ancient custom of concluding feasts with a sprig of mint to soothe the stomach. Science has lent support to this age-old practice, as well as many other healing uses of these herbs, best known as the source of menthol, which flavors candies, gums, toothpastes, and mouthwashes.

The Double Mints

Peppermint and spearmint are both used in herbal healing and have similar effects, but peppermint is the tastier and more potent. It is also the more recent arrival.

Spearmint was the original medicinal mint. Peppermint appeared later, a natural hybrid of spearmint species. But authorities aren't exactly sure which species combined to form peppermint, or when the spicier mint actually appeared. All the mints were considered one plant, mint, until 1696, when British botanist John Ray differentiated them.

Mint was mentioned as a stomach soother in the *Ebers Papyrus*, the world's oldest surviving medical text. From Egypt, mint spread to Palestine, where it was accepted as payment for taxes. In Luke (11:39) Jesus scolds the Pharisees: "You pay tithes of mint and rue . . . but have no care for justice and the love of God."

Mythical Origins

From the Holy Land, mint spread to Greece and entered Greek mythology. It seems Pluto, god of the dead, fell in love with the beautiful nymph, Minthe. Pluto's goddess-wife, Persephone, became jealous and changed Minthe into mint. Pluto could not bring Minthe back to life, but he gave her plant form a fragrant aroma. "Minthe" evolved into the mints' genus, *Mentha*.

Greek and Roman homemakers added mint to milk to prevent spoilage and served the herb after meals as a digestive aid. The Roman naturalist Pliny wrote that mint "reanimates the spirit" and recommended hanging it in sickrooms to assist convalescence. The Greek physician Dioscorides considered mint "heating," and therefore a promoter of lust. Other Greek and Roman herbalists prescribed mint for everything from hiccups to leprosy.

Chinese and Ayurvedic physicians have used mint for centuries as a tonic and digestive aid and as a treatment for colds, cough, and fever.

Medieval German abbess/herbalist Hildegard of Bingen recommended mint for digestion and gout.

Seventeenth-century English herbalist Nicholas Culpeper wrote: "[Mint] is very profitable to the stomach . . . especial to dissolve wind [and] help the colic. . . . It is good to repress the milk in women's breasts . . . and a very powerful medicine to stay women's courses [stop menstrual flow]. It helpeth the biting of a mad dog . . . and is good to wash the heads of young children against all manner of breaking out, sores, and scabs. . . ." But Culpeper disagreed with Dioscorides on mint and sex. Instead of calling it a lust promoter, Culpeper considered it "an especial remedy for venereal [sexual] dreams and pollutions in the night [nocturnal emissions], being applied outwardly to the testicles."

Shortly after Culpeper, peppermint and spearmint were differentiated, and herbalist decided the former was the better digestive aid, cough remedy, and treatment for colds and fever.

Menthol Rubs and Other Uses

Colonists found the Indians using native American mints to treat cough, chest congestion, and pneumonia. The colonists introduced spearmint and peppermint, and the plants quickly went wild.

By the late 19th century, the Eclectics prescribed peppermint for headache, cough, bronchitis, stomach distress, and hysteria (menstrual discomforts), and added it to laxatives to minimize intestinal cramping and disguise their unpleasant taste.

The Eclectics also valued spearmint but considered it "somewhat inferior to peppermint" except for its "superior" ability to treat fever.

Chemists distilled menthol from peppermint oil in the early 1880s. The Eclectic text, *King's American Dispensatory*, touted its "active germicidal properties," and its "considerable anesthetic power" when applied to wounds, burns, scalds, insect bites and stings, eczema, hives, and toothache. The Eclectics also used menthol vapors in inhalants and chest rubs to relieve asthma, hay fever, and morning sickness.

Contemporary herbalists recommend peppermint externally for itching and inflammations, and internally as a digestive aid and treatment for menstrual cramps, motion sickness, morning sickness, colds, cough, flu, congestion, headache, heartburn, fever, and insomnia. Some herbalists consider peppermint and spearmint interchangeable, but most call peppermint more potent. As they do with so many other aromatic herbs, herbalists also recommend these herbs for relaxing herbal baths.

HEALING with the Mints

Both spearmint and peppermint owe their value in healing to their aromatic oils. Peppermint oil is mostly menthol. Spearmint oil contains a similar chemical (carvone). These chemicals have similar properties, but as the herbalists of old believed, menthol is the more potent.

Digestive Aid. Thumbs up for the after-dinner mint. Menthol appears to soothe the smooth muscle lining of the digestive tract, making it an antispasmodic. German and Russian studies show peppermint also may help to prevent stomach ulcers and stimulate bile secretion. Thus, it may confer added benefits as an ingredient in the antacids Tums, Gelusil, BiSoDol, and Phillips' Milk of Magnesia.

Anesthetic. The Eclectics were on the right track about menthol's "considerable anesthetic power." It's an ingredient in many pain-relieving skin creams: Solarcaine, Unguentine, Ben-Gay, and Noxzema Medicated Cream.

Decongestant. Menthol vapors do, indeed, help relieve nasal, sinus, and chest congestion. Menthol is an ingredient in Mentholatum and Vicks VapoRub. Peppermint is a Food and Drug Administration–approved remedy for the common cold, primarily because of its decongestant action.

Infection Prevention. The Eclectics may also have been on the right track about menthol being "actively germicidal." Peppermint oil in the test tube kills several bacteria and the *Herpes simplex* virus, which causes cold sores and genital herpes, findings which lend some credence to peppermint's traditional uses in the treatment of wounds and bronchitis.

Women's Health. Antispasmodics soothe not only the smooth muscle lining of the digestive tract, but other smooth muscles, such as the uterus, as well. Several herbals recommend peppermint as a treatment for morning sickness. *The Toxicology of Botanical Medicines*, however, suggests medicinal concentrations of peppermint may promote menstruation.

Pregnant women who want to try peppermint for morning sickness should stick to dilute, beverage-tea concentrations rather than more potent medicinal infusions. Women with a history of miscarriage should not use this herb while pregnant. Other women may try peppermint to bring on their periods.

Rx for Mints

For wounds, burns, scalds, and herpes, apply a few drops of peppermint oil directly to the affected area.

For a possible decongestant or digestive infusion, use 1 to 2 teaspoons of dried herb per cup of boiling water. Steep 10 minutes. Drink up to 3 cups a day. Peppermint has a sharper taste than spearmint, and it cools the mouth.

In a tincture, take 1/4 to 1 teaspoon up to three times a day.

In an herbal bath, fill a cloth bag with a few handfuls of dried or fresh herb and let the water run over it.

Dilute mint preparations may be given cautiously to children under age 2.

The Safety Factor

As dried plant material, neither spearmint nor peppermint has been reported to cause problems. On rare occasions, however, the sharp, pungent fragrance of concentrated mint oils have caused gagging in young children. If you give mint teas to infants, use dilute infusions.

Alert: If ingested, pure menthol is poisonous. As little as a teaspoon (about 2 grams) can be fatal. Do not ingest pure menthol. Pure peppermint oil has also been found to produce toxic effects, such as cardiac arrhythmias. So stay away from pure peppermint oil, too.

Other Cautions

Peppermint and spearmint are included in the Food and Drug Administration's list of herbs generally regarded as safe. For otherwise healthy nonpregnant, nonnursing adults, they are considered safe in amounts typically recommended.

Mints should be used in medicinal amounts only in consultation with your doctor. If mints cause minor discomforts, such as stomach upset or diarrhea, use less or stop using it. Let your doctor know if you experience unpleasant effects or if the symptoms for which the herb is being used do not improve significantly in two weeks.

Almost Too Easy to Grow

Spearmint is a perennial that reaches 2 feet and spreads by underground root runners. It has the mint family's characteristic square stems with wrinkled, lance-shaped, serrated, 2-inch leaves, and flower spikes with whorls of small white, pink, or lilac flowers, which bloom in midsummer.

Peppermint looks like spearmint, except it grows somewhat taller, spreads by surface runners, has stems with a purplish cast, and has longer, less-wrinkled leaves.

Mints crossbreed so easily, it's often impossible to tell what's sprouting from seeds. The best way to propagate true peppermint or spearmint is to use root cuttings. Any piece of root with a joint or node can produce a plant. Contain your mint bed or plant in containers. In rich, moist, well-drained soil, under full sun or partial shade, spreading mints may become pests.

Frequent cutting encourages bushiness. Leaves may be harvested as they mature. Cut the entire plant within a few inches of the ground when the first flowers appear. Most species become woody after a few years. Dig them out and replant new root cuttings.

MISTLETOE

Christmas Gift for Blood Pressure

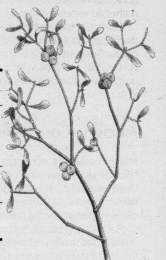

Family: Loranthaceae; all its botanical relatives are called mistletoe

Genus and species: *Viscum album* (European); *Phoradendron serotinum* (American), also known as *P. tomentosum*

Also known as: Viscum, herbe de la croix, lignum crucis

Parts used: Leaves, fruits (berries), young twigs

Mistletoe is best known as the plant under which people kiss at Christmas, a custom with an ironically gruesome origin. As a healing herb, mistletoe is also fraught with irony. One scientific authority calls it "gentle . . . [and] nontoxic." Others call it "poisonous," and insist "all parts of the plant should be regarded as toxic."

The truth lies somewhere in between. Mistletoe is potentially hazardous, but Europeans have used it extensively—and apparently safely—to help treat high blood pressure and cancer.

The Kissing Herb

We owe the herb's association with kissing to Norse mythology. Balder, god of peace, was slain by an arrow made of mistletoe. When his parents, god-king Odin and goddess-queen Frigga, restored him to life, they gave the plant to the goddess of love and decreed that anyone who passed under it should receive a kiss.

Early Christians believed mistletoe was a freestanding tree during Jesus's time and that its wood was used to make the cross. God punished the plant for its role in the crucifixion by turning it into a parasite. This story gave mistletoe its Latin name, *lignum crucis*, wood of the cross, and its French name, *herbe de la croix*.

Ancient Controversy

Mistletoe is a parasitic shrub that grows in trees, rooting into their bark. Hippocrates prescribed the herb for disorders of the spleen, but most other ancient physicians, particularly Dioscorides and Galen, advised limiting this herb to external uses, foreshadowing the current controversy over its safety.

A French medical text of 1682 recommended mistletoe for "falling sickness" (epilepsy), and some herbals still recommend it for convulsions. (Ironically, high doses may *cause* convulsions.)

Seventeenth-century English herbalist Nicholas Culpeper reiterated Hippocrates' recommendation, asserting the herb "doth mollify hardness of the spleen, and helpeth old sores." He also advocated mistletoe for "falling sickness and apoplexy [stroke]," and advised wearing a sprig around the neck to "remedy witchcraft."

Mistletoe Comes to America

Several Indian tribes used American mistletoe to induce abortions and to stimulate contractions during childbirth.

The 19th-century Eclectic text, *King's American Dispensatory*, recommended both European and American mistletoe for epilepsy, typhoid fever, dropsy (congestive heart failure), and "hysterical" (gynecological) complaints: menstrual cramps, menstruation promotion, and relief from postpartum hemorrhage. King's also warned that large amounts "possess toxic properties. Vomiting, catharsis, muscular spasms, coma, convulsions, and death have been reported from eating the leaves and berries."

Koreans use mistletoe tea to treat colds, muscle weakness, and arthritis. Chinese physicians prescribe the dried inner stems as a laxative, digestive aid, sedative, and uterine relaxant during pregnancy.

American Versus European

Somewhere along the line, herbalists came to believe European and American mistletoe had opposite effects. European mistletoe was reputed to reduce blood pressure and soothe the digestive tract, while the American herb was said to raise blood pressure and stimulate uterine and intestinal contractions.

Contemporary herbalists are divided on mistletoe. Some say the two varieties have opposite effects. Others make no distinctions between them. Some consider the herb calming, asserting it reduces blood pressure, quiets the heart, and relaxes the nervous system. Others say it raises blood pressure and stimulates uterine contractions. In *The Herb Book*, John Lust, M.D., calls the berries poisonous: "Children's deaths have been attributed to eating them." In *Weiner's Herbal*, Michael Weiner, Ph.D., disputes this: "There is good reason to believe . . . the reports of adverse effects and even death . . . are incorrect. There was no evidence . . . the plant material ingested was really mistletoe."

HEALING with Mistletoe

Despite the traditional belief that European and American mistletoe have opposite actions, science has found out that they contain similar active chemicals and have similar effects. Mistletoe has the ability to slow the pulse, stimulate gastrointestinal and uterine contractions, and lower blood pressure.

Blood Pressure. Mistletoe contains substances that may raise blood pressure as well as substances that may lower it, but blood pressure reduction appears to predominate. In Germany, where herbal medicine is considerably more mainstream than it is in the United States, mistletoe extract is an ingredient in many medications prescribed to reduce blood pressure. German medical herbalist Rudolph Fritz Weiss, M.D., writes: "Anyone who treats hypertension [high blood pressure] will confirm that mistletoe by mouth has definite benefit. . . . For a gentle antihypertensive drug that is well tolerated . . . and nontoxic in the usual dosage . . . mistletoe is the drug of choice." High blood pressure is a serious condition requiring medical treatment. Use the herb only with the permission and supervision of your doctor.

Immune Stimulant. In one experiment, cells damaged by X-ray radiation regenerated more quickly when exposed to a commercial mistletoe extract (the Swiss drug, Iscador).

Cancer Treatment. Studies going back 25 years show mistletoe impairs the growth of test-tube tumor cells. In Germany, three mistletoe-based chemotherapy agents are administered by injection to treat human cancers. These drugs have reportedly shown significant benefit in treating lung and ovarian tumors. Dr. Weiss writes: "The great advantage offered by mistletoe extracts is that unlike [other chemotherapeutic] drugs, their . . . immunostimulant and tonic effects . . . are nontoxic and well tolerated."

Mistletoe has not been seriously investigated in the United States for cancer treatment, however, because of its reputation as a poison. Ironically, many approved cancer drugs are also toxic.

R$_x$ for Mistletoe

Mistletoe should be used only under the close supervision of a physician who has knowledge of herbs. To treat high blood pressure, Dr. Weiss recommends a tea made of equal parts of mistletoe, hawthorn, and balm. "Infuse 2 teaspoons of the mixture for 5 to 10 minutes. Take 1 cup in the morning and 1 at night." Other herbalists recommend 1 cup a day of an infusion made from 1 teaspoon of freshly dried plant steeped in 1 cup of boiling water for 10 minutes.

In a tincture, the recommended dose for blood pressure control is 5 drops per day.

Mistletoe should not be given to children, and it may have unexpected effects in the elderly.

The Safety Factor

Most authorities on this side of the Atlantic scoff at Dr. Weiss's suggestion that mistletoe is "gentle, nontoxic, and well tolerated." The Food and Drug Administration calls it unsafe and has not approved any mistletoe preparation for treatment of any disease. In Natural Product Medicine, pharmacognosists Ara Der Marderosian, Ph.D., and Lawrence Liberti speak for most American experts when they write: "Mistletoe's use should be discouraged because of the documented toxicity associated with ingestion of all parts of the plant."

How toxic is it? The Eclectics reported coma, convulsions, and deaths from ingestion of large doses of mistletoe leaves and berries. J. M. Kingsbury's classic book, Poisonous Plants of the United States, reported one fatality from an overdose of berries. And Dr. Der Marderosian and Liberti report two mistletoe deaths, one from mistletoe tea intended as a tonic and another from high doses of the herb used to induce abortion.

On the other hand, a recent review of more than 300 cases of mistletoe ingestion in Annals of Emergency Medicine showed no deaths, and a majority of those who ingested the plant—typically its berries—developed no symptoms of poisoning. The investigators concluded that while mistletoe is potentially toxic, adult ingestion of up to three berries or two leaves is unlikely to produce serious poisoning.

Keep It Away from Children

Child fatalities, however, have been reported from as few as two berries. Keep mistletoe out of the reach of children. If you hang it at Christmas, secure it carefully and explain to children that its berries should never be eaten—or remove the berries.

Caution for Women

Mistletoe contains a chemical (tyramine) that may stimulate uterine contractions. Pregnant women should not use it, except possibly at term and only under the supervision of a physician to induce labor.

Mistletoe's abortion-inducing dose is close to its fatal dose. This herb should never be used to terminate pregnancy.

Those taking any MAO inhibitor antidepressant (Marplan, Nardil, Parnate) also should not use mistletoe, because the interaction of these drugs and the herb might cause a serious elevation in blood pressure, resulting in loss of consciousness.

Mistletoe may slow heart rate. People with heart disease or a history of stroke should not use it.

Other Cautions

Mistletoe may be used cautiously in low doses but only under the supervision of a medical professional. For otherwise healthy nonpregnant, nonnursing adults who are not taking MAO inhibitors or other blood pressure medications, mistletoe is thought to be relatively safe when used cautiously in small amounts for brief periods.

Mistletoe should be used in medicinal amounts only in consultation with your doctor. If mistletoe causes minor discomforts, such as stomach upset or diarrhea, use less or stop using it. Let your doctor know if you experience unpleasant effects or if the symptoms for which the herb is being used do not improve significantly in two weeks.

If any symptoms of toxicity develop—nausea, vomiting, diarrhea, headache, decreased heart rate, hallucinations, muscle spasms, or convulsions—seek emergency treatment immediately. At high doses, fatalities typically occur within ten hours of ingestion.

The Christmas Parasite

Both European and American mistletoe are parasitic, branching, woody, evergreen shrubs that live on a large number of trees. The European herb has thin, leathery, tonguelike, 2-inch leaves. The American variety also has leathery leaves, but they are broader and up to 3 inches long. Both plants produce small, sticky white berries, which contain single seeds.

Mistletoe is well adapted to its aerial existence. Its sticky white berries attract birds, which carry them to perches in other trees. The birds eat some but drop others, which stick to the tree bark. Within a few days, the seeds inside newly "planted" mistletoe berries produce tiny roots, which bore their way into the host tree and establish new plants.

Mistletoe is gathered from the wild, not cultivated, but some crafters of mistletoe Christmas products reportedly "plant" the sticky seeds by inserting them into the bark of host trees.

MOTHERWORT

Tranquilizer and Stimulant

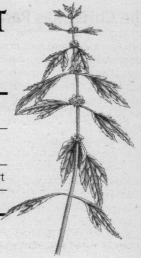

Family: Labiatae; other members include mints

Genus and species: *Leonurus cardiaca*

Also known as: Lion's tail, heartwort

Parts used: Leaves, flowers, stems

otherwort is a misleading name for this healing herb. The herb is more likely to prevent motherhood than promote it. And despite one of its popular names, lion's tail, motherwort won't strengthen the lion-hearted. In fact, it's more apt to turn lions into lambs.

Good Cheer and Long Life

The ancient Greeks and Romans used motherwort for both physical and emotional problems of the heart—palpitations and depression.

In ancient China, motherwort was reputed to promote longevity. According to legend, a youth was banished from his village for a minor crime to a remote valley with a spring surrounded by motherwort. He supposedly lived to be 300.

In Europe, motherwort first became known as a treatment

for cattle diseases. Sixteenth-century herbalist John Gerard called it "a remedy against certain diseases in cattell . . . and for that husbandmen much desire it." Gerard also recommended it for "infirmities of the heart."

Seventeenth-century English herbalist Nicholas Culpeper wrote: "There is no better herb to take meloncholy vapors from the heart . . . and make a merry, cheerful soul." Culpeper viewed this herb primarily as an antidepressant; however, he mentioned, "it is . . . of much use in trembling of the heart [palpitations], and faintings, and swoonings, from whence it took the name cardiaca. . . . It took the name motherwort [because] it settles mothers' wombs . . . and is a wonderful help to women in their sore travail [delivery]. . . . It also provoketh women's courses [menstruation]."

As the centuries passed, herbalists used motherwort in contradictory ways—both to relax the uterus during pregnancy and after childbirth, and to stimulate menstruation and labor. Eventually it came to be viewed as a uterine stimulant.

Colonists introduced motherwort into North America, and the 19th-century Eclectics recommended it as a menstruation promoter and aid to expelling the afterbirth. They also prescribed it as a tranquilizer for "morbid nervous excitement, and all diseases with restlessness [and] disturbed sleep." The Eclectics did not consider it a heart remedy at all.

Contemporary herbalists recommend motherwort as a tranquilizer and for heart palpitations and delayed or suppressed menstruation.

HEALING with Motherwort

Until recently, scientists dismissed motherwort as useless. But studies have indicated that the ancients who named this herb *cardiaca* may have been onto something.

Heart Disease. Test-tube studies in China show motherwort relaxes heart cells, which lends some support to its ancient use in calming palpitations. Other Chinese studies suggest motherwort helps prevent the internal blood clots that trigger heart attack. And Russian researchers suggest the herb contains chemicals that reduce blood pressure. These findings are preliminary, but they support the ancient view that motherwort has a general tonic effect on the heart.

In otherwise healthy adults, occasional heart palpitations are usually no cause for alarm. However, they may also be a sign of disturbances in heart rhythm (cardiac arrhythmia), which is potentially serious and requires professional attention. If you experience frequent palpitations, consult your physician.

If you have high blood pressure or heart disease and would like to incorporate motherwort into your treatment plan, do so only with approval and supervision from your physician.

Tranquilizer. German studies show motherwort has mild sedative action, comparable to valerian, making it potentially effective against insomnia or anxiety.

Women's Health. Not many tranquilizers are also uterine stimulants, but motherwort contains a chemical (leonurine) that encourages uterine contractions, lending support to its traditional use in childbirth and menstruation promotion.

Pregnant women should not use it, except possibly at term and only under the supervision of a physician, to help stimulate labor. For other women, it may help bring on their periods.

Rx for Motherwort

For a possible tranquilizing, uterine stimulating, blood pressure–lowering infusion, use 1 to 2 teaspoons of dried herb per cup of boiling water. Steep 10 minutes. Drink up to 2 cups a day, a tablespoon at a time. Motherwort tastes very bitter. Add sugar, honey, and lemon, or mix it into an herbal beverage tea to improve flavor.

In a tincture, take ½ to 1 teaspoon up to twice a day.

Motherwort should not be given to children under age 2. For older children and people over 65, start with low-strength preparations and increase strength if necessary.

The Safety Factor

Motherwort's possible anticlotting effect means those with clotting disorders should avoid it.

Some people develop a rash from contact with this plant.

The Food and Drug Administration lists motherwort as an herb of "undefined safety." For otherwise healthy nonpregnant, nonnursing adults who do not have clotting disorders and are not taking other sedative, heart, or blood pressure medications, motherwort is considered relatively safe in amounts typically recommended.

Motherwort should be used in medicinal amounts only in consultation with your doctor. If motherwort causes minor discomforts, such as stomach upset or diarrhea, use less or stop using it. Let your doctor know if you experience unpleasant effects or if the symptoms for which the herb is being used do not improve significantly in two weeks.

Harvest Tranquilizing Flowers

Motherwort's perennial root gives rise to stout, square stems tinged with red or violet, which grow to 4 feet. Its lower leaves are sharply lobed, like maple. Its upper leaves are narrow and toothed. Motherwort produces whorls of small white, pink, or red flowers which bloom in summer.

Motherwort grows so easily, it may become a pest. Plant seeds in spring and thin seedlings to 12-inch spacing. Motherwort prefers rich, moist, well-drained soil and full sun but tolerates considerably less ideal conditions. Harvest the entire plant after the flowers blossom.

MULLEIN

A Velvety Soother

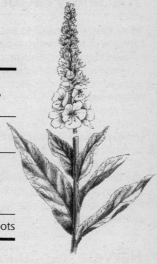

Family: Scrophulariaceae; other members include figwort, foxglove, eyebright

Genus and species: *Verbascum thapsus*

Also known as: Candlewick plant, torches, velvet dock, flannel plant, feltwort, Aaron's rod, shepherd's staff, lungwort

Parts used: Leaves, flowers, and roots

Mullein (it rhymes with sullen) grows everywhere and is hard to miss, yet few who encounter the velvet-leafed weed with its rodlike stem and striking yellow flowers appreciate its place in herbal healing as a treatment for some respiratory complaints.

Candlewick Plant

When dried, mullein burns readily. Before the introduction of cotton, the ancients used its leaves and stems as candle wicks, giving it the name candlewick plant. The dried stems and flowers were also dipped in suet to make them burn longer, hence one popular name, torches.

Ancient cultures around the world considered mullein a magical protector against witchcraft and evil spirits. Like other herbs used in magic, mullein has a long history as a healer. Its botanical family name, the Scrophularia-ceae, is derived from *scrofula*, an old term for chronically

swollen lymph glands, later identified as a form of tuberculosis.

The Greek physician Dioscorides prescribed a decoction
of mullein root in wine as a treatment for "lask and fluxes of
the belly" (diarrhea). During the Middle Ages, the French used
the herb to treat *malandre*, an animal disease that produces
boils on horses' necks. *Malandre* eventually became *malen*, and
finally *mullein*.

Respiratory Remedy

Early on, this herb gained a reputation as a respiratory remedy, which endures to this day. In ancient India, Ayurvedic
physicians prescribed mullein for cough. English herbalist
Nicholas Culpeper wrote that gargling a mullein decoction
"easeth toothache . . . and old cough." And herbalist William
Coles wrote farmers "give it their cattle against cough. . . ."

Colonists introduced mullein into North America, and the
Indians quickly adopted it for coughs, bronchitis, and asthma.
The accepted way to take mullein in early America seems
ridiculous today: People *smoked* it.

The 19th-century Eclectics viewed mullein as a diuretic to
treat water retention and as a stomach and respiratory
soother, with mild pain-relieving and tranquilizing action.
King's American Dispensatory asserted: "Upon the upper portion
of the respiratory tract, its influence is pronounced." The
Eclectics recommended mullein for colds, coughs, asthma,
and tonsillitis, as well as diarrhea, hemorrhoids, and urinary
tract infection.

Contemporary herbalists recommend mullein internally for
coughs, colds, sore throat, and other respiratory complaints,
and externally in a hot vinegar compress for hemorrhoids.

During the late 19th and early 20th centuries, mullein was
listed in the *National Formulary* as a cough remedy, but it
was deleted in 1936 for lack of effectiveness. Nonetheless, in a
1986 survey of folk medicine in Indiana, Purdue researcher
and herb expert Varro Tyler, Ph.D., found mullein "a very
popular Hoosier remedy for all types of respiratory complaints."

HEALING with Mullein

In the test tube, at least, mullein inhibits the growth of the bacteria that causes tuberculosis, so perhaps it was of some value against scrofula. Today it's used mostly to soothe minor respiratory irritation.

Cough and Sore Throat. Mullein contains a substance called mucilage, which swells and becomes slippery as it absorbs water. This probably accounts for its soothing action on the throat. German medical herbalist Rudolph Fritz Weiss, M.D., writes that mullein has a "well-founded reputation as a cough remedy."

Hemorrhoids. Mullein possibly does more than help soothe hemorrhoids. It also contains tannins, which are astringent. And one study showed the herb has anti-inflammatory properties as well.

Diarrhea. Mullein's astringent tannins probably account for its traditional use in treating diarrhea.

R$_x$ for Mullein

For an infusion that can help soothe cough and sore throat and that may help treat diarrhea, use 1 to 2 teaspoons of dried leaves, flowers, or roots per cup of boiling water. Steep 10 minutes. Drink up to 3 cups a day. Mullein tastes bitter; add sugar, honey, and lemon, or mix it into an herbal beverage blend to improve flavor.

To help treat hemorrhoids, apply a compress made with a strong, cooled infusion.

In a tincture, take ½ to 1 teaspoon up to three times a day.

Dilute mullein infusions may be given cautiously to children under age 2 to help soothe persistent coughs.

The Safety Factor

Mullein seeds are toxic and may cause poisoning. There have been no reports, however, of adverse effects from the herb's leaves, flowers, and roots.

Tannins have both pro- and anti-cancer effects. Scientists are not sure which way the balance tilts. Anyone with a history of cancer should not take mullein internally.

The Food and Drug Administration includes mullein in its list of herbs generally regarded as safe. For otherwise healthy nonpregnant, nonnursing adults, mullein is considered safe in amounts typically recommended.

Mullein should be used in medicinal amounts only in consultation with your doctor. If mullein causes minor discomforts, such as stomach upset or diarrhea, use less or stop using it. Let your doctor know if you experience unpleasant effects or if the symptoms for which the herb is being used do not improve significantly in two weeks.

The Fuzzy Plant That Keeps on Giving

Mullein is a hardy biennial that grows almost anywhere in temperate climes. During its first year, it produces a rosette of large, hairy, tongue-shaped, greenish white, 6- to 15-inch leaves, hence many of its common names: velvet dock, flannel plant, and feltwort. In its second year, mullein sends up a solitary, fibrous stem that reaches 3 to 6 feet, the source of such names as Aaron's rod and shepherd's staff. A striking, cylindrical spike of small, dense, yellow flowers develops atop the stem.

Mullein grows easily from seeds in light sandy soil under full sun, but it tolerates other conditions. Sow seeds in spring after danger of frost has passed.

Harvest up to one-third of the leaves during the plant's first year. Harvest the rest the following year before the flowers bloom. Pick the flowers as they open. Harvest the roots during autumn.

Mullein is a prolific self-sower. Many authorities recommend removing the flower head before the seeds ripen to keep it under control.

MYRRH

Thoroughly Modern Mouthwash

Family: Burseraceae; other members include balm of Gilead, bdellium

Genus and species: *Commiphora abyssinica* or *C. myrrha*

Also known as: Balsamodendron

Parts used: The oleo-gum-resin from the stem

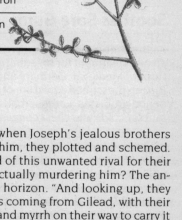

The Bible tells us that when Joseph's jealous brothers decided to dispose of him, they plotted and schemed. How could they get rid of this unwanted rival for their father's affection without actually murdering him? The answer soon appeared on the horizon. "And looking up, they saw a caravan of Ishmaelites coming from Gilead, with their camels bearing gum, balm, and myrrh on their way to carry it down to Egypt" (Genesis 37:25). They sold Joseph to the Ishmaelites.

This is just the first of a dozen biblical references to the hardened, tear-shaped clots of clear or reddish brown aromatic resin that exude from incisions in the bark of a small Middle Eastern tree.

First used by the ancient Egyptians in embalming mixtures, myrrh became the all-purpose biblical aromatic for perfumes, funerals, and insect repellents. Today it may help to repel tooth decay and gum disease.

Mythological Origins

The Greeks traced myrrh's teardrop shape to Myrrha, daughter of the Syrian king Thesis. Myrrha refused to worship Aphrodite, the goddess of love. Angered by this blasphemy, Aphrodite tricked her into committing incest with her father. When Thesis realized what he had done, he threatened to kill his daughter. To save her, the gods transformed her into a myrrh tree, whose teardrop resin recalls the girl's sorrow.

Ancient Greek and Roman physicians used the herb to treat wounds and prescribed it internally as a digestive aid and menstruation promoter.

Soothes Sore Gums

As the centuries passed, myrrh became valued primarily as an oral treatment for bleeding gums, mouth ulcers, and sore throat. Medieval German abbess/herbalist Hildegard of Bingen prescribed a mixture of powdered myrrh and aloe for dental problems. Later herbalists also used it as an expectorant for colds and chest congestion.

America's 19th-century Eclectics considered myrrh an external antiseptic for treatment of "indolent sores and gangrenous ulcers." They prescribed internal use for colds, laryngitis, asthma, bronchitis, indigestion, gonorrhea, sore throat, dental cavities, and bad breath. The Eclectics also warned that large amounts can have violent laxative action and cause sweating, nausea, vomiting, and accelerated heartbeat.

Contemporary herbalists recommend adding powdered myrrh to well-washed wounds as an antiseptic and consider a gargle made from the herb effective against sore throat, colds, sore teeth and gums, coughs, asthma, and chest congestion.

HEALING with Myrrh

Myrrh continues to be used as it has been for 1,000 years, for oral hygiene.

Mouthwash. Myrrh contains tannins, which have an astringent, drawing effect on tissues. Chinese researchers have identified substances in the herb that fight bacteria. And Indian scientists have discovered that the herb has anti-inflammatory action. All of these factors make it useful as a mouthwash. Myrrh tastes bitter but refreshing and may help relieve the inflammation and destroy the bacteria involved in gingivitis, the early form of gum disease. The herb is an ingredient in Odara mouthwash.

Toothpaste. Myrrh is a common ingredient in European toothpastes—it's included to help fight the bacteria that cause tooth decay. Some natural food stores in America carry one brand, Merfluan.

Intriguing Possibility. Myrrh may help prevent heart disease. Preliminary Indian studies suggest it reduces cholesterol. The herb also may help prevent the internal blood clots that trigger heart attack.

Rx for Myrrh

For a mouthwash, steep 1 teaspoon of powdered herb and 1 teaspoon of boric acid in 1 pint of boiling water. Let stand 30 minutes and strain. Use cool.

For an infusion that might help prevent heart disease, use 1 teaspoon of powdered herb per cup of boiling water. Steep 10 minutes. Drink up to 2 cups a day. Myrrh tastes bitter and unpleasant. Add sugar, honey, and lemon, or mix it into an herbal beverage blend to improve flavor.

In a tincture, take 1/4 to 1 teaspoon up to three times a day.

Myrrh should not be given to children under age 2. For older children and people over 65, start with low-strength preparations and increase strength if necessary.

The Safety Factor

Myrrh has not been shown to stimulate uterine contractions, but its traditional use as a menstruation promoter should serve as a red flag to pregnant women.

Large amounts may have violent laxative action and could cause the other symptoms the Eclectics described—sweating, nausea, vomiting, and accelerated heartbeat.

Myrrh is included in the Food and Drug Administration's list of herbs generally regarded as safe. For otherwise healthy nonpregnant, nonnursing adults, myrrh is considered safe in amounts typically recommended.

Myrrh should be used in medicinal amounts only in consultation with your doctor. If myrrh causes minor discomforts, such as stomach upset or diarrhea, use less or stop using it. Let your doctor know if you experience unpleasant effects or if the symptoms for which the herb is being used do not improve significantly in two weeks.

If gum bleeding or tooth or gum pain persists longer than two weeks, consult a dentist.

Healing Drops from Trees

Myrrh is a large shrub or small tree that grows in the Middle East and Ethiopia and Somalia. A pale yellow oil drips from cuts in its dull gray bark and hardens to form teardrop-shaped nuggets of myrrh, which are powdered for use as a healing herb.

NETTLE

Takes the Sting out of Gout

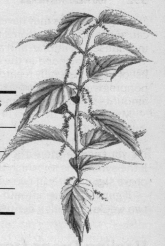

Family: Urticaceae; other members include other nettles

Genus and species: *Urtica dioica*

Also known as: Stinging nettle, common nettle, greater nettle

Parts used: Leaves and stems

Everyone agrees nettle stings hurt, but controversy surrounds the herb's use in healing. One modern herbalist calls nettle "one of the most widely applicable plants we have." Many scientists, however, say the herb "has no pharmacologic value when administered orally."

Nettle is no wonder herb, but externally it may help treat the pain of gout, and internally it may relieve hay fever symptoms and help treat high blood pressure.

Strong as Canvas

Nettle was used in weaving before it became popular in herbal healing. Archeologists have discovered nettle-fabric burial shrouds at Bronze Age sites in Denmark. In *Les Misérables*, one of Victor Hugo's characters calls nettle fabric as strong as canvas. And during World War I, when cotton was in short supply in Germany, nettle cloth was substituted.

Its use in healing also harkens back to the ancient world. Around the 3rd century B.C., Hippocrates' Greek contemporaries prescribed nettle juice externally to treat snakebites and scorpion stings and internally as an antidote to such plant poisons as hemlock and henbane.

Roman soldiers flailed themselves with nettles in cold climates because the herb's sting warmed their skin. This practice, called urtication, evolved into a treatment still used today for the joint stiffness of arthritis and the intense joint pains of gout.

From Nosebleeds to Mother's Milk

Early European herbalists touted nettle tea to treat cough and tuberculosis, and strange as this sounds today, the herb was smoked to treat asthma. Herbalists also prescribed nettle to treat scurvy and stop bleeding, particularly nosebleeds. Somewhere along the way, nettle juice gained a reputation as a hair-growth stimulant, and it remained an ingredient in hair-growth nostrums well into the 19th century.

Seventeenth-century English herbalist Nicholas Culpeper endorsed all the nettle prescriptions which preceded him, and added some of his own: "The decoction of the leaves in wine is singularly good to provoke women's courses [menstruation]."

American Indian women believed drinking nettle tea during pregnancy strengthened the fetus and eased delivery. They also used it to stop uterine bleeding after childbirth. Early settlers adopted this use, and nursing mothers also used nettle to increase their milk production.

The 19th-century Eclectics recommended nettle primarily as a diuretic to treat urinary, bladder, and kidney problems. But *King's American Dispensatory* also called it "an excellent styptic" (blood stopper) and treatment for infant diarrhea, hemorrhoids, and eczema.

Contemporary herbalists recommend nettle as a tonic "to strengthen and support the whole body." Many reiterate all the herb's traditional uses, from milk promotion to hair restoration.

HEALING with Nettle

Nettle won't grow hair, boost milk production, or guarantee easy childbirth, but science lends some support to a few of its age-old uses.

Gout. Some German researchers have shown nettle juice and infusion help relieve the pain of gout. According to German medical herbalist Rudolph Fritz Weiss, M.D., the effect "is not very powerful, but long-term use may give definite clinical results."

Gout sufferer James Duke, Ph.D., an authority on herbal healing for the U.S. Department of Agriculture, agrees nettle helps gout but prefers urtication: "Recently after a painful week, the pills my doctor prescribed had improved but not terminated the gout pain in my elbow. I stung the elbow with nettle. The sting caused momentary forgetfulness of the gout, and be it an effective remedy or coincidence, my gout subsided by nightfall. As a matter of fact, I walked and ran several miles that afternoon with no pain at all."

High Blood Pressure. Nettle also has some diuretic action. In Germany, where herbal medicine is more mainstream than it is in the United States, physicians prescribe nettle in the treatment of high blood pressure. Dr. Weiss writes: "Nettle juice is definitely useful [in] diuretic therapy. It has the advantage of being well tolerated and safe, as distinct from the [pharmaceutical] thiazides [now] so widely used."

High blood pressure is a serious condition requiring professional care. If you'd like to include nettle in your overall treatment plan, do so only with the supervision of your physician.

Nettle may be safer than thiazides, but diuretics deplete the body of potassium, an essential nutrient. If you use nettle frequently, be sure to eat foods high in potassium, such as bananas and fresh vegetables.

Pregnant and nursing women should avoid diuretics.

Congestive Heart Failure. Physicians often prescribe diuretics to combat the fluid accumulation involved in this condition. Heart failure demands professional care. If you'd like to include nettle in your overall treatment plan, do so only with approval from and supervision by your physician.

Hay Fever. A study at the National College of Naturopathic Medicine in Portland indicated that two 300-milligram capsules of freeze-dried stinging nettle provide significant relief from the symptoms of hay fever. These capsules are not available outside research facilities, but you might try an infusion and see if it works for you.

Premenstrual Syndrome. Diuretics help relieve the bloated feeling caused by premenstrual fluid buildup. Women bothered by PMS might want to try some nettle during their premenstrual days.

Scurvy. Nettle is high in vitamin C, which supports its traditional use in treating scurvy.

Intriguing Possibility. One German study suggests stinging nettle juice might relieve symptoms of noncancerous prostate enlargement (benign prostatic hypertrophy).

Rx for Nettle

For juice used to help treat the pain of gout and possibly help with prostate enlargement, process fresh plant material in a juicer.

For a pleasantly warming infusion for possible help in the treatment of high blood pressure, congestive heart failure, and hay fever, use 1 to 2 teaspoons of dried herb per cup of boiling water. Steep 10 minutes. Drink up to 2 cups a day.

In a tincture, use 1/4 to 1 teaspoon up to twice a day.

Nettle should not be given to children under age 2. For older children and people over 65, start with low-strength preparations and increase strength if necessary.

The Safety Factor

This herb's sting is its major problem. If you harvest it, wear strong gloves, a long-sleeved shirt, and long pants.

Herbal folklore is filled with remedies for nettle stings. An age-old recommendation is to rub the affected area with nettle juice. Rubbing with other herbs—rosemary, sage, or mint—also reputedly helps. But the most famous nettle remedy is dock, immortalized in this old British rhyme: "Nettle in, dock out/Dock rub, nettle out." Nonherbal treatments for nettle stings include washing with soap and water, topical hydrocortisone creams (Cort-Aid), and oral antihistamines.

Large doses of nettle tea may cause stomach irritation, burning skin, and urinary suppression.

Some diet programs tout diuretics to eliminate water weight. But weight-control authorities discourage diuretics. Weight lost using diuretics almost invariably returns. The key to permanent weight control is a low-fat, high-fiber diet and regular aerobic exercise.

Nettle stimulates uterine contractions in rabbits. Pregnant women should not use it internally.

Other Cautions

The Food and Drug Administration considers nettle an herb of "undefined safety." For otherwise healthy nonpregnant, nonnursing adults who are not taking other diuretics, nettle is considered relatively safe in amounts typically recommended.

Nettle should be used in medicinal amounts only in consultation with your doctor. If nettle causes minor discomforts, such as stomach upset or diarrhea, use less or stop using it. Let your doctor know if you experience unpleasant effects or if the symptoms for which the herb is being used do not improve significantly in two weeks.

Plants That Burn

Stinging nettle is only one of 500 species of *Urtica*, a name derived from the Latin *uro*, to burn. And burn they do. Just be thankful the Javanese species, U. *urentissima*, doesn't grow in North America. Its burn is reputed to last a year.

Nettle's erect stem grows from a creeping underground rhizome. It has opposite, serrated, dark green, heart-shaped leaves, and male and female flowers grow on separate plants (dioecious). The hairs that give this herb a downy appearance are actually hollow needles attached to sacs filled with irritant chemicals. Brushing against the plant bends the hairs, squeezing the irritants onto the skin of the hapless passerby.

Nettles grow very easily from seeds or root divisions in just about any soil. Plant seeds in spring. Take root divisions in autumn after the leaves have died back.

Harvest the leaves (wearing gloves and protective clothing) before the plants flower in late spring or early summer. Young leaves may be boiled or steamed like spinach and eaten as a vegetable. Boiling or drying eliminates the sting. The fresh tender shoots do not sting and may be used in salads.

Nettles have a reputation for increasing the aromatic oil content of angelica, marjoram, oregano, peppermint, sage, valerian, and other fragrant herbs. Nettles also reputedly help decomposition in compost.

OREGANO

Pizza for Colds

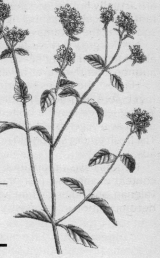

Family: Labiatae; other members include marjoram, mint; Verbenaceae; other members include vervain, teak; Asteraceae; other members include aster; Scrophulariaceae; other members include mullein

Genus and species: Primarily *Origanum vulgare, O. heracleoticum, O. onites,* and *Lippia graveolens,* but also more than 40 other plants

Also known as: Wild marjoram, Mexican wild sage

Parts used: Leaves and stems

To most Americans, oregano is simply the seasoning on pizza. But to botanists, the word *oregano* can be a real headache. More than 40 plants in four botanical families go by the name oregano. For healing, this confusion doesn't matter much. All the plants called oregano taste similar and contain a similar oil, so they probably have similar effects.

Traditional Chinese physicians have used oregano for centuries to treat fever, vomiting, diarrhea, jaundice, and itching skin conditions.

Much More Than a Topping

Europeans used it like marjoram, as an aromatic spice and as a digestive aid, arthritis treatment, expectorant for cough, colds, flu, and chest congestion, and as a menstruation promoter.

America's 19th-century Eclectic physicians considered oregano "a gently stimulant tonic" and menstruation promoter. Other folk healers used oregano oil to treat toothache, relieve arthritis, and grow hair on bald heads.

Contemporary herbalists call oregano an expectorant, digestive aid, mild tranquilizer, and menstruation promoter.

HEALING with Oregano

Oregano won't grow hair on bald heads, but next time you have a cough or bronchitis, try a pizza with extra oregano. (If it doesn't help, at least it will taste good.)

Cough Remedy, Expectorant. All the oreganos contain a volatile oil high in two chemically related expectorants (carvacrol and thymol). They help loosen phlegm and make it easier to cough up, lending credence to the herb's traditional use in colds, flu, and chest congestion.

Digestive Aid. Like most culinary spices, oregano helps soothe the smooth muscle lining of the digestive tract, making it an antispasmodic. It may also help expel parasitic intestinal worms. These attributes lend support to its age-old use as a digestive aid.

Rx for Oregano

For a warm, aromatic, spicy infusion to help settle the stomach after meals or to help treat a cold, use 1 to 2 teaspoons of dried herb per cup of boiling water. Steep 10 minutes. Drink up to 3 cups a day.

Medicinal doses of these herbs should not be given to children under age 2.

The Safety Factor

Antispasmodic herbs often quiet the uterus as well as the digestive tract, but oregano appears to be an exception. The herb has never been scientifically shown to stimulate uterine contractions, but it has a long history as a menstruation promoter. One Oakland, California, pizza parlor enjoys a considerable local reputation for triggering labor in pregnant women at term. Who knows? Maybe it's the oregano. Pregnant women may use culinary amounts, but they should stay away from medicinal preparations.

The medical literature contains no reports of harm from oregano.

For otherwise healthy nonpregnant, nonnursing adults, all the oreganos are considered safe in amounts typically recommended.

Oregano should be used in medicinal amounts only in consultation with your doctor. If oregano causes minor discomforts, such as stomach upset or diarrhea, use less or stop using it. Let your doctor know if you experience any unpleasant effects or if the symptoms for which the herb is being used do not improve significantly in two weeks.

Harvest Your Own Spice

Among the dozens of plants called oregano, authorities generally recommend O. *heracleoticum* as the most flavorful and aromatic. It may be propagated from seeds, cuttings, or root divisions. Seeds are sometimes slow to germinate. For best aroma and flavor, O. *heracleoticum* needs light, well-drained, slightly alkaline soil and full sun. Harvest when the plants begin to bloom.

Another tasty oregano is *Lippia graveolens*. It grows outdoors in the South and Southwest. Elsewhere it must be grown indoors in containers in sunny, south-facing windows. The soil should be well drained but need not be especially rich. Harvest when the plant begins to bloom.

PAPAYA

Tropical Digestive Aid

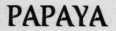

Family: Caricaceae; other members include custard apple

Genus and species: *Carica papaya*

Also known as: Pawpaw, melon tree

Parts used: Fruit, leaves, and latex

Fruit with seeds

Cookbooks warn that Jell-O won't gel if you add pineapple. The same is true if you add papaya, only more so. Both fruits contain digestive enzymes that prevent the proteins in gelatin from solidifying. Papaya's powerful enzymes are key to its healing value as a digestive aid.

Super Meat Tenderizer

Centuries ago, the Caribbean Indians noticed that meat wrapped in papaya's broad leaves becomes more tender. Today papaya extract is the active ingredient in most commercial meat tenderizers.

The Indians also cut incisions into mature but unripe papayas, collected the milky fluid (latex), and applied it to the skin to treat psoriasis, ringworm, wounds, and infections. Caribbean Indian women ate unripe papayas to trigger menstruation, abortion, and labor.

After Europeans introduced papaya into tropical Asia, it quickly became incorporated into healing. Filipinos used a root decoction to treat hemorrhoids. The Javanese believed eating papaya fruit prevented arthritis. The Japanese used the latex to treat digestive disorders. And throughout Asia, the leaves were applied to wounds, and the latex was dabbed onto the cervix at term to stimulate labor.

Papaya was not used in traditional American herbal medicine. But in the last 25 years, as tropical fruits have become widely available, papaya has become quite popular, and the plant's leaves and latex have become available through specialty herb outlets.

Contemporary herbalists recommend papaya fruit and leaf infusions as digestive aids, for stomach upset, and to eliminate intestinal worms. Herbalists suggest applying the leaves and latex externally to wounds.

HEALING with Papaya

Papaya leaf, latex, and fruit contain several digestive enzymes, which account for the herb's action as a digestive aid and its ability to tenderize, that is, predigest, meat. The latex contains the most enzymes, followed by the leaves, and lastly the fruit, though the fruit still contains enough to aid digestion.

Digestive Aid. The most important digestive enzyme in papaya is papain, similar to the human digestive enzyme pepsin, which helps break down proteins. In fact, papain is sometimes called vegetable pepsin. The herb's other enzymes include one similar to human rennin, which breaks down milk proteins, and another similar to pectase, which helps digest starches.

Ulcer Prevention. One animal study shows papaya exerts a direct effect on the stomach, helping to prevent ulcers. Two groups of experimental animals were fed high doses of ulcer-inducing aspirin and steroids. Those fed papaya for six days prior to the ulcer-producing drugs developed significantly fewer ulcers. This finding suggests papaya may prove of special benefit to arthritis sufferers who take high doses of aspirin and to people with inflammatory conditions who take steroids.

Contact Lenses. Papain is an active ingredient in the enzyme cleaning solutions that were developed to be used with soft contact lenses.

Slipped Disks. In 1982 the Food and Drug Administration approved another papaya enzyme, chymopapain, as a treatment for herniated ("slipped") vertebral disks in the back. Injected directly into the affected area, the chymopapain helps dissolve cellular debris.

R$_x$ for Papaya

Papaya fruit is ripe when soft. It tastes similar to cantaloupe. Have some as an appetizer before meals to help digestion.

For a pleasant-tasting infusion that will aid digestion, use 1 to 2 teaspoons of dried leaves per cup of boiling water. Steep 10 minutes. Drink during or after meals, especially those high in protein (red meat and dairy). Do not boil papaya leaves, as boiling deactivates the papain.

Papaya fruit may be given to children under age 2. Papaya leaf tea should be given cautiously.

The Safety Factor

Pregnant women may eat ripe papaya fruit in moderation but should stay away from papaya latex and medicinal doses of the herb's leaves. It was used in many cultures as a menstruation promoter and labor inducer. In addition, one study in which papain was administered orally to experimental animals shows that it causes birth defects and fetal death in animals.

Some allergic reactions, including asthma, have been reported.

Papaya latex may cause stomach inflammation (gastritis).

For otherwise healthy nonpregnant, nonnursing adults, papaya is considered safe in amounts typically recommended.

Papaya should be used in medicinal amounts only in consultation with your doctor. If papaya causes minor discomforts, such as stomach upset, use less or stop using it. Let your doctor know if you experience any unpleasant effects or if the symptoms for which the herb is being used do not improve significantly in two weeks.

Melon Tree

If you're lucky enough to live in the tropics, you can grow your own papaya tree.

Native to the Caribbean and now naturalized throughout the tropics, a papaya tree can reach 25 feet. Its trunk is hollow, with spongy wood and fibrous light-colored bark that is used to make rope. Its leaves are smooth, hand-shaped (palmate), and large, often 2 feet across.

The fruits are yellow-green, pear-shaped melons with tasty orange-yellow pulp. Papayas sold in the United States are typically about the size of large potatoes. But in the tropics, they grow to the size of large honeydews and can weigh up to 10 pounds. That's where the name melon tree comes from.

PARSLEY

More Than Just a Garnish

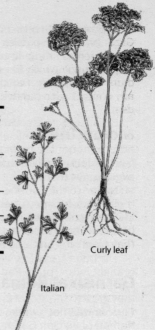

Family: Umbelliferae; other members include carrot, celery, fennel, dill, angelica

Genus and species: *Petroselinum crispum, P. hortense, P. sativum*

Also known as: Rock selinon

Parts used: Leaves, fruits ("seeds"), roots

Curly leaf

Italian

ew herbs are more familiar than parsley. Its lacy sprigs typically adorn restaurant plates—and usually remain uneaten. This is unfortunate, for parsley is nutritious and an effective after-dinner breath freshener. Medicinally, however, this herb is controversial. In *The New Honest Herbal*, Varro Tyler, Ph.D., dismisses it as "essentially worthless." But in the German medical text *Herbal Medicine*, Rudolph Fritz Weiss, M.D., calls it "a major medicinal plant."

Rich in Symbolism

Parsley is one of the first herbs to appear in spring, and it has been used for centuries in the Seder, the ritual Jewish Passover meal, as a symbol of new beginnings.

406

The ancient Greeks, however, saw the herb differently. In Greek mythology, parsley sprang from the blood of Opheltes, infant son of King Lycurgus of Nemea, who was killed by a serpent while his nanny directed some thirsty soldiers to a spring. For centuries, Greek soldiers believed any contact with parsley before battle signaled impending death.

Because of its association with death, parsley was planted on Greek graves. Ironically, this custom led to its rehabilitation. To honor the memory of important figures, the Greeks held athletic contests and crowned the winners with parsley wreaths. Over a few centuries, the herb came to symbolize strength.

But the shadow of bad luck clung to the herb well into the Middle Ages, when some Europeans considered it a Devil's herb, sure to bring disaster upon those who grew it—unless they planted it on Good Friday.

Garnish at Roman Feasts

Parsley was not widely used in ancient medicine, but the Roman physician Galen prescribed it for "falling sickness" (epilepsy) and as a diuretic to treat water retention. The Romans also munched sprigs at banquets to freshen their breath—the origin of the parsley garnish on restaurant plates today.

Medieval German abbess/herbalist Hildegard of Bingen prescribed parsley compresses for arthritis and parsley boiled in wine for chest and heart pain.

Seventeenth-century English herbalist Nicholas Culpeper reiterated Galen's recommendations and added to them, prescribing parsley to "provoke urine and women's courses [menstruation] . . . to expel wind . . . to break the stone [kidney stones] and ease the pains and torments thereof . . . and against cough." Culpeper also recommended parsley compresses for inflamed eyes and black-and-blue marks and suggested the herb "fried with butter and applied to [the] breasts" for nipple soreness as a result of nursing.

Parsley Uses in America

From the 1850s through 1926, parsley was recognized by the United States Pharmacopoeia as a laxative, a diuretic for kidney problems and fluid accumulation due to congestive heart failure, and as a substitute for quinine to treat malaria.

The Eclectic text, King's American Dispensatory, echoed the Pharmacopoeia and chronicled the 1855 isolation of a chemical (apiol) from parsley oil, which it recommended for "menstrual derangements," though high doses caused "intoxication, giddiness, flashes of light, vertigo, and ringing in the ears [tinnitus]."

During the early 20th century, large doses of apiol were used to induce abortion, despite its considerable toxicity.

Contemporary herbalists recommend parsley in cooking as a rich source of vitamins A and C. They suggest the fresh herb as a breath freshener and the infusion or tincture as a diuretic, digestive aid, and gas expeller.

HEALING with Parsley

Parsley root, leaves, and fruit (seeds) all contain the volatile oil, but it is most concentrated in the seeds. Parsley oil contains two major chemicals (apiol and myristicin) with mild laxative and significant diuretic action.

High Blood Pressure. Physicians often prescribe diuretics to treat this condition, and a published study in the American Journal of Chinese Medicine suggests parsley's diuretic action can help control it. In Germany, where herbal medicine is more mainstream than it is in the United States, parsley seed tea is widely prescribed as a diuretic to treat high blood pressure. Further study is needed to determine if parsley does indeed help in the treatment of high blood pressure.

High blood pressure is a serious health problem requiring professional care. If you'd like to include parsley in your overall treatment plan, do so only with the approval of your physician.

Diuretics deplete the body of potassium, an essential nutrient. If you use medicinal parsley preparations frequently, be sure to eat foods high in potassium, such as bananas and fresh vegetables.

Pregnant and nursing women should avoid diuretics.

Congestive Heart Failure. Physicians often prescribe diuretics to combat the fluid accumulation involved in this condition. Heart failure demands professional care. If you'd like to include parsley in your overall treatment plan, do so with the approval and supervision of your physician.

Breath Freshener. Parsley also contains one of the highest levels of chlorophyll of any herb. Chlorophyll is the active ingredient in many breath fresheners (Clorets), thus supporting a use of parsley dating back to Roman times.

Women's Health. Both apiol and myristicin are uterine stimulants. In the former Soviet Union, a preparation called Supetin, which contains 85 percent parsley juice, is used to stimulate uterine contractions during labor.

Pregnant women may eat culinary amounts of parsley, but they should not take medicinal preparations, except at term and under the supervision of a physician to help induce labor. Other women might try some parsley tea to bring on their periods.

Diuretics help relieve the bloated feeling caused by premenstrual fluid buildup. Women bothered by PMS might want to try some parsley during their premenstrual days.

Allergies. A study published in the *Journal of Allergy and Clinical Immunology* shows parsley inhibits the secretion of histamine, a chemical the body produces that triggers allergy symptoms. Parsley's apparent antihistamine action might help those with hay fever or hives.

Fever. Parsley has never been proven effective against malaria, so the *Pharmacopoeia* was incorrect on that score. But apiol has some fever-reducing (antipyretic) properties. Don't count on parsley to take the place of aspirin, but you may want to try it in addition to standard medications.

Intriguing Possibility. Parsley contains psoralen, a chemical best known for inducing photosensitivity. But psoralen shows promise in the treatment of one form of cancer, cutaneous T-cell lymphoma. Although it's premature to believe that parsley can be used to treat cancer, testing this herb against cancer is certainly warranted.

Rx for Parsley

To freshen breath, a few sprigs of fresh parsley usually suffice. For a pleasant-tasting infusion that may help in the management of high blood pressure, heart failure, allergies, fever, or to induce labor, use 2 teaspoons of dried leaves or root, or 1 teaspoon of bruised seeds per cup of boiling water. Steep 10 minutes. Drink up to 3 cups a day.

In a tincture, take ½ to 1 teaspoon up to three times a day.

Medicinal doses of parsley should not be given to children under age 2. For older children and people over 65, start with low-strength preparations and increase strength if necessary.

The Safety Factor

The psoralen in parsley has been known to cause skin rash in agricultural workers who harvest large quantities. Those with sensitive skin should be aware of this possibility.

The Eclectics were right about high doses of parsley oil causing headache, nausea, vertigo, giddiness, hives, and liver and kidney damage. But the medical literature contains no reports of problems from the herb itself.

Other Cautions

Parsley's potential diuretic action should not be used to promote weight loss. Some diet programs tout diuretics to eliminate water weight. But weight-control authorities discourage diuretics. Weight lost using diuretics almost invariably returns. The key to permanent weight control is a low-fat, high-fiber diet and regular aerobic exercise.

For otherwise healthy nonpregnant, nonnursing adults, parsley is generally safe in amounts typically recommended.

If symptoms of toxicity develop, use less or stop using it. Let your doctor know if you experience any unpleasant effects or if the symptoms for which the herb is being used do not improve significantly in two weeks.

Growing Healing Garnishes

Parsley is a small, bright green biennial that reaches 12 inches the first year and up to 3 feet the second year, when it flowers. Parsley has a thick carrotlike taproot and juicy stems terminating in feathery, deeply divided, curly or flat leaves, depending on the variety. Its tiny yellow-green flowers develop on the umbrella-like canopy (umbels) characteristic of the Umbelliferae.

Although it's a biennial, parsley should be cultivated as an annual. The seeds are slow to germinate, often requiring up to six weeks. Sow anytime from early spring to autumn. Parsley can be sown indoors and transplanted, but most authorities recommend outdoor planting with 1/4 inch of soil cover.

Parsley grows best in moist, sandy, well-drained loam with a neutral pH. Thin seedlings to 8-inch spacing. Late-season planting is fine. The herb—even seedlings—usually survives one or two frosts.

Leaves may be harvested once plants have reached about eight inches. Fruits are harvested when they appear full-size and gray-brown. Dig the roots during the autumn of the first year or the spring of the second.

Looks Like Hemlock

Alert: Unless you are an experienced field botanist, do not pick wild parsley. It closely resembles three potentially lethal plants: water hemlock, poison parsley (also known as poison hemlock), and fool's parsley (dog parsley, small hemlock).

PASSION-FLOWER

For Tension and Insomnia

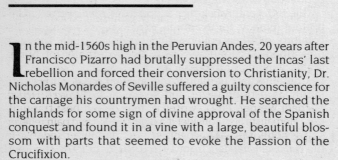

Family: Passifloraceae; other members include granadilla, sweet calabash, Jamaican honeysuckle

Genus and species: *Passiflora incarnata*

Also known as: Maypop, apricot vine, water lemon

Parts used: Leaves

In the mid-1560s high in the Peruvian Andes, 20 years after Francisco Pizarro had brutally suppressed the Incas' last rebellion and forced their conversion to Christianity, Dr. Nicholas Monardes of Seville suffered a guilty conscience for the carnage his countrymen had wrought. He searched the highlands for some sign of divine approval of the Spanish conquest and found it in a vine with a large, beautiful blossom with parts that seemed to evoke the Passion of the Crucifixion.

To Dr. Monardes, the plant's three styles represented the three nails of the Cross. Its ovary looked like a hammer. Its corona evoked the crown of thorns. And its 10 petals suggested the 10 true apostles (the original 12 minus Judas, the betrayer, and Peter, who denied Christ). Monardes christened the vine passionflower.

Some misinformed herbalists recommend passionflower tea as an aphrodisiac, mistaking the Passion of the Cross for another kind of passion. This herb has no sex-stimulant effect. Quite the contrary. It's a potential mild tranquilizer and sedative and may be good for treating anxiety, stress, insomnia, and possibly for prevention of heart attack.

Gulf Coast Cure

The Incas brewed a tonic tea from passionflower. The herb's pleasant taste and its Christian symbolism quickly turned its leaves into a popular item in Europe, where it was used as a tranquilizer and mild sedative.

When colonists settled the American Gulf Coast, they found the Indians there using passionflower tea to soothe their nerves. The Indians also used its crushed leaves in poultices on cuts and bruises. Southerners adopted passionflower as both an ornamental and medicinal vine. But it remained a folk remedy until 1839, when two Gulf Coast Eclectic physicians touted it in the *New Orleans Medical Journal* as a nonnarcotic sedative and digestive aid.

The 19th-century Eclectics adopted passionflower as "an important remedy" for insomnia, restlessness, menstrual discomforts, diarrhea, epilepsy, and whooping cough. They also prescribed passionflower leaf juice externally for burns, scalds, wounds, and toothache.

Contemporary herbalists recommend passionflower primarily as a tranquilizer and sedative. In *Weiner's Herbal*, Michael Weiner, Ph.D., writes it "may be our best tranquilizer." Herbalists also consider it a digestive aid and pain reliever.

Passionflower was recognized as a tranquilizer/sedative in the *National Formulary* from 1916 to 1936. In 1978, the Food and Drug Administration (FDA) banned it from sleep aids for lack of proven effectiveness.

HEALING with Passionflower

The FDA had a reasonable argument in 1978 before this herb had been more extensively researched, but the agency has apparently not kept up with recent findings.

Tranquilizer, Sedative. Passionflower contains substances that are potentially tranquilizing (maltol, ethyl-maltol, and flavonoids), as well as substances that are potentially stimulating (harmala chemicals). Various researchers have concluded the herb has "complex activity" on the central nervous system with an overall mild tranquilizing/sedative effect despite the presence of stimulants. In Europe, passionflower is an ingredient in many tranquilizing and sedative preparations. It's nonnarcotic, so there's no need for a prescription, and there's no possibility of addiction.

Digestive Aid. Passionflower may relax the smooth muscle lining of the digestive tract, making it an antispasmodic, thus lending credence to its traditional use as a digestive aid.

Women's Health. Antispasmodics relax not only the digestive tract but other smooth muscles, such as the uterus, as well, lending credence to passionflower's traditional use for menstrual discomforts.

Wound Treatment. One study suggests passionflower helps relieve pain. Two others show it kills many disease-causing molds, fungi, and bacteria, supporting its Indian and Eclectic use in wound treatment.

Intriguing Possibilities. In animal studies, the harmala chemicals in passionflower open (dilate) the coronary arteries. Blocked coronary arteries result in heart attack, so the herb might help prevention. Heart disease is a serious condition requiring professional care. If you'd like to incorporate passionflower into your overall treatment plan, do so only with the approval and supervision of your physician.

R$_x$ for Passionflower

For possible first aid in the garden, crush a few passionflower leaves and flowers onto minor cuts on the way to washing and bandaging them.

For a pleasant-tasting infusion that may help you relax, fall asleep, or help deal with heart disease, use 1 teaspoon of dried leaves per cup of boiling water. Steep 10 to 15 minutes.

For insomnia, drink a cup before bed. For other uses, drink up to 3 cups a day.

In a tincture, use ¼ to 1 teaspoon up to three times a day.

Passionflower should not be given to children under age 2. For older children and people over 65, start with low-strength preparations and increase strength if necessary.

The Safety Factor

The medical literature contains no reports of harm from passionflower. However, the harmala compounds in passionflower are uterine stimulants. Whole passionflower has not been associated with miscarriage, but prudence suggests pregnant women stay away from an herb with such complex effects on the central nervous system.

Some sources warn passionflower contains cyanide, a potent poison. This is a botanical error. Ornamental blue passionflower (P. *caerulea*) contains the poison. The healing herb, P. *incarnata*, does not. When buying passionflower, check to make sure it's P. *incarnata*.

Other Cautions

For otherwise healthy nonpregnant, nonnursing adults who are not taking other tranquilizers or sedatives, passionflower is considered safe in amounts typically recommended.

Passionflower should be used in medicinal amounts only in consultation with your doctor. If passionflower causes minor discomforts, such as stomach upset or diarrhea, use less or stop using it. Let your doctor know if you experience unpleasant effects or if the symptoms for which the herb is being used do not improve significantly in two weeks.

Divine Vine

Passionflower has a perennial root with fast-growing, climbing, annual tendrils that may reach 30 feet before succumbing to frost. Passionflower's leaves are dull green, 4 to 6 inches long, and deeply divided into three to five lobes with serrated edges. Its sweet-scented white flowers are 3 inches across and tinged with purple. They bloom in May, hence the name maypops, and produce egg-sized yellow or orange edible fruits, the source of the names apricot vine and water lemon.

Passionflower grows easily from seeds, cuttings, or root runners divided in autumn. It prefers rich, slightly acidic, well-watered, well-drained loam in locations with plenty of light but shaded from strong, direct summer sun. The perennial root is hardy but may not survive temperatures below −15°F. The vine tendrils need something to climb—a fence or trellis.

Harvest the leaves around the time the flowers bloom. When generously watered, the fruits are edible and sweet.

PENNYROYAL

Good Herb with a Bad Reputation

Family: Labiatae; other members include mints

Genus and species: *Mentha pulegium* (European); *Hedeoma pulegioides* (American)

Also known as: Pulegium, hedeoma, fleabane, tickweed, mosquito plant, squawmint

Parts used: Leaves and flower tops

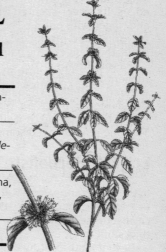

Flower detail

Few healing herbs have a reputation as bad as pennyroyal's—or as undeserved. Critics charge small amounts can be fatal. It is true that as little as 2 tablespoons of pennyroyal *oil* can cause death. But the dried herb is not dangerous. Pennyroyal's highly aromatic leaves and flower tops are a safe decongestant, cough remedy, and digestive aid.

Known as Fleabane

Pennyroyal became popular during the first century after the Roman naturalist Pliny noted the aromatic plant repelled fleas, hence its name, fleabane. When rubbed on the skin or strewn, it also repels other insects, hence such common names as tickweed and mosquito plant.

In addition to its use against fleas, Pliny touted pennyroyal as a cough remedy and digestive aid and recommended hang-

417

ing the plant in sickrooms in the belief its fragrance promoted healing. The Greek physician Dioscorides seconded Pliny's recommendations, adding that pennyroyal stimulates menstruation and helps expel the afterbirth.

During the early Middle Ages, pennyroyal was recommended for truly bizarre purposes. Physician/philosopher Saint Albertus Magnus wrote that by covering drowning bees in its warm ashes, "they shall recover their lyfe after a space of one houre," though it remains unclear why anyone would want to revive drowning bees.

English Herbalists Tout It

In the 16th century John Gerard touted pennyroyal's ancient use as an expectorant: "Penny-royale taken with honey cleanseth the lungs and cleareth the breast from all gross and thick humors."

Seventeenth-century English herbalist Nicholas Culpeper recommended the herb for many other conditions: "Drunk with wine, it is of singular service to those stung or bit by any venomous beast . . . applied to the nostrils with vinegar, it is very reviving [for] fainting . . . being dried and burnt, it strengtheneth the gums, and is helpful for those troubled with the gout . . . being applied as a plaster, it taketh away carbuncles [boils]."

Americans Adopt It

Early American colonists introduced European pennyroyal (M. *pulegium*) into North America, but found the Indians already using the American herb (H. *pulegioides*) for similar uses—externally to dress wounds and repel insects and internally to treat colds, flu, cough, congestion, and to stimulate menstruation and abortion. Folk healers also recommended aromatic pennyroyal garlands for headache and dizziness.

During the early 19th century, Thomsonian herbalists

packed pennyroyal leaves into the nostrils to treat nose-bleeds. After the Civil War, the Eclectics adopted it as a stimulant, fever treatment, digestive aid, and menstruation promoter. Their text, *King's American Dispensatory*, called it "an excellent remedy for the common cold" and recommended it for arthritis, whooping cough (pertussis), "colic in children . . . and hysteria" (menstrual discomforts).

Starting around 1887, the Eclectics were among the first to use pennyroyal oil, which they considered more convenient than the raw herb. They also recognized its potential hazards. *King's* mentioned a case of pennyroyal poisoning caused by ingesting 1 tablespoon.

From 1831 to 1916, pennyroyal was listed in the U.S. *Pharmacopoeia* as a stimulant, digestive aid, and menstruation promoter. From 1916 to 1931, pennyroyal oil was listed as an intestinal irritant and abortion inducer.

Contemporary herbalists advise against taking pennyroyal oil because of its toxicity, but they recommend using the herb externally as an insect repellent and treatment for cuts and burns. They also recommend taking the herb (not the oil) internally for colds, cough, upset stomach, flatulence, anxiety, and menstruation promotion.

Healing with Pennyroyal

Pennyroyal's oil contains one chemical (pulegone) that accounts for its actions as an insect repellent, menstruation promoter, and abortion inducer.

Insect Repellent. Pennyroyal oil is an ingredient in several natural insect repellents. It appears to help repel flies, gnats, mosquitoes, fleas, and ticks.

Decongestant and Cough Remedy. As one of the most aromatic mints, the strong aroma of pennyroyal infusion acts as a decongestant and possible expectorant.

Digestive Aid. Pennyroyal also contains chemicals similar to peppermint's menthol, which may help relax the digestive tract, though pennyroyal's stomach-soothing action is not as strong as peppermint's.

Rx for Pennyroyal

For repelling insects, rub fresh, crushed plant material around the body, or mix pennyroyal tincture into a skin cream and rub that on.

For an herbal pet flea collar, try a pennyroyal garland or a bag of the herb hung from a regular collar.

For an infusion to help treat cough, congestion, or upset stomach, use 1 to 2 teaspoons of dried herb per cup of boiling water. Steep 10 to 15 minutes. Drink up to 2 cups a day. The aroma resembles spearmint, but it's sharper and not quite as inviting. The taste is warm and pleasant, initially bitter with a cool finish.

In a tincture, use 1/4 to 1/2 teaspoon up to twice a day.

Pennyroyal should not be given to children under age 2. For older children and people over 65, start with low-strength preparations and increase strength if necessary.

The Safety Factor

Ever since pennyroyal's abortion-inducing oil was first distilled more than 100 years ago, this herb has been notorious because its oil is so toxic. Pulegone does indeed stimulate uterine contractions. Unfortunately, the dose necessary for abortion is quite close to the lethal dose, a fact that many women have learned the hard way. The British medical journal *Lancet* reported a case of abortion-related pennyroyal oil poisoning as early as 1897, and since then about a dozen similar cases have appeared in the medical literature.

As little as 1/2 teaspoon of pennyroyal oil can produce convulsions, and according to a report in the *Journal of the American Medical Association*, an 18-year-old pregnant woman died within 2 hours after taking 2 tablespoons, despite emergency treatment.

Clearly, women wishing to terminate pregnancy should not use pennyroyal oil. In fact, no one should.

Though small amounts of pennyroyal oil can be fatal, the oil is a superconcentrated extract of the herb. Drinking a few cups of pennyroyal infusion poses no hazard. University of Illinois pharmacognosist Norman Farnsworth, Ph.D., estimates it would take 75 *gallons* of strong pennyroyal infusion to approach a potentially toxic dose of pennyroyal oil.

Other Cautions

For otherwise healthy nonpregnant, nonnursing adults, pennyroyal herb—*not the oil*—is considered relatively safe in amounts typically recommended.

Pennyroyal should be used in medicinal amounts only in consultation with your doctor. If pennyroyal causes minor discomforts, such as stomach upset or diarrhea, use less or stop using it. Let your doctor know if you experience unpleasant effects or if the symptoms for which the herb is being used do not improve significantly in two weeks.

Good Soil Required

Despite their botanical differences, both European and American pennyroyal yield similar oils and are used interchangeably.

The European herb is a perennial that spreads by underground runners. Its square stems grow to about 12 inches. Its opposite, oval leaves are smooth or slightly hairy. Tight whorls of small lilac flowers appear in midsummer.

European pennyroyal may be propagated from root runner divisions in early spring or fall, or by rooting stem cuttings during summer. Both species do best in rich, well-watered, sandy, slightly acidic loam under full sun, though the European herb tolerates partial shade. European pennyroyal needs room to spread. Its runners emerge after it flowers.

American pennyroyal is an annual with square stems that reach 15 inches. Its leaves resemble those of the European variety; however, its summer-blooming flowers tend to be smaller and more bluish.

American pennyroyal must be grown from seeds sown in spring or fall. Cover them with $1/4$ inch of soil. Thin seedlings to about 5-inch spacings.

Harvest the leaves and flower tops of both plants when they are in full bloom. In the autumn, cut them a few inches above the ground and hang them to dry.

PSYLLIUM

Laxative Cholesterol Cutter

Family: Plantaginaceae; other members include about 250 Plantago species, including rib grass

Genus and species: *Plantago psyllium*

Also known as: Fleaseed, plantago, plantain

Parts used: Seeds

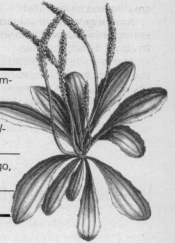

ention psyllium, and most people say, "Huh?" But mention the brand-name laxative Metamucil, and everyone says, "Oh, yes." The fact is, except for a little sweetening, coloring, and flavoring, Metamucil *is* psyllium—the seeds of a hardy plant distributed around the world. Psyllium is among the safest, gentlest laxatives, which earned it a place in herbal healing centuries ago. But recently scientists discovered psyllium also has the remarkable ability to reduce cholesterol.

Psyllium is often called plantain. However, it should not be confused with the other plantain (*Muca paradisiaca*), a palm-like tree that produces a fruit similar to bananas.

Nature's Cure to Nature's Call

For centuries, traditional Chinese and Ayurvedic physicians have used the seeds and leaves of several Asian *Plantago* species

423

to treat diarrhea, hemorrhoids, constipation, urinary problems, and more recently, high blood pressure.

Psyllium entered European folk medicine in the 16th century as a remedy for diarrhea and constipation. Seventeenth-century English herbalist Nicholas Culpeper recommended the seeds for inflammations, gout, hemorrhoids, and sore nipples (mastitis) in nursing mothers.

European physicians eventually adopted psyllium, but it was not widely used on this side of the Atlantic until after World War I. Today, psyllium is one of North America's most popular bulk-forming laxatives—the active ingredient in Metamucil, Fiberall, Hydrocil, Naturacil, Effersyllium, Pro-Lax, and V-Lax.

HEALING with Psyllium

Up to 30 percent of psyllium's seed coat is a water-absorbing substance called mucilage. When exposed to water, psyllium seeds swell to more than ten times their original size and become gelatinous. The herb's mucilage accounts for its use in treating both diarrhea and constipation.

Diarrhea. Psyllium absorbs excess fluid in the intestinal tract and restores normal bulk to stool.

Constipation. Psyllium's bulk-forming action increases stool volume. Larger stools press on the colon wall, triggering the wavelike contractions (peristalsis) we recognize as "the urge." Some cases of constipation also involve hard, dense stools, which are painful to pass. Psyllium's water-absorbing action decreases stool density and helps lubricate its passage. Studies show a teaspoon of psyllium seeds three times a day usually produces significant relief.

Hemorrhoids. Psyllium also provides some relief from the pain, bleeding, and itching of hemorrhoids, according to a report in *Diseases of the Colon and Rectum*, thus supporting Culpeper's recommendation.

Cholesterol Cutter. But the big news these days is the discovery that psyllium may reduce cholesterol. People taking a teaspoon three times a day for eight weeks experience significant decreases in blood cholesterol levels, according to a study in *Archives of Internal Medicine*. The researchers concluded that many people with elevated cholesterol may be able to benefit from the cholesterol-lowering action of psyllium and avoid taking prescription cholesterol-lowering medications.

A similar 12-week study published in the *Journal of the American Medical Association* shows psyllium reduces cholesterol by 5 percent. Heart disease authorities say that for every 1 percent decrease in cholesterol, heart attack risk drops 2 percent. So this 5 percent cholesterol reduction means a 10 percent decrease in heart attack risk.

Psyllium is also safer than the prescription drugs typically prescribed to reduce cholesterol. If you are taking such medication, ask your physician about using the seeds as a substitute for or in conjunction with your current treatment.

Intriguing Possibilities. One study showed psyllium protects experimental animals from intestinal damage from toxic food additives. The psyllium increases the bulk of the animals' stools, so the toxic chemicals have less direct contact with sensitive intestinal tissues and less opportunity to cause harm. Researchers believe this same mechanism explains why a high-fiber diet is associated with reduced risk of colorectal cancer. No studies show that psyllium helps prevent this cancer, the leading cause of cancer deaths among nonsmokers, but the American Cancer Society recommends a diet high in fibers such as psyllium to possibly help prevent this cancer.

Psyllium reduces blood sugar (glucose) levels in experimental animals, suggesting a possible role in human diabetes management.

Rx for Psyllium

For a laxative or cholesterol control, take 1 teaspoon of seeds three times a day with meals and with plenty of water. Psyllium is odorless and almost tasteless, but it has a gritty texture some people find unpleasant. If you take a commercial preparation, follow label directions.

Psyllium should not be given to children under age 2. If your infant or child appears constipated, consult a physician.

The Safety Factor

As a laxative, cholesterol cutter, and possible cancer preventive, psyllium does not work by itself. The seeds swell *only* in the presence of water. If you take psyllium but don't drink more water, you could wind up like the man whose intestine became completely blocked by a large psyllium plug. He required abdominal surgery.

Inhaling dust from psyllium seeds may trigger allergic reaction. As a result, a person who is sensitive to psyllium could later experience allergy symptoms from ingesting it. Severe allergic reactions are extremely rare, but if you have breathing difficulties after ingesting psyllium, seek emergency help immediately.

Psyllium has no history as a menstruation promoter, but other *Plantago* species do. Constipation is a common complaint of pregnancy. Pregnant women should avoid psyllium as well as other laxatives and control constipation by eating other high-fiber foods, such as fruits, vegetables, and whole-grain bread products.

Psyllium should be used in medicinal amounts only in consultation with your doctor. If psyllium causes minor discomforts, such as stomach upset or diarrhea, use less or stop using it. Let your doctor know if you experience unpleasant effects or if the symptoms for which the herb is being used do not improve significantly in two weeks.

Don't Grow It

Psyllium is an annual that reaches 18 inches and produces inconspicuous white flowers in summer that soon give way to a small brown seed pod.

Most of the psyllium used in this country is imported from France. Although available from specialty seed houses, psyllium is not usually grown as a garden herb. It looks like a weed and, if the seed pods are not harvested before they break open, the wind scatters the seed—a major problem when you consider that each pod contains up to 15,000 seeds and that the plant grows aggressively.

RASPBERRY

Premier Pregnancy Herb

Family: Rosaceae; other members include rose, apple, almond, strawberry

Genus and species: *Rubus idaeus, R. strigosus*

Also known as: Hindberry, bramble

Parts used: Leaves, fruits

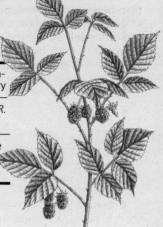

For more than 2,000 years, raspberry was considered a minor healer, a footnote under blackberry. But since the 1940s, it has emerged from blackberry's shadow and virtually replaced it in herbal healing—all because it has become *the* herb for pregnant women.

The Also-Ran Herb

The ancient Greeks, Chinese, Ayurvedics, and American Indians used raspberry and blackberry interchangeably, as a treatment for wounds and diarrhea.

Seventeenth-century English herbalist Nicholas Culpeper recommended raspberry as "very binding" (astringent) and good for "fevers, ulcers, putrid sores of the mouth and secret parts [genitals] . . . spitting blood [tuberculosis] . . . piles [hemorrhoids], stones of the kidney . . . and too much flowing of women's courses [heavy menstrual flow]."

The Eclectic text, *King's American Dispensatory*, continued the long tradition of considering raspberry a footnote under blackberry, which it recommended as being "of much service in dysentery . . . pleasant to the taste, mitigating suffering, and ultimately effecting a cure."

Contemporary herbalists recommend raspberry for diarrhea and to treat nausea and vomiting, especially the morning sickness of pregnancy. One herbalist goes so far as to call raspberry a "panacea during pregnancy . . . allaying morning sickness, preventing miscarriage, [and] erasing labor pains."

HEALING with Raspberry

Raspberry won't "erase labor pains," and it's no "panacea during pregnancy," but science has shown it to be of some value for pregnant women.

Pregnancy. In 1941, raspberry emerged from blackberry's shadow when an animal study published in the British medical journal *Lancet* showed it contains a "uterine relaxant principle." Over the next 30 years, several other studies confirmed this finding, and today physicians in England and Europe prescribe a number of raspberry preparations for morning sickness, uterine irritability, and threatened miscarriage. The herb is also included in many herbal pregnancy blends sold in the United States.

Diarrhea. Raspberry leaves contain tannins, which are astringent and help explain its traditional use as a diarrhea treatment.

Intriguing Possibilities. One animal study shows raspberry helps reduce blood sugar (glucose), suggesting possible value in diabetes management.

Another shows raspberry root tannins of value in treating a rare form of cancer.

Rₓ for Raspberry

For a pleasantly astringent, sweet infusion to treat diarrhea or the discomforts of pregnancy, use 1 to 2 teaspoons of dried herb per cup of boiling water. Steep 10 to 15 minutes. Drink as needed.

In a tincture, take ½ to 1 teaspoon up to three times a day.

Parents may use dilute raspberry tea cautiously to treat infant diarrhea.

The Safety Factor

Standard medical advice warns pregnant women against taking *any* drugs during pregnancy because of the possibility of harming the fetus. Raspberry used medicinally is an exception to this rule, although it should only be used with the consent and supervision of an obstetrician. Raspberry has been widely recommended for decades as a uterine relaxant, and there are no reports in the medical literature of any problems with it. Women with a history of miscarriage may find it especially valuable. On the other hand, prudence dictates using the lowest effective dose. Start with a weak infusion and increase the concentration if necessary.

Tannins have both pro-and anti-cancer action. Pregnant women with a history of cancer should discuss using raspberry with their physicians.

Other Cautions

For otherwise healthy adults, raspberry is safe in amounts typically recommended.

Raspberry should be used in medicinal amounts only in consultation with your doctor. If raspberry causes minor discomforts, such as stomach upset or diarrhea, use less or stop using it. Let your doctor know if you experience unpleasant effects or if the symptoms for which the herb is being used do not improve significantly in two weeks.

Berry Good Fruit

Raspberry's perennial invasive roots produce a dense spreading mass of thorny biennial stems, which can grow to 10 feet, with serrated, lance-shaped leaves, small white summer-blooming flowers, and hanging clusters of tart red berries, which become very sweet as they ripen.

Raspberry bushes grow so vigorously and invasively, they quickly become impenetrable pests. Rooting them out is quite difficult. Even when cleared, stray root fragments send up new shoots. Make sure your raspberries are well contained.

Plant 1/2-inch root cuttings in a few inches of soil. Raspberry grows best under full sun in loose, rich, well-drained soil amended with manure or compost.

Harvest leaves any time. Mature fruits appear in summer. For ease of harvesting the berries, train branches along supports. Prune mercilessly.

RED CLOVER

Possible Cancer Herb

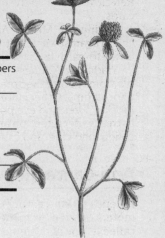

Family: Leguminosae; other members include beans, peas

Genus and species: *Trifolium pratense*

Also known as: Trifolium, purple clover, sweet clover, cow clover

Parts used: Flower tops

Red clover is one of the world's oldest agricultural crops, cultivated as forage since prehistoric times. The ball-shaped flowers of the three-leafed herb have been used almost as long in herbal healing. For the last 100 years, red clover has been touted as a cancer treatment. Meanwhile, many contemporary scientists say red clover is useless against cancer. Some studies do show some antitumor action, however.

The Suit of Clubs

Because of its importance in early agriculture, red clover has a long history as a religious symbol. The ancient Greeks, Romans, and the Celts of pre-Christian Ireland all revered it. Early Christians linked the plant to the Trinity, and some say red clover is the model for Ireland's symbol, the shamrock.

Red clover was also the model for the suit of clubs in playing cards.

During the Middle Ages, red clover was considered a charm against witchcraft. In the Far East, herbalists had more down-to-earth uses for red clover.

Traditional Chinese physicians have long used red clover blossoms as an expectorant. Russian folk healers recommend it for asthma. Other cultures have used it externally in salves for skin sores and eye problems and internally as a diuretic to treat water retention and as a sedative, anti-inflammatory, cough medicine, and cancer treatment.

Anti-Cancer Reputation

America's 19th-century Eclectic physicians were great promoters of red clover. Their text, *King's American Dispensatory*, called it "one of the few remedies which favorably influences pertussis [whooping cough] . . . possess[ing] a peculiar soothing property." The Eclectics recommended red clover for cough, bronchitis, and tuberculosis but waxed truly enthusiastic about the herb as a cancer treatment: "It unquestionably retards the growth of carcinomata."

During the late 19th and early 20th centuries, red clover was the major ingredient in many patent medicines known as Trifolium Compounds. The most popular, produced by the William S. Merrell Chemical Co. of Cincinnati, was a combination of red clover and several other herbs. Manufacturers claimed Trifolium Compounds were tonics and treatments for skin diseases, syphilis, and scrofula (tuberculosis of the lymph nodes). In 1912, the American Medical Association's Council on Pharmacy and Chemistry attacked Trifolium Compounds, saying "We have no information to indicate they possess medicinal properties." Nonetheless, red clover continued to be listed for skin diseases in the *National Formulary* until 1946. Red clover was also one of the herbs in ex–coal miner Harry Hoxsey's controversial alternative cancer treatment (see page 23).

Contemporary herbalists recommend red clover externally

as a treatment for eczema and psoriasis and internally as a digestive aid, and expectorant for coughs, bronchitis, and whooping cough. Some continue to recommend it for cancer.

HEALING with Red Clover

Red clover doesn't get much respect among many herbal experts. The Food and Drug Administration (FDA) says, "There is not sufficient reason to suspect it of any medicinal value." And in *The New Honest Herbal*, Varro Tyler, Ph.D., dismisses claims that red clover helps treat cancer as "simply not factual."

Cancer. On the other hand, researchers from the National Cancer Institute (NCI) have found antitumor properties in the herb. NCI researchers felt compelled to investigate the plant after their own Jonathan Hartwell, Ph.D., published a monograph in *The Journal of Natural Products* in which he pointed out that 33 different cultures around the world use red clover to treat cancer. That amounts to a whole lot of people agreeing that the herb has anti-cancer action.

And sure enough, NCI researchers emerged from their laboratories with confirmation that red clover contains four antitumor compounds, including daidzein and genistein.

In addition, red clover contains significant amounts of the antioxidant chemical tocopherol, a form of vitamin E that has been shown to help prevent breast tumors in animals, according to James Duke, Ph.D., herbal medicine authority for the U.S. Department of Agriculture.

These findings are still preliminary, and red clover should not be considered a treatment for cancer at this time. But for those with cancers not aggravated by estrogen (nonestrogen-dependent tumors), red clover may hold some promise. Ask your physician about using it in addition to your regular treatment.

Women's Health. Several studies show that in large quantities, red clover acts like the female sex hormone estrogen. As a result, it might help relieve some menopausal symptoms, though women taking postmenopausal estrogen replacement therapy should discuss using it with their physicians.

Intriguing Possibility. One study showed red clover effective against several bacteria in the test tube, including the one that causes tuberculosis, which lends some credence to the Eclectics' use of this herb in treating TB.

Rx for Red Clover

For a pleasantly sweet infusion, use 1 to 3 teaspoons of dried flower tops per cup of boiling water. Steep 10 to 15 minutes. Drink up to 3 cups a day.

In a tincture, use $1/2$ to $1 1/2$ teaspoons up to three times a day.

Medicinal red clover preparations should not be given to children under age 2. For older children and people over 65, start with low-strength preparations and increase strength if necessary.

The Safety Factor

Women taking birth control pills should consult their physicians before using this herb. Estrogens are used to treat some prostate cancers but also may accelerate the growth of estrogen-dependent breast and gynecological tumors. Estrogen also increases risk of internal blood clots (thromboembolism) and inflammation of blood vessels (thrombophlebitis). Those with a history of these disorders or heart disease or stroke should use red clover cautiously if at all. The medical literature contains no reports of harm from red clover.

Other Cautions

The FDA includes red clover in its list of herbs generally regarded as safe. For otherwise healthy nonpregnant, nonnursing adults who do not have estrogen-dependent cancers or a history of heart disease, stroke, thromboembolism, or thrombophlebitis, red clover is considered relatively safe in amounts typically recommended.

Red clover should be used in medicinal amounts only in consultation with your doctor. If red clover causes minor discomforts, such as stomach upset or diarrhea, use less or stop using it. Let your doctor know if you experience any unpleasant effects or if the symptoms for which the herb is being used do not improve significantly in two weeks.

For the Clover Lover

Red clover is a perennial that grows to 2 feet. Its leaves are arranged in groups of three. Its fragrant, edible, red or purple ball-shaped flowers are composed of many tiny florets.

Because it's a legume, red clover adds nitrogen to the soil, and its deep roots help break up compacted soil. Plant seeds in spring or fall. In sunny conditions, this herb thrives in a variety of moist, well-drained soils but does not grow well in sand or gravel. Harvest the flowers when the tops are fully in bloom.

RED PEPPER

Medically, It's HOT!

Family: Solanaceae; other members include potato, tomato, eggplant, tobacco, nightshade

Genus and species: *Capsicum annuum, C. frutescens*

Also known as: Hot pepper, cayenne chili pepper, African pepper, Tabasco pepper, Louisiana long (and short) pepper, Guinea pepper, bird pepper, capsicum; green and red bell pepper, paprika, and pimiento are all milder varieties of *C. annuum*

Parts used: Fruit

The fiery taste and bright color of red pepper make it one of the world's most noticeable spices. Recently, this herb has become as hot in healing as it is on the tongue. Extracts of red pepper have proved remarkably effective at relieving certain types of severe, chronic pain. It also may aid digestion.

Although it's been a culinary staple in Asia since ancient times, it was unknown in Europe until Columbus returned with it from his first voyage to the New World.

Don't Call It Cayenne

The term *cayenne* comes from the Caribbean Indian word *kian*. Today Cayenne is the capital of French Guiana. But ironically, only a tiny fraction of the U.S. red pepper supply comes from South America or the Caribbean. Most comes from India and

437

Africa. Tabasco (Louisiana pepper) grows along the Gulf Coast of the United States. Because so little red pepper comes from around Cayenne, the American Spice Trade Association considers *cayenne* a misnomer and says this herb should be called red pepper.

Too Hot to Handle

Seventeenth-century English herbalist Nicholas Culpeper wrote that immoderate use of red pepper "inflames the mouth and throat so extremely it is hard to endure," and warned it "might prove dangerous to life." But when used sparingly, he claimed the herb was of "considerable service" to "help digestion, provoke urine, relieve toothache, preserve the teeth from rottenness, comfort a cold stomach, expel the stone from the kidney, and take away dimness of sight." Culpeper urged women to mix red pepper, gentian, and bay laurel oil in cotton, and insert it vaginally to "bring down the courses" (menstruation). But he warned that "if [it] be put into the womb after delivery, it will make [the woman] barren forever."

During the 18th century, red pepper was mixed with snuff to boost the inhaled tobacco's kick. Herbalist Phillip Miller warned against this, saying the combination caused "such violent fits of sneezing as to break the blood vessels in the head."

In India, the East Indies, Africa, Mexico, and the Caribbean, red pepper enjoys a long history as a digestive aid. But this use never caught on among Europeans, who have traditionally believed that hot spices cause stomach ulcers.

American Foot Warmer

The first North American to advocate red pepper in healing was Samuel Thomson, creator of Thomsonian herbal medicine, which enjoyed considerable popularity before the Civil War. Thomson believed most disease was caused by cold and cured by heat, so he prescribed "warming" herbs extensively, and red pepper was chief among them.

After the Civil War, America's Eclectic physicians called red pepper *capsicum* and recommended it externally for arthritis and muscle soreness and internally as a digestive stimulant and treatment for colds, cough, fever, diarrhea, constipation, nausea, and toothache. The Eclectics also advised adding red pepper to socks to treat cold feet, a use echoed in some herbals today.

The Eclectics considered red pepper invaluable in the treatment of delirium tremens, the combination of hallucinations and violent tremors common among advanced alcoholics: "Capsicum is the very best agent that can be used in delirium tremens. It enables the stomach to take and retain food. The best form is in a tea or strong beef soup. There is no danger of overdose as a [large] quantity may be swallowed with evident pleasure and without ill results."

American folk healers have also recommended dusting children's hands with powdered red pepper to stop thumb sucking and nail biting.

Contemporary herbalists prescribe capsules of cayenne powder for colds, gastrointestinal and bowel problems, and as a digestive aid. Externally, they recommend cayenne plasters for arthritis and muscle soreness.

HEALING with Red Pepper

Modern science has supported this herb's traditional uses as a digestive aid and pain reliever. Red pepper owes its heat and its value in herbal healing to one chemical found in its fruit—capsaicin.

Digestive Aid. Red pepper assists digestion by stimulating the flow of both saliva and stomach secretions. Saliva contains enzymes that begin the breakdown of carbohydrate, while stomach secretions (gastric juices) contain acids and other substances that further digest food.

In cultures with bland cuisine, such as traditional American meat-and-potatoes cooking, people often believe highly spiced foods damage the stomach and contribute to ulcers. This is not the case. In a study published in the *Journal of the American Medical Association*, researchers used a tiny video camera to examine subjects' stomach linings after both bland meals and meals liberally spiced with jalapeño peppers. They reported no difference in stomach condition and concluded: "Ingestion of highly spiced meals by normal individuals is not associated with [gastrointestinal] damage."

Diarrhea. Like many culinary spices, red pepper has antibacterial properties, possibly explaining traditional claims that it helps relieve infectious diarrhea.

Chronic Pain. For centuries, herbalists have recommended rubbing red pepper into the skin to treat muscle and joint pains. Medically, this is known as using a counterirritant—a treatment that causes minor superficial pain and distracts the person from the more severe, deeper pain. Several capsaicin counterirritants are available over-the-counter, among them Heet, Stimurub, and Omega Oil.

Recently, however, red pepper has been shown to possess real pain-relieving (analgesic) properties for certain kinds of chronic pain. For reasons still not completely understood, capsaicin interferes with the action of "substance P," the chemical in the peripheral nerves that sends pain messages to the brain. Several recent studies all showed capsaicin so effective at relieving a particular type of chronic pain, two over-the-counter capsaicin creams, Zostrix and Axsain, have won Food and Drug Administration (FDA) approval.

Shingles. Zostrix is the most effective treatment yet for the severe chronic pain following the disease known as shingles, or herpes zoster. Shingles is an adult disease caused by the same virus that causes chicken pox in children. The virus remains dormant in the body until later in life when, for unknown reasons, it reappears in some people as shingles, causing a rash on one side of the body that progresses from red bumps to blisters to crusty pox resembling chicken pox. In otherwise healthy adults, shingles clears up by itself within three weeks. But some people—typically the elderly or those with other illnesses, particularly Hodgkin's disease—suffer severe, chronic pain, a condition that doctors call post-herpetic neuralgia. Now, thanks to capsaicin, they don't have to suffer as much.

Diabetic Foot Pain. Capsaicin's pain-relieving ability has also led to its use in treating the severe ankle and foot pain known as burning foot syndrome, which affects approximately half of all diabetics. In one study, 71 percent of diabetics reported significant relief after four weeks. The FDA recently approved a capsaicin preparation, Axsain, for use in treating this condition.

Cluster Headaches. A report in *Environmental Nutrition* showed capsaicin also helps relieve the pain of cluster headaches, extremely severe pain on one side of the head. In this study, cluster headache sufferers rubbed a capsaicin preparation inside their nostrils and outside their nose. Within five days, 75 percent reported less pain and fewer headaches. They also reported burning nostrils and a runny nose, but these side effects subsided within a week.

Intriguing Possibility. Red pepper may help cut cholesterol and prevent heart disease, according to two studies done in India and the United States. While it is too early to recommend red pepper as a means of lowering cholesterol and treating heart disease, this common kitchen spice may someday have a role to play in these areas.

Rx for Red Pepper

In food, season to taste, but err on the side of caution. A little too much can set the mouth on fire.

For an infusion to aid digestion and possibly help reduce risk of heart disease, use 1/4 to 1/2 teaspoon per cup of boiling water. Drink it after meals.

For external application to help treat pain, mix 1/4 to 1/2 teaspoon per cup of warm vegetable oil and rub it into the affected area.

Red pepper should not be given to children under age 2. For older children, start with a small amount and use more if necessary. People over 65 often suffer a loss of taste-bud and skin-nerve sensitivity and may require more than younger adults.

The Safety Factor

Chopping red peppers may burn the fingertips, a condition dubbed Hunan hand because it was first identified in a man who was preparing a Hunan Chinese recipe that called for chopping many of the fiery fruits. He wound up in an emergency room with severe hand pain.

Red pepper does not wash off the hands easily. (Washing in vinegar removes it best.) Even with careful washing, the pungent herb may remain on the fingertips for hours and cause severe eye pain if contaminated fingers touch the eyes. Use rubber gloves when chopping red peppers.

One French study shows that red pepper boosts resistance to infection. Some bacteria-fighting spices can be sprinkled on cuts to help prevent infection, but don't do this with red pepper. It burns terribly.

Red pepper has not been linked to menstruation promotion since the 17th century, but some research suggests the herb's stems and leaves—not the more typically used powdered fruits—stimulate uterine contractions in animals. Pregnant women and those wishing to conceive should stick to the powdered fruits.

Other Cautions

Red pepper is on the FDA's list of herbs generally regarded as safe. For otherwise healthy nonpregnant, nonnursing adults, red pepper is considered safe in the small amounts typically recommended.

Red pepper should be used in medicinal amounts only in consultation with your doctor. If red pepper causes minor discomforts, such as stomach upset, diarrhea, or burning during bowel movements, use less or stop using it. Let your doctor know if you experience unpleasant effects or if the symptoms for which the herb is being used do not improve significantly in two weeks.

Harvest Some Heat

Red pepper is a shrubby, tropical perennial with shiny, pendulous, leathery fruits. It grows best in tropical or subtropical areas but also prospers in south-facing windows and greenhouses.

In southern states, seeds may be sown after danger of frost has passed. Farther north, sow seeds indoors in flats eight weeks before the final frost date, then transplant. Space seedlings 12 inches apart.

Red pepper prefers rich, well-watered, sandy soil and full sun, but it tolerates some shade. When harvesting ripened fruit, be careful not to break the stems, or they may spoil. To dry red peppers, hang them in a warm, dry place. Drying takes several weeks.

RHUBARB

More Than Pie Filling

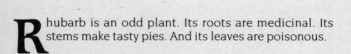

Family: Polygonaceae; other members include buckwheat

Genus and species: *Rheum officinale, R. palmatum;* garden rhubarb, *R. rhaponticum* has similar but less powerful action

Also known as: Rheum, or Chinese, Himalayan, Turkish, or medicinal rhubarb

Parts used: Roots

Rhubarb is an odd plant. Its roots are medicinal. Its stems make tasty pies. And its leaves are poisonous.

Powerful Asian Laxative

Chinese physicians have used rhubarb root since ancient times. They prescribed it externally as a treatment for cuts and burns and internally in small amounts for dysentery. They also discovered that *large* amounts have powerful laxative action and promote menstruation. Over the centuries, the Indians, Russians, and Europeans adopted rhubarb as a healing herb and discovered their own native species have similar, though less powerful effects.

Seventeenth-century English herbalist Nicholas Culpeper endorsed rhubarb's laxative action: "This herb purges downward." He also recommended it externally as "a most effectual remedy to heal scabs and running sores." In addition,

444

Culpeper claimed rhubarb "heals jaundice . . . provokes urine . . . is very effectual for reins [gonorrhea] . . . and helps gout, sciatica . . . toothache . . . the stone [kidney stones] . . . and dimness of sight."

Later herbalists repudiated most of Culpeper's recommendations and returned to prescribing small doses of rhubarb root for diarrhea and larger doses as a laxative.

Widely Used for Dysentery

America's 19th-century Eclectics used rhubarb primarily to treat diarrhea and dysentery. *King's American Dispensatory* noted its effectiveness for constipation but said "it sometimes produces griping [cramping]." The Eclectics also considered the herb helpful in treating "hepatic derangement" (liver problems) and delirium tremens.

Bacterial dysentery was a common—and often fatal—disease in British East Africa between the World Wars. In 1921, Nairobi-based physician R. W. Burkitt wrote in *Lancet* that he'd treated it with rhubarb almost exclusively for three years: "I know of no remedy in medicine which has such a magical effect. No one who has ever used rhubarb would dream of using anything else . . . in this dreadful tropical scourge."

Contemporary herbalists are divided on rhubarb. Some recommend low doses for diarrhea and large doses for constipation. Others simply recommend it as a laxative.

HEALING with Rhubarb

The ancient Chinese appear to have been right about rhubarb's dual effects.

Diarrhea. Studies show small amounts of this herb help treat diarrhea.

Constipation. Large amounts have powerful laxative action. Rhubarb contains similar laxative chemicals (anthraquinones) as those found in buckthorn, cascara sagrada, and senna.

Anthraquinone laxatives should be used only as a last resort to treat constipation. First, eat more fresh fruits and vegetables, drink plenty of water, and get more exercise. If that doesn't work, try a bulk-forming laxative such as psyllium (see page 423). If you still need help, try cascara sagrada (see page 144), generally regarded as the gentlest anthraquinone. After that, try rhubarb—or buckthorn (see page 132) or senna (see page 484)—in consultation with a physician.

Women's Health. Some animal studies suggest rhubarb stimulates uterine contractions, lending some credence to its use in China as a menstruation promoter. Thus, pregnant women should try to avoid it. Other women might try it to begin their periods.

Rx for Rhubarb

For diarrhea, make a decoction by gently boiling ½ teaspoon of powdered root per cup of water for 10 minutes. Take 1 tablespoon at a time periodically, up to 1 cup per day. Rhubarb tastes bitter and unpleasant.

In a tincture, use ¼ teaspoon per day.

For constipation, make a decoction by boiling 1 to 2 teaspoons of powdered root per cup of water for 10 minutes. Take 1 tablespoon at a time, up to 1 cup per day.

In a tincture, use ½ to 1 teaspoon a day.

Rhubarb should not be given to children under age 2. For older children and people over 65, start with low-strength preparations and increase strength if necessary.

The Safety Factor

Alert: Because of rhubarb's powerful action, laxative amounts should not be used by those with chronic intestinal problems, such as ulcers or colitis.

Pregnant and nursing women should not use anthraquinone laxatives.

Laxative amounts of rhubarb should not be used for more

than two weeks, because over time, it causes lazy bowel syndrome, an inability to move stool without chemical stimulation.

Rhubarb stems are used in pie fillings, but the plant's leaf blades contain oxalic acid, which is poisonous, causing burning in the mouth and throat, nausea, vomiting, weakness, and other symptoms. Fatalities have occurred.

Rhubarb may color the urine bright yellow or red.

Other Cautions

For otherwise healthy nonpregnant, nonnursing adults who are not taking other laxatives, rhubarb is considered relatively safe in amounts typically recommended when used for brief periods.

Rhubarb should be used in medicinal amounts only in consultation with your doctor. If rhubarb causes minor discomforts, such as stomach upset or diarrhea, use less or stop using it. Let your doctor know if you experience unpleasant effects or if the symptoms for which the herb is being used do not improve significantly in two weeks.

It's Really Big

Medicinal rhubarb is a large, leafy perennial that reaches 10 feet. Its root is thick and branching, brown on the outside and yellow inside. Its stems are round, hollow, and jointed and terminate in branching spikes of numerous small flowers. The medicinal species are not garden herbs.

Garden rhubarb reaches only 3 feet. It has thick roots, reddish outside, yellow inside, and purple stems. Garden rhubarb is considered less potent in herbal healing. If you use it medicinally, start with the amounts recommended above, but be prepared to adjust them upward.

Garden rhubarb requires a dormant period in winter and does not do well in the South, where winters are warm. Sow seeds or root cuttings 4 feet apart in late spring in deeply dug, well-watered beds under full sun or partial shade. Add compost and mulch in winter.

Harvest stems for pies the second year, roots the fourth.

ROSE

Helpful Hints

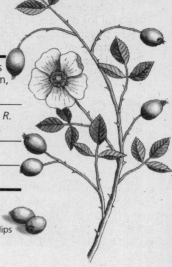

Family: Rosaceae; other members include raspberry, blackberry, plum, peach, almond

Genus and species: *Rosa canina, R. rugosa, R. centifolia*

Also known as: Hipberry

Parts used: Fruits ("hips")

Hips

Prized since the dawn of history, the rose is queen of the flowers. But in herbal healing, this plant becomes noteworthy only after the velvety petals have fallen away, revealing the cherry-sized fruits, or hips.

Rose hips contain vitamin C, but authorities disagree on how much. Some herbalists call rose hips "one of the best natural sources" of vitamin C. Scientific sources scoff at this claim, asserting it would take more than a dozen cups of rose hip tea to provide the recommended daily allowance and a lot more to help treat colds and flu.

While herbalists have generally overstated this herb's vitamin C content, it still may be of some benefit for colds and flu.

Medicine Flowers

Roses were a favorite of the ancient Egyptians, who used the fragrant petals as air fresheners and rose water as perfume.

In Greece, Hippocrates recommended rose flowers mixed with oil for diseases of the uterus. India's traditional Ayurvedic physicians have long considered rose petals cooling and astringent, leading to their use in poultices to treat skin wounds and inflammations. The Ayurvedics also used rose petals and rose water as a laxative.

Western herbalists echoed Ayurvedic uses of the herb. Medieval German abbess/herbalist Hildegard of Bingen recommended rose hip tea as the initial treatment for just about every illness. Seventeenth-century English herbalist Nicholas Culpeper called the herb "binding and restringent [astringent]" and wrote it "strengthens the stomach, prevents vomiting, stops tickling coughs, . . . [is] good against all kinds of fluxes [diarrhea] . . . [and is] of great service in consumptions [tuberculosis]."

As the centuries passed, European herbalists recommended dried rose petal tea for headache, dizziness, mouth sores, and menstrual cramps.

Vitamin C Revival

Americans have always loved roses. They were among the first flowers planted around the White House. But American herbalists considered the rose only a minor healing herb. The 19th-century Eclectic physicians did not use rose petals at all. They beat the hips into a pulp and used it as a base for making pills containing other medicines.

Roses almost disappeared from early 20th-century herbals. Then came the discovery of vitamin C in the 1930s and the finding that rose hips may contain appreciable amounts.

Contemporary herbalists are unanimous in their praise of rose hips as a source of America's favorite vitamin. One best-selling herbal claims: "Rose hips are rich in vitamin C, richer by far than oranges ounce for ounce. Some people say we should make rose hip tea a part of our daily diet." Because of its vitamin C content, herbalists tout rose hips for colds and flu. Some also recommend the herb as a mild laxative.

HEALING with Rose

There's nothing wrong with making rose hips a part of your daily diet, but don't count on the bright red fruits—or the prepackaged teas containing them—to supply all the vitamin C you need, especially if you use the vitamin to try to treat the common cold and flu.

Rose hips contain a significant amount of vitamin C. However, the drying process destroys from 45 to 90 percent of it, and infusions extract only about 40 percent of what's left. That still leaves a fair amount of vitamin C, but considerably less than most herbals promise.

Many companies that manufacture vitamin C claim their products are "made from rose hips." In fact, none are made exclusively from rose hips. In commercial "rose hip" vitamin C preparations, the hips are combined with ascorbic acid from other sources.

Colds and Flu. Some scientific studies have supported the use of vitamin C to help relieve the symptoms and decrease the duration of the common cold. The studies that show positive benefit—including those published in the *Canadian Medical Association Journal* and the *New England Journal of Medicine*—call for using 2,000 milligrams a day or more from the moment the first cold symptoms appear until all symptoms disappear.

That's a lot of vitamin C—considerably more than the current Recommended Daily Allowance (USRDA) of 60 milligrams a day. It would be impractical to obtain this much vitamin C from rose hip preparations alone.

But rose hip tea can help boost cold and flu sufferers' overall vitamin C intake. In addition, hot liquids may help relieve the sore throat, nasal congestion, and cough associated with colds and flu, and they warm the throat, which may help impair viral replication. (Cold viruses reproduce best at around 95°F.)

Rx for Rose Hips

For a pleasant-tasting, mildly astringent infusion that may help in the treatment of colds and flu, use 2 to 3 teaspoons of dried, chopped hips per cup of boiling water. Steep 10 minutes. Drink as needed.

In a tincture, use 1/2 to 1 teaspoon as needed.

Dilute rose hip infusions may be given to children under age 2.

The Safety Factor

High doses of vitamin C cause diarrhea in some people. High doses also strain the kidneys. This is not a problem for people with healthy kidneys, but those with kidney disease should consult their physicians before taking large amounts of rose hips.

Rose hips are included in the Food and Drug Administration's list of herbs generally regarded as safe. For otherwise healthy nonpregnant, nonnursing adults, rose hips are safe in amounts typically recommended.

Consult a physician if cold or flu symptoms do not improve significantly in two weeks, if a fever develops toward the end of a cold or flu, or if a cold- or flu-related cough brings up brown or red phlegm.

Harvest the Hips

Roses have been bred for every climate. "Old roses" are generally more fragrant than newer hybrids, but they have less-showy, faster-wilting flowers. Consult a nursery for the variety best suited to your conditions and desires. Enjoy the flowers, then harvest and dry the hips.

ROSEMARY

The Tasty Natural Preservative

Family: Labiatae; other members include mints

Genus and species: *Rosmarinus officinalis*

Also known as: Rosemarine, incensier (French)

Parts used: Leaves

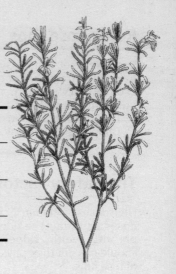

Thousands of years before refrigeration, ancient peoples noticed that wrapping meats in crushed rosemary leaves preserved them and imparted a fresh fragrance and pleasing flavor. To this day, the herb remains a favorite in meat dishes, and its preservative ability is the basis for its use in herbal healing.

Rosemary's ability to preserve meats led to the belief that it helped preserve memory. Greek students wore rosemary garlands to assist their recall. As the centuries passed, the herb was incorporated into wedding ceremonies as a symbol of spousal fidelity and into funerals to help survivors to remember the dead. In *Hamlet*, Ophelia gives Hamlet a sprig, saying, "There's rosemary . . . for remembrance."

Symbol of Love

During the Middle Ages, rosemary's association with weddings evolved into its use as a love charm. If a young person tapped another with a rosemary twig containing an open blossom, the couple would supposedly fall in love.

Placed under one's pillow, the aromatic herb was believed to repel bad dreams. Planted around one's home, it was reputed to ward off witches.

But by the 16th century, planting rosemary around the home became a bone of contention in England, where the belief developed that it signified a household where the woman ruled. Men were known to rip out rosemary plants as evidence that they—not their wives—ruled the roost.

The ancients used rosemary as they used all aromatic, preservative herbs—for head, respiratory, and gastrointestinal problems. Traditional Chinese physicians mixed it with ginger and used it to treat headache, indigestion, insomnia, and malaria.

Hungary Water

In 1235, Queen Elizabeth of Hungary became paralyzed. According to legend, a hermit soaked a pound of rosemary in a gallon of wine for several days, then rubbed it on her limbs, curing her. Rosemary/wine combinations became known as Queen of Hungary's Water and were used externally for centuries for gout, dandruff, baldness prevention, and skin problems. (As the centuries passed, pennyroyal and marjoram were incorporated into what became known as Hungary Water.)

The French hung rosemary around sickrooms and in hospitals as a kind of healing incense, calling it *incensier*. As recently as World War II, French nurses burned a mixture of rosemary leaves and juniper berries in hospital rooms as an antiseptic.

Little Used in America

Colonists brought rosemary to North America, and an early medical guide, *The American New Dispensatory*, recommended the herb's leaves, flowers, and Hungary Water for use "in nervous and menstrual affections, for strokes, paralysis, and dizziness."

Oddly, those great proponents of botanical medicine, the Eclectics, had little use for rosemary. Their text, *King's American Dispensatory*, noted its use as a digestive aid and menstruation promoter but declared it "seldom used except as a perfume."

Central American folk healers use rosemary oil as an insect repellent and menstruation promoter.

Contemporary herbalists say rosemary stimulates the circulatory, digestive, and nervous systems. They recommend it for headache, indigestion, depression, muscle pain, as a gargle to treat bad breath, externally to prevent premature baldness, and in baths for relaxation.

HEALING with Rosemary

Rosemary may not guarantee A's on exams, marital fidelity, or vivid memories of the dear departed, but the ancients were right about its ability to preserve meats.

Food Poisoning Preventive. Meats spoil in part because their fats oxidize and turn rancid. Rosemary and its oil contain chemicals that are strongly antioxidant. In fact, rosemary's preservative power compares favorably with the commercial food preservatives, BHA and BHT.

Rosemary's preservative action may help prevent food poisoning on your next picnic. Mix the crushed leaves generously into hamburger meat and tuna, pasta, and potato salads.

Digestive Aid. Like most culinary herbs, rosemary may help relax the smooth muscle lining of the digestive tract (making it an antispasmodic). The ancients appear to have been on the right track when they used it as a digestive aid.

Decongestant. Like other aromatic herbs, rosemary may help relieve nasal and chest congestion caused by colds, flu, and allergies.

Infection Prevention. Rosemary contains chemicals that may help fight infection-causing and food-spoiling bacteria and fungi. For minor cuts in the garden, press some fresh, crushed leaves into the wound on the way to washing and bandaging it.

Women's Health. Antispasmodics soothe not only the digestive tract but other smooth muscles, such as the uterus, as well. As an antispasmodic, rosemary should theoretically calm the uterus, but Italian researchers have discovered that it does exactly the opposite.

Pregnant women should steer clear of medicinal preparations of this herb. Other women may try the herb to bring on their periods.

Rx for Rosemary

For a pleasantly aromatic infusion to settle the stomach or clear a stuffed nose, use 1 teaspoon of crushed herb per cup of boiling water. Steep 10 to 15 minutes. Drink up to 3 cups a day.

In a tincture, use 1/4 to 1/2 teaspoon up to three times a day.

Dilute rosemary preparations may be given cautiously to children under age 2.

The Safety Factor

In culinary amounts, rosemary poses no dangers. But even small amounts of rosemary oil may cause stomach, kidney, and intestinal irritation. Larger doses may cause poisoning.

Rosemary is included in the Food and Drug Administration's list of herbs generally regarded as safe. For otherwise healthy nonpregnant, nonnursing adults, rosemary is safe in amounts typically recommended.

Rosemary should be used in medicinal amounts only in consultation with your doctor. If rosemary causes minor discomforts, such as stomach upset or diarrhea, use less or stop using it. Let your doctor know if you experience unpleasant effects or if the symptoms for which the herb is being used do not improve significantly in two weeks.

Pretty Garden Accent

Rosemary is a woody, pine-scented, evergreen perennial with needlelike leaves. It reaches 3 feet in the United States and produces small, pale blue flowers in summer. Creeping rosemary (R. *prostratus*) is widely used in the Western United States as a groundcover and cascade over garden walls.

Rosemary can be grown from seeds, but germination can be a problem and seedlings are slow to develop, which is why most herb growers prefer to start with cuttings. If you sow seeds, plant them in spring 6 inches apart. Plant cuttings in sandy soil, leaving only one-third of each twig showing.

Rosemary prefers light, sandy, well-drained soil and full sun. Overwatering may cause root rot. Rosemary usually survives zero-degree winter temperatures without special care. If you live where temperatures dip lower, mulch plants each autumn or grow the herb in pots, bring them indoors each winter, and keep in a south-facing window.

Cut twigs and strip the leaves anytime after plants have become established.

SAFFRON

Expensive, but Worth It

Family: Iridaceae; other members include iris, gladiolus, crocus

Genus and species: *Crocus sativus*

Also known as: Saffron crocus or Spanish saffron, but not American saffron, which is safflower

Parts used: Stigmas (part of the pistil)

Blossom

Saffron is the yellow-gold spice that for centuries was literally worth its weight in gold. It still is, costing around $500 an ounce. Like the price of gold, saffron's value in herbal healing has fluctuated. But its value may be on the rise again because of its potential to help reduce some risk factors for heart disease, the nation's leading cause of death.

75,000 Flowers to the Pound

The Arabs introduced saffron into Spain around the 8th century, and that country has been a major exporter ever since. Saffron's violet, lilylike flowers contain three yellow-orange stigmas, the part with economic value. Used as a dye, spice, medicine, and perfume, saffron stigmas have been in great demand since ancient times. It takes about 75,000 flowers to yield 1 pound of saffron. You don't have to be an economist to understand why this herb has always been so expensive.

Because of its value, saffron has a long history of adulteration. The adulterant of choice has always been safflower, also a source of yellow-red dyes and variously known as fake saffron, dyer's saffron, and bastard saffron.

Egyptian Aromatic

Saffron was a favorite of the ancient Egyptians. The nobility wore robes dyed with saffron, anointed themselves with saffron perfumes, ate foods spiced with the herb, and used it like other aromatics to treat head, respiratory, and gastrointestinal complaints.

India's traditional Ayurvedic physicians considered saffron a circulatory stimulant, kidney and liver remedy, cholera treatment, menstruation promoter and aphrodisiac. Chinese physicians prescribed it for depression, menstrual complaints, and complications of childbirth.

Despite its cultivation in Moorish Spain, saffron was rare in northern Europe until after the Crusades. But by the 14th century, it had become so popular as a dye, spice, perfume, and medicine that spice merchants throughout the continent were known as saffron grocers.

Under the Doctrine of Signatures—the medieval belief that plants' physical appearances revealed their healing value—anything yellow was linked to the liver's yellow bile and considered good for that organ. Folk healers recommended saffron for jaundice. They also used it to treat insomnia and cancer.

Highly Regarded, Widely Touted

Herbalist John Gerard called saffron a lifesaver: "For those at death's doure and almost past breathing, saffron bringeth breath again."

Seventeenth-century English herbalist Nicholas Culpeper considered it "elegant . . . exhilerating . . . and useful. . . . It strengthens the heart exceedingly . . . [Saffron] is particularly serviceable in disorders of the breast . . . and hysteric [menstrual] depressions. It strengthens the stomach, helps digestion, cleanses the lungs, and is good in coughs." But for all his praise, Culpeper also considered saffron potentially hazardous: "When the dose is too large, it produces a heaviness of the head and sleepiness. Some have fallen into convulsive laughter, which ended in death."

In 1851, scientists isolated the herb's most active constituent, crocetin, which America's 19th-century Eclectics prescribed as a menstrual remedy, menstruation promoter, and treatment for childhood fevers. But America's botanical physicians considered saffron "too costly" and noted the herb was so frequently adulterated, preparations called saffron could not be relied upon to contain the herb.

Contemporary herbalists recommend saffron as a sedative, expectorant, sexual stimulant, pain reliever, digestive aid, and menstruation promoter.

HEALING with Saffron

Culpeper may have been right when he said saffron "strengthens the heart exceedingly." The herb is indeed expensive, but it costs a lot less than some clot-dissolving drugs injected directly into the heart to treat heart attack (up to $2,000 per dose) or bypass surgery (approximately $25,000). People who use enough saffron might actually *save* money in the end, because it may help control some risk factors for heart disease.

Cholesterol. Several animal studies show injected crocetin produces significant cholesterol decreases. Of course, people who ingest whole saffron orally may not receive the same benefit as animals injected with the herb's active constituent. Population studies, however, support the herb as a protector against human heart disease. Certain populations in Spain have little heart disease (or stroke) despite a relatively high-fat diet. Some experts credit the liberal use of olive oil in cooking. But an article in the British medical journal *Lancet* argued for saffron—also used liberally in Spanish cuisine—as the more important protective factor.

Artery-Clogging Deposits. Crocetin also increases the amount of oxygen in blood. Some researchers suggest this additional oxygen slows the growth of the artery-clogging plaque deposits involved in heart disease.

Blood Pressure. Animal research in China shows saffron reduces blood pressure, and in the United States, crocetin is used to treat high blood pressure in cats. These findings suggest it may help control another important risk factor in human heart disease.

Women's Health. Saffron may stimulate the uterus, lending some credence to its traditional use in menstruation promotion. Pregnant women should not use medicinal amounts. Other women may try it to trigger their periods.

R℩ for Saffron

For potential heart disease prevention or menstruation promotion, use 12 to 15 stigmas (threads) per cup of boiling water. Steep 10 minutes. Take up to 1 cup a day. Saffron tastes pleasant and richly aromatic, but it becomes bitter in large amounts.

Medicinal doses of saffron should not be given to children under age 2. For older children and people over 65, start with low-strength preparations and increase strength if necessary.

The Safety Factor

Crocetin has been used to induce abortion. Unfortunately, it's toxic in large amounts. Fatalities have been reported in women attempting to terminate pregnancy.

The medical literature contains no reports of harm from recommended amounts of this herb, however.

Saffron is included in the Food and Drug Administration's list of herbs generally regarded as safe. For otherwise healthy nonpregnant, nonnursing adults, saffron is considered safe in amounts typically recommended.

Saffron should be used in medicinal amounts only in consultation with your doctor. If saffron causes minor discomforts, such as stomach upset or diarrhea, use less or stop using it. Let your doctor know if you experience any unpleasant effects or if the symptoms for which the herb is being used do not improve significantly in two weeks.

Save the Stigmas

Saffron grows from a bulb called a corm. It's a perennial, showy ornamental that rarely grows taller than 18 inches. Saffron has no true stem. What appears to be the stem is actually the tubular portion of the flower envelope (corolla), which is surrounded by leaves resembling blades of grass.

Plant corms in the fall or spring, 3 inches deep with the root side down in light, well-drained soil under full sun. Allow 6 inches between plants. The flowers bloom briefly in late summer or early fall. Carefully collect the three-pronged stigmas and allow them to dry. Store them in a sealed glass vial in a cool, dry place.

SAGE

Herb for the Wise

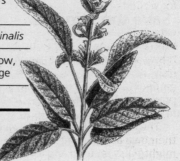

Family: Labiatae; other members include mints

Genus and species: *Salvia officinalis*

Also known as: Garden, meadow, Spanish, Greek, or Dalmatian sage

Parts used: Leaves

Close your eyes and imagine Thanksgiving turkey stuffing. Chances are the warm, rich aroma comes from sage. Thousands of years before the Pilgrims stuffed the first Thanksgiving turkey, people all over the world were celebrating the healing powers of this aromatic herb. The generic name for sage, *Salvia*, comes from the Latin word meaning "to heal."

Sage was used to treat so many maladies, it gained a reputation as a panacea, prompting herb expert Varro Tyler, Ph.D., to write: "If one consults enough herbals . . . every sickness known to humanity will be listed as being cured by sage." Sage is no cure-all, but research shows this herb has some value as an antiperspirant, preservative, wound treatment, and digestive aid.

The Immortality Herb

The ancient Greeks and Romans first used sage as a meat preservative. They also believed it could enhance memory, like another powerful preservative, rosemary. But sage gained a much broader medicinal reputation. The Roman naturalist Pliny prescribed it for snakebite, epilepsy, intestinal worms, chest ailments, and menstruation promotion. The Greek physician Dioscorides considered it a diuretic and menstruation promoter and recommended sage leaves as bandages for wounds.

Around the 10th century, Arab physicians believed sage extended life to the point of immortality. After the Crusades, this belief showed up in Europe, where students at the medieval world's most prestigious medical school in Salerno, Italy, recited: "Why should a man die who grows sage in his garden?" The same thought evolved into a medieval English proverb: "He that would live foraye [forever]/ Must eat sage in May."

The French called the herb *toute bonne*, "all's well," and had their own adage: "Sage helps the nerves, and by its powerful might/Palsy is cured and fever put to flight." Charlemagne ordered sage grown in the medicinal herb gardens on his imperial farms.

Widely Prescribed

Around the year 1000, an Icelandic herbal recommended sage for bladder infections and kidney stones. German abbess/herbalist Hildegard of Bingen prescribed sage for headache and gastrointestinal and respiratory ailments from the common cold to tuberculosis.

During the 16th century, Dutch explorers introduced sage to the Chinese, who prized it so highly they gladly traded 3 pounds of their own tea for each pound of the new European healer. Chinese physicians used sage to treat insomnia, depression, gastrointestinal distress, mental illness, menstrual complaints, and nipple inflammation (mastitis) in nursing mothers.

India's traditional Ayurvedic physicians used Indian sage similarly. They also prescribed it for hemorrhoids, gonorrhea, vaginitis, and eye disorders.

Herbalist John Gerard called sage "singularly good for the head and brain. It quickeneth the senses and memory, strengtheneth the sinews, restoreth health to those that have palsy, and taketh away shaky trembling of the members." Seventeenth-century English herbalist Nicholas Culpeper seconded Gerard, and recommended sage "boiled in water or wine to wash sore mouths and throats, cankers, or the secret parts [genitals] of man or woman."

America Embraces the Herb

Colonists introduced sage into North America, where it was widely used by folk healers to treat insomnia, epilepsy, measles, seasickness, and intestinal worms.

America's 19th-century Eclectics used sage primarily to treat fever. They also prescribed sage poultices for arthritis and the tea as "a valuable anaphrodisiac [sexual depressant] to check excessive venereal desires . . . used in connection with moral . . . and other aids, if necessary."

As late as the 1920s, U.S. medical texts recommended sage tea as a gargle for sore throat and sage leaf poultices for sprains and swellings.

Modern herbalists recommend sage externally for wounds and insect bites, as a gargle for bleeding gums, sore throat, laryngitis, tonsillitis, and in an infusion to reduce perspiration, terminate milk production, and treat dizziness, depression, menstrual irregularity, and intestinal upsets.

HEALING with Sage

Toute bonne overstates things a bit, but sage contains an aromatic oil with some value in herbal healing. The oil has one unique property that sets sage apart from all other healing herbs—it reduces perspiration.

Antiperspirant. Several studies show sage cuts perspiration by as much as 50 percent, with the maximum effect occurring 2 hours after ingestion. This effect helps explain how sage developed a reputation for treating fever, which causes profuse sweating, and for drying up mothers' milk. Today a sage-based antiperspirant (Salysat) is marketed in Germany.

Wound Treatment. Sage is active against several infection-causing bacteria in the test tube, lending some credence to its age-old use in treating wounds. Modern physicians would not recommend bandaging wounds with sage leaves as did Dioscorides, but for cuts and scrapes in the garden, you may want to crush some sage leaves into the wound on the way to washing and bandaging it.

Preservative. Meats spoil in part because their fats turn rancid (oxidize). Like rosemary, sage contains powerful antioxidants, which slow spoilage. The antioxidants in sage, comparable to the commercial preservatives BHA and BHT, support its traditional use as a preservative.

Sage's preservative action may help prevent food poisoning on your next picnic. Mix it generously into hamburger meat and tuna, pasta, and potato salads.

Digestive Aid. Like most culinary spices, sage may help relax the smooth muscle lining of the digestive tract (making it an antispasmodic). This property lends support to the herb's traditional use in gastrointestinal complaints.

Diabetes. One German study shows sage reduces blood sugar (glucose) levels in diabetics who drink the infusion on an empty stomach. Diabetes is a serious condition requiring professional care. If you'd like to include sage in your overall management plan, discuss the herb with your physician.

Sore Throat. Sage contains astringent tannins, which account for its traditional use in treating canker sores, bleeding gums, and sore throat. In Germany, where herbal healing is more mainstream than it is in the United States, physicians recommend a hot sage gargle for sore throat and tonsillitis.

Women's Health. Some studies suggest sage oil may stimulate the uterus, possibly explaining its traditional use in menstruation promotion. Pregnant women should not take medicinal doses. Other women might try it to bring on their periods.

Rx for Sage

For garden first aid, crush some fresh leaves into cuts and scrapes on the way to thoroughly washing and bandaging them.

For an infusion to settle the stomach, or possibly help manage diabetes, use 1 to 2 teaspoons of dried leaves per cup of boiling water. Steep 10 minutes. Drink up to 3 cups a day. This may also be used as a gargle. Sage tastes warm, pleasantly aromatic, and somewhat pungent.

In a tincture, take 1/2 to 1 teaspoon up to three times a day. It might also help reduce wetness if you perspire a lot.

Medicinal doses of sage should not be given to children under age 2. For older children and people over 65, start with low-strength preparations and increase strength if necessary.

The Safety Factor

The medical literature contains a few reports of inflammation of the lips and lining of the mouth associated with ingestion of sage tea.

Sage contains relatively high levels of one toxic chemical (thujone). In large amounts, thujone causes a variety of symptoms culminating in convulsions, but the heat of sage infusions eliminates much of the chemical, so the risk from recommended amounts of sage infusion is negligible.

Alert: Sage oil might cause toxicity and should not be ingested.

Other Cautions

Sage is included in the Food and Drug Administration's list of herbs generally regarded as safe. For otherwise healthy nonpregnant, nonnursing adults, sage is considered relatively safe in amounts typically recommended.

Sage should be used in medicinal amounts only in consultation with your doctor. If sage causes minor discomforts, such as lip or mouth inflammation, use less or stop using it.

Let your doctor know if you experience any unpleasant effects or if the symptoms for which the herb is being used do not improve significantly in two weeks.

Sage Advice for the Garden

Sage is a perennial, branching, evergreen shrub that reaches about 3 feet. It has square, woolly, woody stems near its base, which become herbaceous toward the top. Its 2-inch leaves are oval, velvety, and gray-green with long stalks. Depending on the species, sage's small, summer-blooming flowers are pink, white, blue, or purple.

Sage is not related to the West's sagebrush, but the latter was so named because of its vaguely sagelike aroma.

Sage may be propagated from seeds or cuttings. Germination takes a few weeks. Sow seeds $1/2$ inch deep in spring. It takes about two years to grow good-size plants from seeds, which is why many authorities recommend planting 4-inch cuttings taken in the fall for use the following spring.

Sage grows well in almost any soil but requires good drainage and full sun. Water well until plants have become established, after which they require less water. Sage should be replaced every three or four years because plants become woody and less productive. If your winter temperatures fall below zero, mulch your sage in fall.

Harvest leaves before the flower buds open by cutting the plant back to 4 inches aboveground. Discard the stems and leaf stalks. Dry the herb, then store it in airtight containers.

ST.-JOHN'S-WORT

Possible AIDS Treatment

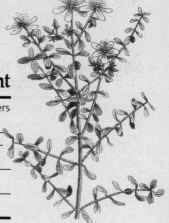

Family: Hypericaceae; other members include rose of Sharon

Genus and species: *Hypericum perforatum*

Also known as: Hypericum

Parts used: Leaves and flowers

St.-John's-wort has been used in herbal healing for more than 2,000 years, most notably for its ability to speed wound healing. And only recently scientists have gathered some evidence on the herb's possible effectiveness as an immune system stimulant.

But its most exciting potential medical use was discovered in 1988, when researchers at New York University and the Weizmann Institute found it has "dramatic" activity against a family of viruses that includes HIV (human immunodeficiency virus), which causes acquired immune deficiency syndrome (AIDS). Since then, some AIDS patients have reported "positive results" with the herb.

Saint's Beheading

The leaves and flowers of St.-John's-wort contain special glands that release a red oil when pinched. Early Christians named the plant in honor of John the Baptist, because they believed it released its blood-red oil on August 29, the anniversary of the saint's beheading. (*Wort* is Old English for plant.)

In the first century, the Roman naturalist Pliny prescribed St.-John's-wort in wine as a cure for the bites of poisonous snakes. And the Greek physician Dioscorides recommended it externally for burns and internally as a diuretic, menstruation promoter, and treatment for sciatica and recurring fevers (malaria). The Greeks and Romans also believed the herb was a protector against witches' spells.

Christians adopted the pagan belief that St.-John's-wort repelled evil spirits and burned it in bonfires on St. John's Eve to purify the air, drive away evil spirits, and ensure healthy crops. This poem from around 1400 summed up the popular view:

> St.-John's-wort doth charm all witches away
> If gathered at midnight on the saint's holy day.
> Any devils and witches have no power to harm
> Those that gather the plant for a charm.
> Rub the lintels with that red juicy flower;
> No thunder nor tempest will then have the power
> To hurt or hinder your house; and bind
> Round your neck a charm of a similar kind.

"A Most Precious Remedy"

Under the Doctrine of Signatures—the medieval belief that herbs' physical appearance revealed their healing value—red plants were believed to be good for wounds, and "the juicy red flower" of St.-John's-wort was no exception. In the 16th century John Gerard recommended it as a "most precious remedy for deepe wounds," and wrote the herb "provoketh urine and is right good against stone in the bladder."

The first *London Pharmacopoeia* in 1618 advised chopping St.-John's-wort flowers, immersing them in oil, and placing the mixture in the sun for three weeks. The resulting tincture was a standard treatment for wounds and bruises for several hundred years.

Seventeenth-century English herbalist Nicholas Culpeper

called St.-John's-wort "a singular wound herb; boiled in wine and drank, it healeth inward hurts or bruises; made into an ointment, it opens obstructions, dissolves swellings, and closes up the lips of wounds. . . . [It] helpeth all manner of vomiting and spitting blood [tuberculosis]."

Treatment for Wounds

Early colonists introduced St.-John's-wort into North America but found the Indians using the native American herb in much the same way Europeans used the Old World plant—as a tonic and treatment for diarrhea, fever, snakebite, wounds, and skin problems.

Nineteenth-century botanical medicine authority Charles Millspaugh, M.D., touted St.-John's-wort's value as a wound treatment during the Civil War.

Throughout the 19th century, homeopathy was as popular as orthodox medicine, and homeopaths prescribed the herb for a variety of ailments: wounds, asthma, bites, sciatica, diarrhea, hemorrhoids, and certain forms of paralysis. Contemporary homeopaths continue this tradition.

America's 19th-century Eclectic physicians also considered St.-John's-wort a useful wound treatment and tetanus preventive and advocated the whole herb as a treatment for "hysteria" (menstrual discomforts) because of its "undoubted power over the nervous system and spinal cord."

A Question About Blisters

Contemporary herbalists are divided on St.-John's-wort because in 1977 the Food and Drug Administration declared it unsafe. After eating large quantities, cattle often become overly sensitive to the sun (photosensitization) and develop severe sunburn with blistering. Several sources say the same is true for humans, especially those with fair skin.

One recent herbal says: "Internal use of St.-John's-wort should be avoided." Some herbals say those with fair skin should use St.-John's-wort cautiously, but that other people don't have to worry. Meanwhile, most herbals either ignore the issue or dismiss it, saying the plant has been used safely in herbal healing for more than 2,000 years.

Herbalists unconcerned about the safety issue recommend St.-John's-wort externally for wound treatment and internally for sciatica, insomnia, menstrual cramps, headache, colds, chest congestion, and as a tranquilizer.

HEALING with St.-John's-Wort

St.-John's-wort has been intensively researched, mostly in Germany and the former Soviet Union. It contains high concentrations of some potential immune-modulating chemicals, known as flavonoids. St.-John's-wort also contains another substance, hypericin, that has antiviral and antidepressive action. Other studies show antibacterial, antifungal, and anti-inflammatory effects.

AIDS. One of St.-John's-wort's most exciting effects is hypericin's apparent activity against the AIDS virus.

A study published in the *Proceedings of the National Academy of Sciences* shows the herb has "dramatic activity and little toxicity" against viruses similar to HIV, the AIDS virus, in test-tube and animal tests. Mice were infected with viruses that cause leukemia, then given a single injection of St.-John's-wort extract. It "totally prevented disease." The herb was equally effective when the mice received it orally. Preliminary laboratory tests indicated similar action against the HIV virus. The herb also crosses the blood/brain barrier, which is important in AIDS treatment because the virus often attacks the brain.

These findings caused some excitement among AIDS researchers, some of whom launched studies to test St.-John's-wort in people with AIDS. As this book goes to press, those studies have not been completed. Since early 1989, however, the newsletter *AIDS Treatment News* has published case reports and surveys of AIDS sufferers, some of whom have experienced "significant improvement" using St.-John's-wort, including increased immune function, weight gain, improved appetite, and greater energy.

Such reports are heartening, but like all anecdotal information, they must be viewed cautiously. Until the scientific studies have been completed and replicated, St.-John's-wort cannot be considered an AIDS treatment. Nonetheless, preliminary results look promising.

AIDS patients enrolled in St.-John's-wort studies do not use the bulk herb but rather a "standardized extract." Standardization is crucial to the scientific acceptability of research results.

Wound Healing. Several studies have supported St.-John's-wort's traditional use in wound healing. The hypericin and other antibiotic chemicals in the herb's red oil may help prevent wound infection. In addition, the plant's potential immune-stimulating flavonoids help reduce wound inflammation. One German study showed that compared with conventional treatment, a St.-John's-wort ointment substantially cut the healing time of burns and caused less scarring. (This product is not available in the United States.)

Antidepressant. Hypericin appears to interfere with the activity of a chemical in the body known as monoamine oxidase (MAO), making it an MAO inhibitor. MAO inhibitors are an important class of antidepressant drugs. In a small German study, 15 women in treatment for depression obtained significant relief after taking St.-John's-wort, including increased appetite, greater interest in life, improved feelings of self-worth, and more normal sleep patterns. But St.-John's-wort is not an instant antidepressant. According to German medical herbalist Rudolph Fritz Weiss, M.D., the effect "does not develop quickly. . . . [It takes] two or three months."

R$_x$ for St.-John's-Wort

For AIDS treatment, consult a physician for help in obtaining the standardized extracts or in getting enrolled in a clinical trial of the substance.

For wound treatment, apply crushed leaves and flowers to the affected area after you have cleaned it with soap and water.

For an infusion to help treat depression and possibly stimulate the immune system, use 1 to 2 teaspoons of dried herb per cup of boiling water. Steep 10 to 15 minutes. Drink up to 3 cups a day. St.-John's-wort tastes initially sweet, then bitter and astringent.

In a tincture, use 1/4 to 1 teaspoon up to three times a day.

St.-John's-wort should not be given to children under age 2. For older children and people over 65, start with low-strength preparations and increase strength if necessary.

The Safety Factor

In combination with certain foods and drugs, MAO inhibitors may cause dangerously increased blood pressure (hypertensive crisis). Symptoms include headache, stiff neck, nausea, vomiting, and clammy skin. In recommended amounts, St.-John's-wort is not as powerful as pharmaceutical MAO-inhibitors. Nonetheless, those using the herb should follow certain precautions. While using St.-John's-wort, do not take amphetamines, narcotics, the amino acids tryptophan and tyrosine, diet pills, asthma inhalants, nasal decongestants, or cold or hay fever medications. In addition, don't drink beer, wine, or coffee, or eat salami, yogurt, chocolate, fava beans, or smoked or pickled items.

Shun the Sun

In livestock fed St.-John's-wort, the hypericin concentrates near the skin and causes blistering sunburn.

Laboratory animals injected with large doses of hypericin have died after exposure to sunlight.

The scientific consensus is that in recommended doses, whole St.-John's-wort causes little if any photosensitization except in fair-skinned people, who are generally more sensitive to sunlight. Those taking St.-John's-wort (like those taking the antibiotic tetracycline, another photosensitizing drug) should make an effort to stay out of the sun.

AIDS patients report the herb is relatively nontoxic, but some have reported drowsiness, sun sensitivity, nausea, and diarrhea.

Other Cautions

The FDA can't make up its mind about St.-John's-wort. After declaring it unsafe in 1977, the agency partially reversed its ruling and now allows the herb in vermouths.

For otherwise healthy nonpregnant, nonnursing adults who do not have hypertension and are not taking MAO inhibitors or any medications that interact adversely with them, St.-John's-wort is considered safe in amounts typically recommended. It should only be used, however, with the consent and supervision of a physician.

St.-John's-wort should be used in medicinal amounts only in consultation with your doctor. If St.-John's-wort causes headache, stiff neck, or nausea, use less or stop using it. If symptoms persist, consult your physician promptly.

Flowers That "Bleed"

St.-John's-wort is a woody, invasively spreading perennial that reaches 2 feet and has an aroma reminiscent of turpentine. Its leaves are dotted with glands that produce a red oil. Its striking star-shaped flowers bloom bright yellow in summer. They also contain the leaf oil, and when pinched, turn red.

St.-John's-wort is best propagated from root divisions in spring or fall. It grows in almost any well-drained soil under full sun or partial shade. Contain the herb to control its spread. Although it is a perennial, St.-John's-wort is not particularly long lived. Replant it every few years.

Harvest the leaves and flower tops as the plants bloom. Dry them and store in airtight containers.

SARSAPARILLA

A Sexy Reputation

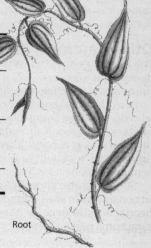

Family: Liliaceae; other members include lily

Genus and species: *Smilax officinalis, S. febrifuga,* and other *Smilax* species

Also known as: Mexican, Vera Cruz, Honduran, Jamaican, American, and Ecuadoran sarsaparilla

Parts used: Rhizome and roots

Root

You probably thought the cowboy asked the saloon keeper to "Give me a sarsaparilla" because he didn't want whiskey. But cowboys who ordered sarsaparilla usually had more than refreshment in mind. The herb was among the most widely used 19th-century treatments for syphilis, and cowboys often ordered it after visiting the local brothel.

Scientists now say sarsaparilla has no benefit against syphilis, and many dismiss the herb as medically useless. But studies suggest it may have some benefit as a diuretic.

Linked to Syphilis

The ancient Greeks and Romans considered European sarsaparilla an antidote to poisons. But the herb was not popular in herbal healing until the 16th century, when Spanish explorers discovered the Caribbean species, a prickly (*zarza*) vine (*parra*) that was small (*illa*). That description became our word *sarsaparilla*. Caribbean and North American Indians used the herb to treat skin conditions, urinary complaints, and as a tonic to keep one young and vigorous, both physically and sexually.

In 1494 an epidemic of unusually virulent syphilis swept Europe, killing thousands, rather like the AIDS epidemic today. Europeans considered the disease an import from the New World, and they looked to herbs from across the Atlantic to treat it. They focused on sarsaparilla.

The conquistadors began shipping Mexican sarsaparilla back to Spain around 1530, and by 1600 it was widely used throughout Europe as a strengthening tonic and treatment for syphilis. Sarsaparilla and syphilis have been entwined ever since.

Sarsaparilla enjoyed a meteoric rise in popularity. Seventeenth-century English herbalist Nicholas Culpeper called it the treatment of choice for "the French disease," the English name for syphilis. Echoing the ancients, he wrote: "If the juice of the berries be given to a new-born child, it shall never be hurt by poison." Culpeper also recommended sarsaparilla for eye problems, head colds, gas pains, pimples, and "all manner of aches in the sinews or joints."

By 1800, many physicians denounced sarsaparilla as completely ineffective against syphilis, but their words fell on deaf ears. Mid–19th-century trade records indicate Britain imported upward of 150,000 pounds a year, much of it for treatment of syphilis.

"Blood Purifier"

In 19th-century America, sexually transmitted diseases were never mentioned in polite conversation. Nonetheless, syphilis was quite prevalent, and physicians experimented with many herbs and patent medicines to treat it. These treatments were known euphemistically as "blood purifiers." One of the most popular was Ayer's sarsaparilla, marketed for "disorders of the liver, stomach, kidneys, as well as tuberculosis, tumors, rheumatism, female weakness, sterility, pimples, and syphilis."

Sarsaparilla was listed in the U.S. P*harmacopoeia* as a syphilis treatment from 1820 to 1882, but after the Civil War, the anti-sarsaparilla bandwagon gained momentum, and by the late 19th century, most physicians dismissed it as worthless.

Although there is no scientific research to back up these traditional uses, contemporary herbalists continue to recommend sarsaparilla for colds, coughs, fevers, and gout. Some say it contains the male sex hormone testosterone. None recommend it for syphilis.

HEALING with Sarsaparilla

For an herb once so popular, it's amazing how little research has been done on sarsaparilla. Most studies date from the 1930s to early 1950s, and few have been replicated. Nonetheless, scientists have turned up some benefits. Sarsaparilla contains chemicals (saponins) with diuretic action, which possibly account for its long association with the genitals.

Syphilis. Western investigators insist sarsaparilla is useless against syphilis. But unconfirmed reports from China suggest it may help. Perhaps the Chinese—and 500 years of herbalism—are completely wrong. Or perhaps 19th-century physicians were right when they observed that sarsaparilla takes a long time to show benefit. The question deserves investigation because syphilis has been on the upswing in the United States in recent years.

High Blood Pressure. Physicians often prescribe diuretics for high blood pressure. High blood pressure is a serious condition requiring professional care. If you'd like to include sarsaparilla in your overall treatment plan, do so only with the approval and supervision of your physician.

Diuretics deplete the body of potassium, an essential nutrient. If you use sarsaparilla frequently, be sure to eat foods high in potassium, such as bananas and fresh vegetables.

Congestive Heart Failure. Physicians often prescribe diuretics to combat the fluid accumulation involved in this condition. Heart failure demands professional care. If you'd like to include sarsaparilla in your overall treatment plan, discuss it with your physician.

Women's Health. Pregnant and nursing women should not use diuretics. But as a diuretic, sarsaparilla might provide some relief for women bothered by premenstrual bloating (fluid retention).

Intriguing Possibilities. Preliminary studies from around the world have reported sarsaparilla helps treat psoriasis and leprosy.

Dead-End File. Saponins bear some chemical resemblance to the male sex hormones testosterone and anabolic steroids. Some writers have claimed sarsaparilla contains testosterone. It does not.

Sarsaparilla has also enjoyed some popularity among body builders who believe it contains anabolic steroids, which they take against medical advice to increase their muscle mass. Sarsaparilla contains no anabolic steroids.

Rx for Sarsaparilla

For a diuretic decoction, use 1 to 2 teaspoons of powdered root per cup of water. Bring to a boil and simmer for 10 to 15 minutes. Drink up to 3 cups a day. Sarsaparilla tastes initially sweetish, then unpleasant.

In a tincture, take ¼ to ½ teaspoon up to three times a day.

Sarsaparilla should not be given to children under age 2. For older children and people over 65, start with low-strength preparations and increase strength if necessary.

The Safety Factor

Some diet programs tout diuretics to eliminate water weight. But weight-control authorities discourage diuretics. Weight lost

using diuretics almost invariably returns. The key to permanent weight control is a low-fat, high-fiber diet and regular
aerobic exercise.

Large amounts of sarsaparilla saponins may cause a burning sensation in the mouth and throat, as well as stomach
and intestinal irritation.

Other Cautions

Sarsaparilla is included in the Food and Drug Administration's list of herbs generally regarded as safe. For otherwise healthy nonpregnant, nonnursing adults, sarsaparilla is
considered relatively safe in amounts typically recommended.

Sarsaparilla should be used in medicinal amounts only in
consultation with your doctor. If sarsaparilla causes minor
discomforts, such as burning in the mouth or stomach upset,
use less or stop using it. Let your doctor know if you experience unpleasant effects or if the symptoms for which the herb
is being used do not improve significantly in two weeks.

Caribbean Vine

Sarsaparilla is not a garden herb in the United States. It's a
perennial, climbing, woody, prickly-stemmed vine with
pointed, generally oval-shaped leaves. Its flowers are dioecious (male and female on different plants), small, and green,
yellow, or bronze. The medicinal parts, the rhizome and long,
slender roots, are underground.

SAVORY

Subtle Soother for Children

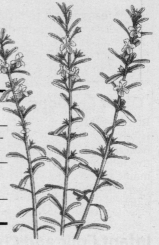

Family: Labiatae; other members include mints

Genus and species: *Satureja hortensis* (summer), *S. montana* (winter)

Also known as: Bean herb, white thyme

Parts used: Leaves

With a spicy aroma and flavor reminiscent of thyme, savory is widely used in sausages, stuffings, soups, and bean dishes. Like other aromatic culinary herbs, savory has been used since ancient times as a cough remedy and stomach soother. But compared with its mint cousins, savory's action is less powerful. Adults might prefer peppermint, but savory can be used safely and confidently for children's coughs, colds, and tummy aches.

A Tale of Two Herbs

Summer savory is a low-growing annual. Winter savory is an equally diminutive perennial. Purists insist the summer herb has a sweeter, more delicate aroma; however, today most cooks and herbalists use them interchangeably. But this was not always the case—especially in the bedroom.

For reasons lost to history, the ancient Romans linked summer savory to the mythological satyrs—the lustful, half-man, half-goat creatures who threw debauched orgies in honor of Dionysus, god of wine. As a result, the Roman naturalist Pliny called summer savory an aphrodisiac and the winter herb a sex depressant. Not surprisingly, summer savory was more popular.

The Romans introduced summer savory throughout Europe, where it quickly became a popular spice. Germanic tribes loved its flavor in beans and called it bean herb (*bohnendraut*). To this day, Germans regard savory as an effective remedy for the downside of beans, flatulence. The Germanic Saxons who settled in Britain thought savory made every food taste, well, savory, which is how it got its English name.

Infant Colic and Childhood Ailments

By the 17th century, summer savory had shed its association with lust. The summer and winter varieties began to be used interchangeably and called simply "savory." Nicholas Culpeper wrote it "expels wind from the stomach and bowels and is good for asthma and other affections of the breast. Neither is there a better remedy for the colic and iliac passion [upset stomach]." He also recommended savory as a stimulant to "quicken the dull spirits." Externally, Culpeper touted savory poultices for sciatica and "palsied members" (paralyzed limbs).

Colonists introduced savory into North America, where it was widely used as a digestive aid and cough, cold, and diarrhea remedy, especially for children. The 19th-century Eclectics also distilled the herb's oil and used it like clove oil to treat toothache.

Contemporary herbalists generally confine their recommendations to indigestion and diarrhea. But some still suggest summer savory as a sexual stimulant, especially for women, even though there has been no scientific research to back this up.

HEALING with Savory

Savory contains an expectorant (cineole) and chemicals that soothe the digestive tract.

Digestive Aid. Although these chemicals make it appropriate as a digestive aid, scientists agree with traditional herbalists that savory is less powerful than most of the mints. Its gentler action confirms its traditional use for childhood ailments.

R$_x$ for Savory

For an infusion to treat childhood cough, colds, and stomach upset, use 1 to 2 teaspoons of dried herb per cup of boiling water. Steep 10 minutes. Give up to 3 cups a day. Savory tastes pleasant, like thyme, only more peppery. Adults may use 4 teaspoons of herb per cup.

In a tincture, use ½ teaspoon up to three times a day for children and 1 teaspoon for adults.

The Safety Factor

The medical literature contains no reports of harm from either summer or winter savory.

Savory is included in the Food and Drug Administration's list of herbs generally regarded as safe. For otherwise healthy nonpregnant, nonnursing adults, savory is safe in amounts typically recommended.

Savory should be used in medicinal amounts only in consultation with your doctor. Let your doctor know if you experience any unpleasant effects or if the symptoms for which the herb is being used do not improve significantly in two weeks.

Savor Your Savory

Annual summer savory reaches 18 inches. It has hairy, purplish stems, narrow, lance-shaped leaves, and small white or pink flowers, which bloom from midsummer through the first frost. Winter savory is a compact, woody, perennial bush that grows to 12 inches. Its leaves are similar to those of its summer cousin, only darker green, and its flowers, which bloom from mid to late summer, are white or lavender.

Both are easy to grow from seeds or cuttings, and both grow well in containers. Summer savory grows in most moist, well-drained soils. Sow seeds no more than 1/8 inch deep under full sun and thin seedlings to 10-inch spacing. Water frequently.

Winter savory is slower to germinate. It prefers lighter, drier soil. Do not overwater. Although it is a perennial, it may not survive New England and midwest winters. Even in warm areas it is short-lived and must be replaced every few years.

Leaves of both species may be harvested when plants reach 6 inches. When they flower, cut them near the ground, dry them, then strip the leaves. Store in airtight containers in a cool, dry place.

SENNA

A Powerful Laxative

Family: Caesalpinioideae; other members include brazilwood

Genus and species: *Cassia senna,* *C. acutifolia* (Alexandrian and Khartoum), *C. angustifolia* (Indian or Tinnevelly), *C. marilandica* (American)

Also known as: Cassia

Parts used: Leaflets, seed pods

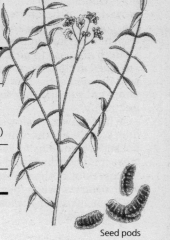

Seed pods

S enna is a powerful laxative—so powerful, in fact, that many authorities call it a cathartic. Arab physicians first wrote of its bowel-stimulating action in the 9th century, but their descriptions suggest it had been widely used for centuries from the Middle East to India.

Senna was introduced into European herbal healing before the Crusades and has been widely used ever since.

Internal Cleanser

Seventeenth-century English herbalist Nicholas Culpeper, who came close to prescribing every herb for every ill, could not resist claiming senna "cleanses the stomach, purges melancholy and phlegm from the head, brain, lungs, heart, liver, and spleen, cleansing those parts of evil humour; strengthens the senses, procures mirth, purifies the blood [treats venereal disease], and is also good in chronic agues [fevers]." Other herbalists generally recommended senna only as a laxative.

The American Indians recognized native American senna's laxative action but used it primarily to treat fever. The 19th-century Eclectics, influenced by Indian medicine, called senna "very useful in all forms of febrile [fever-producing] diseases in which laxative action is desired."

Contemporary herbalists all tout senna's laxative action but warn of its terrible taste and side effects—primarily intestinal cramps.

Not for Toast

Both senna and cinnamon come from trees with peelable bark, in Arabic, *quetsiah*, meaning to cut, which became *cassia* in English. Both are sometimes called cassia today. But these two herbs have very different actions and should not be confused.

HEALING with Senna

Senna does not treat fever, nor does it "purge melancholy and procure mirth." Quite the contrary. If you're not careful with this herb, you'll live to regret using it.

Laxative. Like aloe, buckthorn, and cascara sagrada, senna contains chemicals that stimulate the colon (anthraquinones). The herb is an ingredient in many over-the-counter laxatives: Fletcher's Castoria, Gentlax, Sennexon, Senokap, Senolax, Black Draught, Innerclean Herbal Laxative, and Dr. Caldwell's Senna Laxative.

Senna and the other anthraquinone laxatives, however, should be considered a last resort for constipation. First, increase the fiber in your diet, drink more fluids, and exercise more. If that doesn't work, try the bulk-forming laxative, psyllium (see page 423). If that doesn't help, try a gentler anthraquinone, cascara sagrada (see page 144). And if you still need relief, try senna in consulation with your physician.

Rx for Senna

Because of senna's disgusting taste, herbalists generally discourage using the plant material and instead recommend over-the-counter products containing it.

Those game enough to try the unprocessed herb can brew an infusion from 1 to 2 teaspoons of dried leaves per cup of boiling water. Steep 10 minutes. Drink up to 1 cup a day in the morning or before bed for no more than a few days. The taste of senna is nauseating; add sugar, honey, and lemon, and mix it with such taste-masking herbs as anise, fennel, peppermint, chamomile, ginger, coriander, cardamon, and licorice.

Some sources say the pods have milder action. Steep four pods in a cup of warm water for 6 to 12 hours. Drink up to 1 cup a day in the morning or before bed for no more than a few days.

In a tincture, use $\frac{1}{2}$ to 1 teaspoon in the morning or before bed for no more than a few days.

Senna should not be given to children under age 2. For older children and people over 65, start with a low-strength preparation and increase strength if necessary.

The Safety Factor

Senna's powerful action means it should not be used by those with chronic gastrointestinal conditions, such as ulcers, colitis, or hemorrhoids.

Pregnant and nursing women should not take senna.

Senna should never be used for more than two weeks because over time it causes lazy bowel syndrome, which is an inability to move stool without chemical stimulation.

Large amounts of senna cause diarrhea, nausea, and severe cramps with possible dehydration.

Long-term use may cause enlargement of the fingertips (clubbing). An article in *Lancet* described this effect in a woman who had taken up to 40 senna laxative tablets a day for

15 years. Her fingers returned to normal when she stopped using the herb.

Senna leaves may cause a skin rash in sensitive individuals.

Other Cautions

The Food and Drug Administration considers senna an herb of "undefined safety." For otherwise healthy nonpregnant, nonnursing adults, senna is considered relatively safe when used only occasionally in amounts typically recommended.

Senna should be used in medicinal amounts only in consultation with your doctor. If senna causes cramping, use less or stop using it. Let your doctor know if you experience unpleasant effects or if the symptoms for which the herb is being used do not improve significantly in two weeks.

Rare in the United States

Senna is not a garden herb in the United States. It's a small, woody shrub that reaches 3 feet and has branching stems, pointed leaves, and seeds encased in a leathery pod. The species generally used in herbal medicine is grown in the Tennevelly region of India, near the subcontinent's southern tip. One species grows in the eastern United States, however.

SHEPHERD'S PURSE

Not Exactly Empty

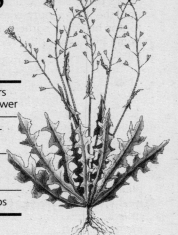

Family: Cruciferae; other members include cabbage, broccoli, cauliflower

Genus and species: *Capsella bur-sapastoris*

Also known as: Lady's purse, rattle pouches, rattle weed

Parts used: Leaves and flower tops

S hepherds never get much respect. In the ancient world, theirs was a humble calling. And in the Old West, cattle ranchers looked down on "sheep herders." So perhaps we should not be surprised that the herb named for shepherds has shared a similar fate.

Sadly Rejected

More than 300 years ago, Nicholas Culpeper wrote: "Few plants possess greater virtues than this, and yet it is utterly disregarded." And as recently as 1988, the British scientific herb guide, *Potter's New Cyclopaedia of Botanical Drugs*, bemoaned the lack of research into its effects. No one is interested, some authorities say, because this common weed is medically worthless. But the few scientific studies done to date have revealed some intriguing possibilities for treating bleeding and inducing labor.

Ancient Greek and Roman physicians recommended shepherd's purse seeds as a laxative. But it was not widely used until the 16th century, when an Italian physician promoted it to stop bleeding, particularly to eliminate blood in the urine. Some physicians adopted the plant, but most others dismissed it as worthless.

The Pilgrims introduced shepherd's purse into North America, where it quickly became a weed. Folk herbalists used it to stop bleeding, while physicians generally dismissed it as useless.

Fresh or Dried?

The Eclectic text, King's American Dispensatory, attempted to explain the shepherd's purse controversy by observing "the fresh herb is decidedly more active than the dried." King's called it "very efficient" for treating bloody urine and recommended it to stop excessive menstrual flow, and to treat diarrhea, dysentery, and bleeding hemorrhoids.

During World War I, when other blood stoppers were in short supply, wounded soldiers were given shepherd's purse tea.

Contemporary herbalists recommend dried shepherd's purse— not the fresh herb—internally for bloody urine, nosebleeds, bleeding after childbirth, and diarrhea, and externally as an astringent to treat wounds and hemorrhoids.

HEALING with Shepherd's Purse

This herb won't set the herbal healing world on fire, but it may help some people with gastrointestinal disorders, women with heavy menstrual flow, or pregnant women waiting to go into labor—if they can stomach its taste.

Bleeding. Shepherd's purse contains substances that hasten the coagulation of blood, according to an article in the British journal Nature. German medical herbalist Rudolph Fritz Weiss, M.D., writes it "definitely has haemostatic [blood-stopping] properties . . . [but they are] not very great."

First-aid authorities recommend treating bleeding with sustained pressure on the wound. Blood in phlegm, urine, or stool requires prompt professional treatment. Shepherd's purse is no substitute for standard treatments. However, people with ulcers, colitis, Crohn's disease, or bleeding disorders or women with heavy menstrual flow might try shepherd's purse in consultation with their physicians, and see if it helps.

Labor Inducer. Shepherd's purse also contains some substances that may help stimulate uterine contractions as effectively as the drug oxytocin (Pitocin). Oxytocin is often given to trigger labor. Pregnant women should not use shepherd's purse, except at term and in consultation with their physicians.

Astringent. The herb also has some minor anti-inflammatory astringent action, lending some credence to its traditional uses for wounds and hemorrhoids.

Rx for Shepherd's Purse

To possibly help stop bleeding or hasten labor, use 1 teaspoon of dried herb per cup of boiling water. Steep 10 minutes. Drink up to 2 cups a day. The taste of shepherd's purse is biting and unpleasant. Add sugar, honey, and lemon, or mix it with an herbal beverage blend to improve flavor.

In a tincture, use 1/4 to 1/2 teaspoon up to twice a day.

Shepherd's purse should not be given to children under age 2. For older children and people over 65, start with low-strength preparations and increase strength if necessary.

The Safety Factor

If this herb does in fact stop bleeding, no one is sure exactly how. It might strengthen blood vessel walls. Or it might stimulate clotting. Internal blood clotting may trigger heart disease, stroke, or thromboembolism. Those with a history of these conditions should not take shepherd's purse.

To use shepherd's purse externally on wounds or hemorrhoids, soak a clean cloth in either an infusion or tincture. The medical literature contains no reports of harm from this herb.

Other Cautions

For otherwise healthy nonpregnant, nonnursing adults who have no history of heart attack, stroke, or thromboembolism, shepherd's purse is considered relatively safe in amounts typically recommended.

Shepherd's purse should be used in medicinal amounts only in consultation with your doctor. If shepherd's purse causes minor discomforts, such as stomach upset or diarrhea, use less or stop using it. Let your doctor know if you experience any unpleasant effects or if the symptoms for which the herb is being used do not improve significantly in two weeks.

Don't Let the Contents Spill

Shepherd's purse is a foul-smelling annual that reaches 18 inches. Its slender stem rises from a rosette of deeply toothed leaves similar to dandelion. The stem bears a few small leaves and terminates in small white flowers. The fruits are wedge-shaped seed pods, containing literally thousands of yellow seeds, hence the herb's names.

Shepherd's purse grows easily from seeds planted in spring under full sun. It prefers well-drained sandy loam but tolerates most North American soils. If unchecked, it can become a garden and lawn pest. To avoid this, clip the seed pods before they open. The young leaves have a peppery taste and may be added to soups and stews or eaten like spinach.

Harvest the leaves and flower tops as the flowers open.

SKULLCAP

All-American Tranquilizer

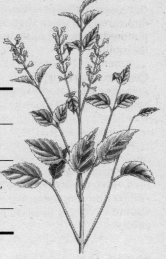

Family: Labiatae; other members include mints

Genus and species: *Scutellaria lateriflora*

Also known as: Skullcap, Virginia skullcap, Quaker bonnet, hoodwort, helmet flower, mad dog weed

Parts used: Leaves

For an herb reputed to calm people down, skullcap has caused considerable controversy. One respected herbalist calls this blue-flowered North American native "perhaps the most widely relevant tranquilizer" in medicine. But skeptics dismiss it as "nearly worthless and essentially inactive."

The truth is, skullcap's traditional use as a tranquilizer may have some merit.

Mad Dog Weed

For centuries, Chinese physicians have used Asian skullcap (S. *baikalensis*) as a tranquilizer/sedative and treatment for convulsions.

Skullcap was first brought to the attention of physicians in the West in 1772 as a cure for rabies. A New England physician claimed that his experiments proved the herb prevented and cured the much dreaded "hydrophobia." Over the next hundred years, herbalists used skullcap as a digestive aid and tranquilizer.

America's 19th-century Eclectic physicians recommended the herb primarily as a tranquilizer/sedative for insomnia and nervousness, and for treatment of "intermittent fever" (malaria), convulsions, and delirium tremens of advanced alcoholism.

Skullcap entered the U.S. *Pharmacopoeia* in 1863 as a tranquilizer. It remained there until 1916, when it moved to the *National Formulary*, the pharmacists' reference, where it remained until 1947.

Contemporary herbalists recommend skullcap as a tranquilizer for insomnia, nervous tension, premenstrual syndrome, and drug and alcohol withdrawal. Some say it treats fever and convulsions.

HEALING with Skullcap

American scientists are almost unanimous in their condemnation of skullcap. They've never gotten over those old, mistaken claims that it treats rabies. The Food and Drug Administration's (FDA) current official assessment echoes the 1943 edition of *The Dispensatory of the United States*, which stated: "Skullcap is as destitute of medicinal properties as a plant may be. When taken internally it produces no obvious effects and probably is of no remedial value."

Tranquilizer, Sedative. Of course, 1943 was a long time ago. Since then, some European and Russian researchers have lent support to skullcap's traditional use as a tranquilizer. European medical experts now accept skullcap's potential usefulness as a tranquilizer and sedative, and it is used in many commercial sleep preparations that are widely available in Europe.

Intriguing Possibility. Two Japanese animal studies showed skullcap increases levels of "good" cholesterol (high-density lipoproteins or HDLs). As HDLs increase, the risk of heart attack decreases. These findings suggest the herb may potentially help prevent human heart disease and some strokes.

Chinese physicians claim to have treated hepatitis successfully with the herb. It's too early to tout skullcap for this potentially serious liver disease, but the herb deserves further research.

Rx for Skullcap

For a tranquilizing infusion, use 1 to 2 teaspoons of dried herb per cup of boiling water. Steep 10 to 15 minutes. Drink up to three times a day. Skullcap tastes bitter; adding honey, sugar, and lemon or mixing it with an herbal beverage blend will improve flavor.

Skullcap should not be given to children under age 2. For older children and people over 65, start with low-strength preparations and increase strength if necessary.

The Safety Factor

There are no reports of toxicity from skullcap infusions, but large amounts of the tincture can cause confusion, giddiness, twitching, and possibly convulsions.

The FDA lists skullcap as an herb of "undefined safety." For otherwise healthy nonpregnant, nonnursing adults, skullcap is considered relatively safe in amounts typically recommended.

Skullcap should be used in medicinal amounts only in consultation with your doctor. If skullcap causes minor discomforts, such as stomach upset or diarrhea, use less or stop using it. Let your doctor know if you experience unpleasant effects or if the symptoms for which the herb is being used do not improve significantly in two weeks.

Sedatives from the Garden

Many skullcap species grow in Europe, but the American herb is the one used in herbal healing. It's sometimes called Virginia skullcap, but it grows all over the United States and southern Canada.

Skullcap is a slender, 2-foot, branching, square-stemmed perennial with opposite, serrated leaves. The flowers have two lips. The upper lip includes an elongated caplike appendage, which is the source of most of the herb's popular names.

Skullcap may be propagated by seeds or root divisions planted in early spring. Thin seedlings to 6-inch spacing. Skullcap grows in any well-drained soil under full sun and requires little care. Although it is a perennial, skullcap rarely lives longer than three years.

Harvest the leaves in midsummer.

SLIPPERY ELM

An Early American Favorite

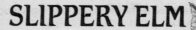

Family: Ulmaceae; other members include nettles

Genus and species: *Ulmus rubra, U. fulva*

Also known as: Red elm, Indian elm

Parts used: Inner bark

Dried bark

No food or drug of today comes close to matching the place of honor slippery elm held in 18th- and 19th-century America. Great elm forests covered the East, and even in cities, the versatile bark was always close at hand.

A Bark for All Reasons

Soaked in water and wrapped around meats, the bark retarded spoilage in the days before refrigeration. Coarsely ground and mixed with water, it turned into a spongy mass and was molded into bandages to cover wounds and made into pill-like coverings for unpleasant-tasting medicines. Ground and mixed with water or milk, slippery elm bark turned into a soothing, nutritious food similar to oatmeal, which was used to treat sore throat, cough, colds, and gastrointestinal ailments and to feed infants and hospital patients. Slippery elm sore throat lozenges were a fixture in home medicine cabinets, and the herb was the nation's leading home remedy for anything in need of soothing.

Slippery elm is still listed in the *National Formulary*, the pharmacists' reference, and health food stores still sell lozenges containing the herb. But our once-great elm forests have been decimated by Dutch elm disease, and both our landscape and our herbal healing heritage are poorer as a result.

Bark for Broken Bones

First-century Greek physician Dioscorides prescribed bathing in a European elm bath to speed the healing of broken bones. His prescription survived more than 1,500 years. In the 17th century, English herbalist Nicholas Culpeper wrote: "The decoction being bathed in, heals broken bones . . . [and] is excellent [for] places . . . burnt with fire. The leaves bruised, applied, and being bound thereon with its own bark heal wounds." Culpeper also claimed elm root decoction restored hair on bald scalps.

Colonists found the Indians using American slippery elm bark as a food and treatment for wounds, sore throat, cough, inflamed nipples (mastitis), and many other ailments. The colonists adopted these uses and developed many more, including applying slippery elm poultices to bring boils to a head.

America's early 19th-century Thomsonian herbalists recommended slippery elm tea as a laxative gentle enough for children, and Thomsonian midwives lubricated their hands with the slippery bark before performing internal examinations.

Elm Stick Law

Indian women inserted slippery elm sticks to induce abortion, and white women adopted the practice, which caused many deaths from uterine infection and hemorrhage. As a result, several state legislatures passed laws forbidding the sale of slippery elm bark in pieces longer than 1 1/2 inches.

By the Civil War, slippery elm was being used to treat syphilis, gonorrhea, and hemorrhoids. America's Eclectic physicians called it "very valuable" and suggested "a tablespoon of the powder boiled in milk affords a nourishing diet for infants newly weaned, preventing the bowel complaints to which they are subject. Some physicians consider the constant use of it, during and after the seventh month of gestation, as advantageous in facilitating an easy delivery."

Contemporary herbalists recommend slippery elm bark externally to cover wounds and soothe skin problems and internally as a tea to treat sore throat, cough, diarrhea, ulcers, colitis, and other gastrointestinal complaints.

HEALING with Slippery Elm

Even the Food and Drug Administration calls this herb "an excellent demulcent" (soothing agent).

Wounds. Slippery elm bark contains special cells that expand into a spongy mass in the presence of liquid. Applied to thoroughly cleaned wounds, it dries to form an herbal bandage.

Cough, Sore Throat, Digestive Complaints. Slippery elm decoction helps soothe the throat and digestive tract.

Women's Health. Slippery elm decoction has a long history of use by pregnant women, and the medical literature contains no reports of problems. The active constituent, mucilage, should not harm the fetus. If you have a history of problematic pregnancy, however, consult your physician before using it.

Dead-End File. Slippery elm has never been shown to speed the healing of broken bones.

Rx for Slippery Elm

For a poultice to bandage wounds, stir enough water into powdered bark to make a paste and apply to the affected area.

For a soothing decoction, use 1 to 3 teaspoons of powdered herb per cup of water. Blend a little water in first to prevent lumpiness. Bring to a boil and simmer for 15 minutes. Drink up to 3 cups a day. Slippery elm has only a slight taste and a mild aroma reminiscent of maple.

Slippery elm may be given cautiously to children under age 2.

The Safety Factor

Allergic reactions are possible. Otherwise, the medical literature contains no reports of slippery elm causing harm.

For otherwise healthy adults, slippery elm is safe in amounts typically recommended.

Slippery elm should be used in medicinal amounts only in consultation with your doctor. Let your doctor know if you experience unpleasant effects or if the symptoms for which the herb is being used do not improve significantly in two weeks. If wounds become increasingly warm, red, painful, or inflamed, consult a physician.

A Tree That Shades and Soothes

Slippery elm is a stately tree that reaches 60 feet. Its trunk bark is brown, but its branch bark is whitish. Its leaves are broad, rough, hairy, and toothed. Check local nurseries to see if this tree can be grown in your area.

TARRAGON

Toothache Treatment

Family: Compositae; other members include daisy, dandelion, marigold

Genus and species: *Artemisia dracunculus*

Also known as: French or Russian tarragon, estragon, dragon herb

Parts used: Leaves

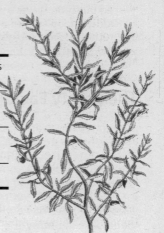

Tarragon is best known as the main seasoning in béarnaise sauce, but like all aromatic herbs, it also has a long history in herbal healing. Unlike most other aromatics, however, it fell from healing fashion in the 17th century and has only recently been rediscovered as an oral anesthetic with some potential for the prevention of heart disease.

Pilgrim's Plant

The ancient Greeks knew chewing tarragon numbs the mouth and used it to treat toothache. They also figured that its anesthetic power—not to mention its wide-ranging root runners—made it the herb of choice to relieve the discomforts of traveling.

Roman naturalist Pliny wrote that the herb prevents fatigue on long journeys. And during the Middle Ages, pilgrims placed tarragon sprigs in their shoes.

Oddly enough for an herb that numbs the mouth, around the 10th century, Arab physicians recommended tarragon as an appetite stimulant.

Under the Doctrine of Signatures—the medieval belief that an herb's appearance reveals its medicinal value—tarragon's serpentine roots were considered a sign it could cure snakebite. Over the centuries, the belief expanded to include the bites of rabid dogs. But by the 17th century, this belief had faded.

Later, herbalists virtually abandoned tarragon because it loses most of its aromatic healing oil as it dries. Even America's 19th-century Eclectic physicians, who prized botanical drugs, had no use for it.

Few contemporary herbalists value tarragon except in French cooking. Those who do recognize it reiterate its traditional uses as a diuretic, appetite stimulant, digestive aid, and treatment for toothache.

HEALING with Tarragon

Tarragon is no wonder herb, but it deserves a place in herbal healing. Its active component is its oil; however, drying largely destroys it, so either fresh or frozen leaves or comparatively large amounts of dried leaves must be used.

Anesthetic. Tarragon oil contains an anesthetic chemical, eugenol, which is the major constituent of anesthetic clove oil, supporting its age-old use for toothache. Tarragon provides only temporary relief of oral pain, however. If toothache persists, consult a dentist.

Infection Prevention. Like many culinary herbs, tarragon oil fights disease-causing bacteria in the test tube. For garden first aid, press some fresh crushed tarragon leaves onto wounds on the way to washing and bandaging them.

Intriguing Possibilities. Tarragon oil contains a chemical (rutin) that strengthens capillary walls. Animal studies show rutin helps prevent the artery-narrowing plaque deposits closely associated with heart disease and some strokes. Tarragon's impact on plaque prevention in human arteries is a matter of conjecture, but it just might help.

An animal study published in the *Journal of the National Cancer Institute* suggests rutin also has some antitumor activity.

R$_x$ for Tarragon

For temporary relief of oral pain, chew fresh leaves as needed.

For garden first aid, apply fresh, crushed leaves to the affected area.

For a pleasant, licorice-flavored infusion that may help in the prevention of heart disease, use 1 to 2 teaspoons of fresh or frozen herb per cup of boiling water. Steep 10 to 15 minutes. Drink up to 3 cups a day.

In a tincture, use ½ to 1 teaspoon up to three times a day.

Medicinal doses of tarragon should not be given to children under age 2. For older children and people over 65, start with low-strength preparations and increase strength if necessary.

The Safety Factor

Tarragon contains another chemical, estragole, that in large amounts produces tumors in mice. Tarragon has never been associated with human cancer, but until its effects are clarified, those with a history of cancer should probably not use medicinal amounts.

Otherwise, the medical literature contains no reports of tarragon causing harm.

Tarragon is included in the Food and Drug Administration's list of herbs generally regarded as safe. For otherwise healthy nonpregnant, nonnursing adults, tarragon is considered safe in amounts typically recommended.

Tarragon should be used in medicinal amounts only in consultation with your doctor. If tarragon causes minor discomforts, such as stomach upset or diarrhea, use less or stop using it. Let your doctor know if you experience unpleasant effects or if the symptoms for which the herb is being used do not improve significantly in two weeks.

Go for the French

Tarragon comes in two varieties, Russian and French. The former has less oil—and therefore, less flavor and medicinal value—so tarragon almost always implies the French plant.

Russian tarragon may be grown from seeds, but the more desirable French variety must be propagated from cuttings or root divisions. Divide the roots in spring and plant 1-inch pieces of their tips. Or take cuttings in summer. Thin plants to 2-foot spacing.

French tarragon is a perennial with a creeping, serpentine root, and stems that reach 2 feet. Its leaves look like a larger version of rosemary. This herb rarely flowers, and if it does, the fruits are sterile.

Tarragon grows best in rich, well-drained soil under full sun. Make sure the roots do not become waterlogged. If your winter temperatures drop below the teens, mulch well each fall. Divide tarragon roots every few years to retain plants' vigor.

Tarragon leaves bruise easily. Harvest them carefully in early summer. Because tarragon loses medicinal value when dried, freeze the fresh herb or preserve it in vinegar.

TEA

World's Most Popular Healer

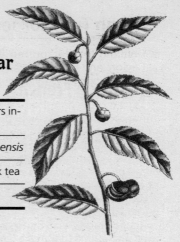

Family: Theaceae; other members include camellia

Genus and species: *Camellia sinensis*

Also known as: Green tea, black tea

Parts used: Leaves

Tea is the world's second most popular beverage (after water) and the world's most widely used herbal medicine. Most people drink it as a mild stimulant, but this herb also may help treat diarrhea, prevent tooth decay, and act as a bronchial decongestant.

Tea Time Goes Way Back

Tea has been used in Chinese medicine for at least 3,000 years to treat headache, diarrhea, dysentery, colds, cough, asthma, and other respiratory problems.

By the 8th century, it was a favorite in India and Indonesia. The Dutch East India Company first brought it to Holland in 1610, and by 1640, black tea had become popular with the English upper class. They drank it as an afternoon stimulant around 4 o'clock, which is still known as tea time.

The Chinese called black tea *pekho*, and the British adopted the term as *pekoe*. They considered the beverage so divine, they named it tea from the Greek *thea*, meaning goddess.

Tough Time for Tea

Demand for tea spurred England's colonization of India, Ceylon, and Hong Kong. By the late 18th century, tea was an integral part of English culture, and around the world, the English simply would not tolerate any threat to their tea supply. In 1773, the British Parliament levied a tax on tea imported into her North American colonies. Outraged by this price hike, the residents of Massachusetts rioted. They stormed tea ships in Boston harbor and dumped enormous quantities of the herb overboard. The Boston Tea Party helped trigger the American Revolution.

In Europe and North America, tea has always been used primarily as a stimulant beverage. Herbalists also adopted all of its Chinese medical uses. Folk healers still recommend tea for headache, diarrhea, colds, coughs, and respiratory problems.

Ironically, few contemporary herbals even mention the world's most popular healing herb. In fact, most people don't even consider tea an herb. They typically ask, "Would you like coffee, tea, or herbal tea?" Of course, coffee and tea are herbs, so all these beverages are herbal teas.

HEALING with Tea

Tea contains three stimulant chemicals—caffeine, theobromine, and theophylline—that help account for some of its uses in herbal healing.

Colds, Congestion, Asthma. All the stimulants in tea are bronchodilators that ease breathing by opening the bronchial passages, thus supporting its traditional use in respiratory problems. Physicians often prescribe pharmaceutical preparations of theophylline to treat asthma.

Diarrhea. Tea contains astringent tannins, which help account for its binding action in diarrhea.

Tooth Decay. Tea is also a good source of fluoride, which helps prevent tooth decay. Both green and black teas contain more fluoride than fluoridated water, according to a report published in the *University of California, Berkeley, Wellness Letter*. The tannins in tea also may help fight the bacteria that cause tooth decay.

Radiation. Among the tannins in tea are substances called catechins, that may help prevent tissue damage from radiation. One study shows tea helps keep radioactive strontium 90 out of bone marrow. This means it may help prevent cancer in people who have been exposed to nuclear fallout. And some experiments show tea helps prevent leukemia in animals exposed to radiation.

Intriguing Possibility. Coffee may raise cholesterol, but an animal study published in the *Journal of Nutrition Science* shows tea may lower it. The herb may have a similar effect in people.

Tannins have some antiviral action, and Chinese reports claim tea helps treat hepatatis. Hepatitis is a serious disease that requires professional care, but during convalescence, tea does no harm, and it might do some good.

Rₓ for Tea

For a pleasantly bitter infusion that may prevent tooth decay, help ease breathing, or help treat diarrhea, use 1 to 2 teaspoons of dried herb per cup of boiling water. Steep 10 to 15 minutes. Drink up to 3 cups a day.

Weak tea preparations may be given cautiously to children under age 2. For older children and people over 65, start with low-strength preparations and increase strength if necessary.

The Safety Factor

A cup of tea contains about half as much caffeine as a cup of brewed coffee. Caffeine is a classically addictive drug that causes nervousness, restlessness, insomnia, and many other potentially problematic effects (see "Coffee" on page 182).

Many studies show tannins have both pro- and anti-cancer effects. Tannins' role in human cancers, if any, remains unclear; however, population studies show unusually high rates of throat cancer among some peoples who drink large amounts of tea. On the other hand, the tea-loving British show no increased risk of throat cancer. Authorities generally agree that the British custom of adding milk to tea exerts a protective effect. The milk neutralizes the tannins. So you might want to do as the Brits do—take your tea with milk.

Other Cautions

For otherwise healthy nonpregnant, nonnursing adults, tea is considered safe in amounts typically recommended.

Caffeine has been linked, however, to an increased risk of birth defects. Pregnant women should not consume it. Large amounts of tea may cause gastrointestinal upsets.

Tea should be used in medicinal amounts only in consultation with your doctor. If tea causes minor discomforts, such as stomach upset, use less or stop using it. Let your doctor know if you experience unpleasant effects or if the symptoms for which the herb is being used do not improve significantly in two weeks.

Always Imported

Tea is not a garden herb in North America. It is cultivated primarily in India, Sri Lanka, and Indonesia. Tea is a small evergreen tree that grows to 30 feet in the wild. In cultivation, however, it is pruned into a bushy shrub. Its leaves are processed into both green and black (pekoe) tea. Green tea is simply the dried leaf. Black tea is dried and then fermented.

THYME

Tried and True

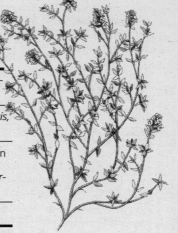

Family: Labiatae; other members include mints

Genus and species: *Thymus vulgaris, T. serpyllum*

Also known as: Common or garden thyme (*T. vulgaris*); Wild, creeping, mother, and mother of thyme (*T. serpyllum*)

Parts used: Leaves and flower tops

arsley, sage, rosemary, and . . . Listerine? Or perhaps Vicks VapoRub. Thyme is commonly found in the kitchen herb cabinet, but millions of Americans stock this herb's oil in their medicine chest as well. Its use in mouthwashes and decongestants is no coincidence. Thyme has a long history of use as an antiseptic, cough remedy, and digestive aid.

Herbed Sacrificial Lamb

Like several other aromatic kitchen herbs, thyme was used as a meat preservative in ancient times. It was sprinkled on sacrificial animals to make them more acceptable to the gods. Thyme was introduced into cooking as an offshoot of its meat-preserving action. The Romans also used it medicinally as a cough remedy, digestive aid, and treatment for intestinal worms.

Charlemagne ordered thyme grown in all his imperial gardens for both its culinary and medicinal value. Medieval German abbess/herbalist Hildegard of Bingen considered it the herb of choice for skin problems, anticipating its later use as an antiseptic.

Signs of Courage

During the Middle Ages, thyme became linked to courage. It was fashionable for noblewomen to embroider sprigs of thyme on scarves and give them to favorite knights departing for the Crusades.

As the centuries passed, thyme was used as an antiseptic during plagues, and those troubled by "melancholia" (depression) were advised to sleep on thyme-stuffed pillows.

Early anatomists named the lymph gland in the chest the thymus because it reminded them of a thyme flower.

Sixteenth-century herbalist John Gerard recommended thyme for leprosy and to "cure sciatica . . . pains in the head . . . [and] falling sickness [epilepsy]."

Later, English herbalist Nicholas Culpeper called thyme "excellent for nervous disorders . . . headaches . . . and a certain remedy for that troublesome complaint, the nightmare." He claimed it "provokes the terms [menstruation], gives safe and speedy delivery to women in travail [labor], and brings away the after-birth." Culpeper also recommended thyme as "a noble strengthener of the lungs . . . an excellent remedy for shortness of breath. . . . It purges the body of phlegm . . . comforts the stomach much and expels wind."

Thymol Antiseptic Oil

By the late 17th century, apothecary shops were selling thyme oil as a topical antiseptic under the name oil of origanum. In 1719, German chemist Caspar Neumann extracted thyme oil's active constituent, which he called camphor of thyme. In 1853, French chemist M. Lallemand named it *thymol*, its name today.

From the mid-19th century through World War I, thymol enjoyed great popularity as an antiseptic. The American Eclectic physicians' text, *King's American Dispensatory*, extolled it: "Thymol is considered by many to be superior to carbolic acid [the antiseptic made famous in 1867 by the father of antiseptic surgery, Joseph Lister]. It prevents putrefaction and arrests it when it has commenced. . . . Dissolved in water, it forms an invaluable disinfectant [for] sick rooms." The Eclectics also prescribed thyme infusion for headache, gastrointestinal upsets, "hysteria" (menstrual cramps), and as a menstruation promoter.

World War Crisis

World War I caused a major thymol crisis. Most of the world's supply was distilled in Germany, and when the British and French declared war on Germany, they had to scramble to overcome a terrible shortage of the suddenly vital battlefield antiseptic. Thymol has since been replaced by more potent germ fighters, but it remains an ingredient in several antiseptic mouthwashes, including Listerine.

Contemporary herbalists recommend thyme externally for wound disinfection and internally for indigestion, sore throat, laryngitis, cough, whooping cough, and nervousness.

HEALING with Thyme

Thyme's aromatic oil contains two chemicals—thymol and carvacol—that account for its medicinal value. Both chemicals have preservative, antibacterial, and antifungal properties. They also have expectorant properties and may be useful as digestive aids.

Antiseptic. Thyme fights several disease-causing bacteria and fungi in the test tube, supporting its traditional use as an antiseptic, though infusions of the dried herb are nowhere near as powerful as the oil or distilled thymol. Still, for garden first aid, you can crush some fresh leaves into minor cuts and scrapes on the way to washing and bandaging them.

Digestive Aid. Some studies show thymol and carvacol relax the smooth muscle tissue of the gastrointestinal tract, making thyme an antispasmodic. This action of these chemical constituents lend support to thyme's traditional use as a digestive aid.

Women's Health. Antispasmodics relax not only the digestive tract but other smooth muscles, such as the uterus, as well. Small amounts may help relieve menstrual cramps, lending credence to the Eclectic physicians' use of this herb. But in large amounts, thyme oil and thymol are considered uterine stimulants.

Pregnant women may use thyme as a culinary spice, but they should avoid large amounts and should not use the herb's oil.

Cough Remedy. German researchers have lent support to thyme's traditional use as a phlegm-loosener (expectorant), and in Germany today, where herbal medicine is considerably more mainstream than it is in the United States, thyme preparations are frequently prescribed to relax the respiratory tract and treat cough, whooping cough, and emphysema. German medical herbalist Rudolph Fritz Weiss, M.D., writes: "Thyme is to the trachea [windpipe] and the bronchi what peppermint is to the stomach and intestines."

Rx for Thyme

For garden accidents, crush fresh leaves into the wound on the way to washing and bandaging it. Once wounds have been thoroughly washed, apply a few drops of thyme tincture as an antiseptic.

For an infusion to help settle the stomach, soothe a cough, or possibly help relieve menstrual symptoms, use 2 teaspoons of dried herb per cup of boiling water. Steep 10 minutes. Drink up to 3 cups a day. Thyme tastes pleasantly aromatic with a faint clovelike aftertaste.

In a tincture, take ½ to 1 teaspoon up to three times a day.

Medicinal preparations of thyme should not be given to children under age 2. For older children and people over 65, start with low-strength preparations and increase strength if necessary.

The Safety Factor

Use the herb, not its oil. Even a few teaspoons of thyme oil can be toxic, causing headache, nausea, vomiting, weakness, thyroid impairment, and heart and respiratory depression.

One animal study showed thyme suppresses thyroid activity in rats. Those with thyroid conditions should consult their physicians before taking medicinal doses.

Thyme and thyme oil may cause a rash in sensitive individuals.

Other Cautions

The Food and Drug Administration includes thyme in its list of herbs generally regarded as safe. For otherwise healthy nonpregnant, nonnursing adults who do not have thyroid problems, thyme is considered safe in amounts typically recommended.

Thyme should be used in medicinal amounts only in consultation with your doctor. If thyme causes minor discomforts, such as headache or nausea, use less or stop using it. Let your doctor know if you experience unpleasant effects or if the symptoms for which the herb is being used do not improve significantly in two weeks.

Time to Grow Thyme

Thyme is an aromatic, perennial, many-branched, ground-cover shrub that reaches about 12 inches. It has small, opposite, virtually stalkless leaves and lilac or pink flowers that bloom in midsummer.

This hardy herb can be propagated from seeds, cuttings, and root divisions. Seeds require a temperature around 70°F to germinate and often do best when started indoors. For cuttings, snip 3-inch pieces from stems with new growth and place them in wet sand. Roots should appear in about two weeks. The best time for root division is in spring. Uproot a plant carefully, preserving as much of its root soil as possible. Divide it in half or thirds and replant the divisions 12 inches apart in moist soil.

Once established, thyme requires little care. It prefers well-drained soil on the dry side. Clumps tend to become woody after a few years. To prevent this, roots should be divided periodically. Wetting thyme leaves during watering reduces their fragrance. Thyme survives frost, but in areas with cold winters, use mulch. Thyme may be killed if winter temperatures drop below 10°F.

Harvest the leaves and flower tops just before the flowers bloom. Dry and store them in airtight containers to preserve the herb's oil.

TURMERIC

Healing with Curry

Family: Zingiberaceae; other members include ginger

Genus and species: *Curcuma longa*

Also known as: Curcuma

Parts used: Roots

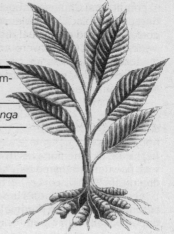

Turmeric is a recent addition to most American spice racks, but it's been a mainstay in Indian curries for thousands of years. Its arrival here is good news for our palate *and* our health.

Turmeric's healing benefits are still largely unknown in North America, but it helps aid digestion, may fight intestinal parasites, may protect the liver, may help prevent heart disease, and may one day play a role in the treatment of cancer.

Whole-Body Cleanser

Turmeric held a place of honor in India's traditional Ayurvedic medicine. A symbol of prosperity, it was considered a cleansing herb for the whole body. Medically, it was used as a digestive aid and treatment for fever, infections, dysentery, arthritis, and jaundice and other liver problems.

514

Traditional Chinese physicians also used turmeric to treat liver and gallbladder problems, stop bleeding, and treat chest congestion and menstrual discomforts.

The ancient Greeks were well aware of turmeric, but unlike its close botanical relative, ginger, it never caught on in the West as either a culinary or medicinal herb. It was, however, used to make orange-yellow dyes.

Turmeric Paper

In the 1870s, chemists discovered turmeric's orange-yellow root powder turned reddish brown when exposed to alkaline chemicals. This discovery led to the development of "turmeric paper," thin strips of tissue brushed with a decoction of turmeric, then dried. During the late 19th century, turmeric paper was used in laboratories around the world to test for alkalinity. Eventually, it was replaced by litmus paper, which is still used today.

American chemists used turmeric paper, but not even the botanically oriented 19th-century Eclectic physicians had much use for turmeric itself, except to add color to medicinal ointments.

Maude Grieve's influential *Modern Herbal*, published in 1931, said turmeric was "once a cure for jaundice," then dismissed it as "seldom used in medicine except as a coloring."

Few contemporary herbalists recommend turmeric. The ones who do advocate it to treat fever, relieve pains and chest congestion, and restore menstrual regularity.

HEALING with Turmeric

Western herbalists, wake up. Turmeric is a healer.

Turmeric has been revered in India for thousands of years, so it should come as no surprise that Indians have conducted most of the research into the healing chemical it contains—curcumin.

Wound Treatment. Like many culinary herbs, turmeric

helps retard food spoilage because it has antibacterial action. To help prevent bacterial wound infections, sprinkle a bit on cuts and scrapes after they have been thoroughly washed.

Digestive Aid. Turmeric also helps stimulate the flow of bile, which helps digest fats, supporting its traditional use as a digestive herb.

Intestinal Parasites. Turmeric fights protozoans in laboratory tests, lending some credence to its traditional use in treating dysentery.

Liver Protection. One animal study showed curcumin has a protective effect on liver tissue exposed to liver-damaging drugs, lending support to the herb's traditional use in liver ailments. If you drink alcohol regularly, and/or take frequent high doses of certain pharmaceutical drugs, including the common pain reliever, acetaminophen (Tylenol), you may be at risk for liver damage. Ask your physician about using turmeric to protect your liver.

Arthritis. Several studies show curcumin has anti-inflammatory action, lending some credence to its traditional use in treating arthritis. This effect may also help relieve wound inflammation.

Heart Protection. One animal study showed that like its botanical relative, ginger, turmeric may help reduce cholesterol. Another study showed it helps prevent the internal blood clots that trigger heart attack and some strokes. Animal results cannot necessarily be applied to people, but in recommended amounts, turmeric is a tasty spice that does no harm, and these studies suggest it might do some good.

Intriguing Possibilities. Recently, curcumin has also been shown to have some anti-cancer activity. A report published in *Cancer Letters* says it inhibits the growth of lymphoma tumor cells. And research at Rutgers University shows curcumin helps prevent tumor development in animals.

Dead-End File. The Chinese used turmeric to stimulate menstruation, but no research to date has identified any effect on the uterus.

Rx for Turmeric

To treat minor wounds, wash them with soap and water, then sprinkle on some powdered herb and bandage.

For an infusion to help aid digestion and possibly help promote heart health, use 1 teaspoon of turmeric powder per cup of warm milk. Drink up to 3 cups a day. These infusions may also offer a measure of protection to the liver and help ease the inflammation of arthritis. Turmeric tastes pleasantly aromatic, but in large amounts, it becomes somewhat bitter.

Medicinal turmeric preparations should not be given to children under age 2. For older children and people over 65, start with low-strength preparations and increase strength if necessary.

The Safety Factor

One animal study showed the herb reduces fertility. This experiment has not been replicated, and its implications for human fertility, if any, remain unclear. But those trying to conceive and those with fertility problems should probably not use medicinal amounts.

Turmeric's potential anticlotting effect might cause problems for those with clotting disorders. If you have a blood-clotting problem, discuss this herb's anticlotting effect with your physician before using medicinal preparations.

Unusually large amounts of turmeric may cause stomach upset.

Other Cautions

Turmeric is on the Food and Drug Administration's list of herbs generally regarded as safe. For otherwise healthy non-pregnant, nonnursing adults who are not taking anticoagulant medications, turmeric is considered safe in amounts typically recommended.

Turmeric should be used in medicinal amounts only in

consultation with your doctor. If turmeric causes minor discomforts, such as heartburn or stomach upset, use less or stop using it. Let your doctor know if you experience unpleasant effects or if the symptoms for which the herb is being used do not improve significantly in two weeks.

An Indian Import

Turmeric is not a garden herb in North America. Grown from India to Indonesia, it's a perennial with pulpy, orange, tuberous roots that grow to about 2 feet in length. The aerial parts, which reach 3 feet, include large, lilylike leaves, a thick, squat, central flower spike, and funnel-shaped yellow flowers.

UVA URSI

The Urinary Antiseptic

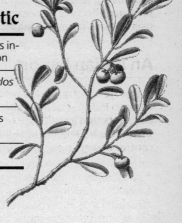

Family: Ericaceae; other members include heath, azalea, rhododendron

Genus and species: *Arctostaphylos uva-ursi*

Also known as: Bearberry, bear's grape, upland cranberry, arbutus

Parts used: Leaves

U va ursi has been used as a diuretic and urinary antiseptic for more than 1,000 years by cultures as widely separated as the Chinese and American Indians. Today it is an ingredient in most herbal diuretics and urinary remedies and many weight-loss formulas. Even herbal conservative Varro Tyler, Ph.D., calls it "a modestly effective urinary antiseptic and diuretic."

But uva ursi may *not* be effective if consumers eat certain foods while taking it—information some herbals fail to mention.

The Mark of Marco Polo

The Roman physician Galen used uva ursi's astringent leaves to treat wounds and stop bleeding. But this herb was largely ignored by Western herbalists until the 13th century, when

Marco Polo reported Chinese physicians using it as a diuretic to treat kidney and urinary problems. Polo's famous travelogue repopularized uva ursi in Europe as a urinary and kidney remedy.

Uva ursi's association with the kidney was strengthened by the medieval Doctrine of Signatures—the idea that a plant's physical appearance revealed its healing virtues. The herb grew in rocky, gravelly places, and at the time kidney stones were called gravel.

Kinnikinnik

North American colonists found the Indians had independently discovered uva ursi's use as a urinary remedy. Native Americans also mixed its leathery leaves with tobacco and created the smoking mixture, kinnikinnik.

Uva ursi was incorporated into the U.S. *Pharmacopoeia* in 1820 as a urinary antiseptic and remained there until 1936. Chemists isolated the herb's active constituent, arbutin, in 1852.

The 19th-century Eclectics recommended the herb for diarrhea, dysentery, gonorrhea, bed-wetting, and "chronic affections of the kidneys and urinary passages."

Today homeopaths recommend a microdose of uva ursi for incontinence, blood in the urine, and kidney and urinary tract infections.

Contemporary herbalists continue to recommend uva ursi for kidney and urinary problems.

HEALING with Uva Ursi

In the urinary tract, the arbutin in uva ursi is chemically transformed into an antiseptic chemical, hydroquinone, according to several studies. In addition, the herb contains diuretic chemicals, including ursolic acid, powerful astringents (tannins), and a chemical that helps promote the growth of healthy new cells, allantoin.

Urinary Ailments. Together, the actions of uva uri's active chemicals support its age-old use in urinary tract infections (UTIs), and other urinary ailments.

Some herbalists report uva ursi has cured UTIs unresponsive to pharmaceutical antibiotics. This is certainly possible, but scientific sources say pharmaceutical antibiotics are generally more effective. For mild urinary symptoms, try uva ursi as herbal first aid. For urinary problems requiring professional care, use the herb in addition to standard therapies.

But there's an important catch to using uva ursi. To receive the greatest antiseptic benefit, the urine must be alkaline, which means you must avoid acidic foods and supplements, such as sauerkraut, citrus fruits and their juices, and vitamin C, while taking it.

Women's Health. Diuretics may provide relief from the premenstrual bloating that bothers many women. Pregnant and nursing women should not use diuretics, however. Uva ursi also stimulates uterine contractions in animal studies, making it even more off-limits to pregnant women.

High Blood Pressure. Physicians often prescribe diuretics to treat high blood pressure. High blood pressure is a serious condition requiring professional care. If you have it and would like to include uva ursi in your overall treatment plan, do so only with the supervision of your physician.

Diuretics deplete the body of potassium, an essential nutrient. If you use them regularly, increase your consumption of foods high in potassium, such as bananas and fresh vegetables.

Congestive Heart Failure. Physicians often prescribe diuretics to treat this condition, which involves serious fatigue of the heart. Congestive heart failure requires professional care. If you would like to include uva ursi in your overall treatment plan, discuss using the herb with your physician.

Wound Healing. Uva ursi's allantoin may help spur wound healing. Allantoin is the active ingredient in several over-the-counter skin creams, such as Herpicin-L Cold Sore Lip Balm, for relief of oral herpes, and Vagimide Cream, for irritation associated with vaginal infections.

Diarrhea. The astringent tannins in uva ursi are binding and help relieve diarrhea.

Rx for Uva Ursi

For wound treatment, apply fresh, crushed leaves to minor cuts and scrapes after they have been thoroughly washed with soap and water. Or dip a clean cloth in a decoction and apply the compress to the affected area.

To minimize the unpleasantly astringent taste of this high-tannin herb, soak the leaves in cold water overnight. Then, for a decoction to help treat urinary symptoms or diarrhea, simmer 1 teaspoon per cup of boiling water for 10 minutes. Drink up to 3 cups a day.

In a tincture, use ¼ to 1 teaspoon up to three times a day.

Uva ursi should not be given to children under age 2. For older children and people over 65, start with low-strength preparations and increase strength if necessary.

The Safety Factor

Uva ursi often turns urine a dark green. Do not become alarmed.

Herbal weight-loss formulas typically contain diuretics. Uva ursi is the diuretic most often used. Because they boost urine production, diuretics temporarily eliminate some water weight. Weight lost using diuretics almost invariably returns, however. Weight-control experts do not recommend diuretics. The keys to permanent weight control include a low-fat, high-fiber diet, and regular aerobic exercise.

Some herb conservatives warn against using uva ursi because they say it causes vomiting, ringing in the ears, and convulsions. The source of this warning is one study reported in 1949, which did not use bulk uva ursi but rather very large amounts of its isolated antiseptic chemical, hydroquinone. Recommended doses of the whole herb are considered safe, but if nausea or ringing in the ears develops, use less or stop using the herb.

High in Tannins

Uva ursi has such high levels of tannins that it has been used to tan leather. Large doses of tannins may cause stomach upset.

Tannins also have both pro- and anti-cancer action. Some authorities warn against their use, but tannins' role in human cancers, if any, remains unclear. However, those with a history of cancer should either add milk, which appears to neutralize tannins, or not use large amounts.

Other Cautions

The Food and Drug Administration lists uva ursi as an herb of "undefined safety." For otherwise healthy nonpregnant, nonnursing adults, uva ursi is considered relatively safe in amounts typically recommended.

Uva ursi should be used in medicinal amounts only in consultation with your doctor. If uva ursi causes minor discomforts, such as nausea, use less or stop using it. Let your doctor know if you experience unpleasant effects or if the symptoms for which the herb is being used do not improve significantly in two weeks.

Better to Buy Bearberry

Ancient Mediterranean bears must have loved the bright red, mealy, currant-size berries of this delicate, branching, perennial groundcover, because both its generic name, *Arctostaphylos*, from the Greek, and its Latin-rooted specific name, *uva ursi*, mean bear's berry. The plant is often called bearberry in English. Not the berries but the leaves are used in herbal healing, however.

Uva ursi grows throughout the temperate world. It has a long, fibrous root, woody stems and branches, inch-long, leathery, evergreen, paddle-shaped leaves and tiny white flowers tinged with red. The plant rarely grows taller than a few inches and prefers a dry, rocky, or sandy habitat.

Uva ursi is typically propagated from cuttings. Be patient. This plant takes an unusually long time to root. It's more convenient simply to buy small plants from a specialty herb nursery.

Uva ursi does poorly in rich soil. It prefers poor, gravelly, acidic soil, under full sun or partial shade. Keep your uva ursi patch well weeded until the plants have become established. It does not transplant well. Once established, uva ursi spreads to become a hearty, attractive groundcover, which can survive temperatures of −50°F.

Harvest leaves in autumn before the first frost. Because of their leathery texture, they are difficult to air dry. Spread them in a single layer and dry them in your oven.

VALERIAN

You're Getting Sleepy . . .

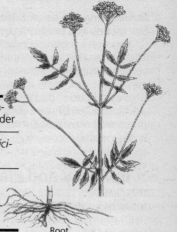

Family: Valerianaceae; other members include spikenard, Jacob's ladder

Genus and species: *Valeriana officinalis*

Also known as: Garden valerian, phu, all-heal

Parts used: Rhizome and root

Root

Back in the 13th century, the elders of Hamelin, Germany, decided to rid their town of rats. They contracted with an itinerant flute player, one Pied Piper, whose music attracted the rodents, allowing him to lead them out of town. But when the Pied Piper returned for his fee, the elders of Hamelin refused to pay him. In revenge, he used his flute to charm Hamelin's children away forever.

In modern versions of this story, the Pied Piper's powers are entirely musical. But early German folklore credits him with being an accomplished herbalist as well. In addition to his hypnotic flute playing, the Pied Piper charmed both the rats and the children with hypnotic valerian root. (Valerian can, indeed, charm rats—and cats. It contains chemicals similar to those in catnip.)

Fu Means P-U

Valerian has a disagreeable odor, and ancient Greek and Roman authorities, including Dioscorides, Pliny, and Galen all called it *fu*. The term *Valeriana* first appeared around the 10th century, derived from the Latin *valere*, to be strong.

Dioscorides recommended valerian as a diuretic and antidote to poisons. Pliny considered it a pain reliever. Galen prescribed it as a decongestant. By the time the plant's name became valerian, early European herbalists considered it a panacea and also called it *all-heal*. The German abbess/herbalist Hildegard of Bingen recommended the herb as a tranquilizer and sleep aid about 100 years before the Pied Piper used it as a hypnotic.

For Epilepsy and Plague

During the late 1500s, valerian's popularity grew after an Italian physician claimed he cured himself of epilepsy using it. In 1597, herbalist John Gerard wrote that in Scotland "no broth or physic [medicine] . . . be worth anything" if it did not include valerian. Gerard recommended the herb enthusiastically for chest congestion, convulsions, bruises, and falls.

Seventeenth-century English herbalist Nicholas Culpeper added several recommendations: "The decoction of the root . . . is of special virtue against the plague. . . . [It] provokes women's courses [menstruation] . . . is singularly good for those troubled with cough . . . is excellent [for] any sores, hurts, or wounds. . . ." Later, European herbalists considered the herb a digestive aid and treatment for "hysteria" (menstrual discomforts).

Tranquilizer Par Excellence

Early colonists discovered several Indian tribes using the pulverized roots of native American valerian to treat wounds. Indian use of the herb brought it to the attention of Samuel Thomson, the founder of Thomsonian medicine, which was popular before the Civil War. Thomson called valerian "the best nervine [tranquilizer] known."

Valerian entered the U.S. *Pharmacopoeia* as a tranquilizer in 1820 and remained there until 1942. It was listed in the *National Formulary*, the pharmacists' guide, until 1950.

The 19th-century Eclectics prescribed it as a "calmative . . . for epilepsy . . . mild spasmodic affections . . . [and] hypochondria." However their text, *King's American Dispensatory*, warned against using large doses because they caused "restlessness, agitation, giddiness, nausea, and visual illusions."

During World War I, Europeans afflicted with "overwrought nerves" from artillery bombardment frequently took valerian.

Contemporary herbalists generally agree with David Hoffmann's *Holistic Herbal*, which calls valerian "one of the most useful relaxing herbs." Today's herbalists recommend it for nervousness, anxiety, insomnia, headache, and intestinal cramps.

In West Germany, where herbal medicine is considerably more mainstream than it is in the United States, valerian is the active ingredient in more than 100 over-the-counter tranquilizers and sleep aids, some of which are specially formulated for children, a use the Pied Piper would probably endorse.

HEALING with Valerian

All parts of valerian contain chemicals that appear to have sedative properties known as valepotriates, but they occur in highest concentration in the roots. The valepotriates are insoluble in water. Many valerian sleep aids are water-based, meaning they cannot contain more than traces of these chemicals, leading some herb critics to dismiss valerian as worthless.

But in 1981, researchers discovered several water-soluble chemicals with apparent sedative properties in valerian, supporting the herb's age-old use as a tranquilizer and sleep aid.

Sedative. In one experiment, researchers gave 128 insomnia sufferers either 400 milligrams of valerian root extract or a look-alike placebo. Those taking the herb showed significant improvement in sleep quality without morning grogginess. Other experiments have produced similar results.

Some researchers have compared valerian to benzodiazepines such as Valium. However, valerian is a much milder and safer sedative.

- Valium can become an addictive drug. Regular users may develop a tolerance and require increasing amounts to obtain the desired effect. When the drug is withdrawn, they may develop withdrawal symptoms including restlessness, insomnia, headache, nausea, and vomiting. Although a psychological dependence may develop, valerian is not addictive and discontinuation produces no withdrawal symptoms.
- Valium's effects are exaggerated by simultaneous use of alcohol and barbiturates. The combination is often used in suicide attempts. Valerian's sedative effect is not significantly exaggerated by alcohol and barbiturates.
- Valium often causes morning grogginess. Unusually large amounts of valerian may cause morning grogginess, but recommended amounts do not.
- Finally, children born to women who used Valium while pregnant suffer an increased risk of cleft palate. Valerian has not been linked to birth defects.

Blood Pressure. Animal studies show valerian reduces blood pressure. Animal results do not necessarily apply to people, but if you have high blood pressure get your physician's approval and supervision before incorporating it into your overall treatment plan.

Intriguing Possibilities. Animal studies suggest valerian has anticonvulsant effects, lending some credence to its traditional use in treating epilepsy.

And several reports show the herb has some antitumor effects similar to those of nitrogen mustard. One day it may play some role in cancer treatment.

Rx for Valerian

For a potential sedative infusion that might also help reduce blood pressure, use 2 teaspoons of powdered root per cup of water. Steep 10 to 15 minutes. Drink 1 cup before bed. Valerian tastes unpleasant. Add sugar, honey, and lemon, or mix it with an herbal beverage blend to improve flavor.

In a tincture, take 1/2 to 1 teaspoon before bed.

Valerian should not be given to children under age 2. For older children and people over 65, start with low-strength preparations and increase strength if necessary.

The Safety Factor

Large amounts may cause headache, giddiness, blurred vision, restlessness, nausea, and morning grogginess.

Valerian is included in the Food and Drug Administration's list of herbs generally regarded as safe. For otherwise healthy nonpregnant, nonnursing adults who are not taking other tranquilizers or sedatives, valerian is considered safe in amounts typically recommended.

Valerian should be used in medicinal amounts only in consultation with your doctor. If valerian causes minor discomforts, such as headache or stomach upset, use less or stop using it. Let your doctor know if you experience unpleasant effects or if the symptoms for which the herb is being used do not improve significantly in two weeks.

Protect from Cat Attack

Medicinal valerian is a hardy perennial that reaches about 5 feet. Its medicinal roots consist of long, cylindrical fibers issuing from its rhizome. Its stem is erect, grooved, and hollow. Valerian leaves are fernlike. Tiny flowers—white, pink, or lavender—develop in umbrella-like clusters and bloom from late spring through summer. When dried, valerian roots have an unpleasant odor, described by American herbalist Michael Moore as "the smell of dirty socks."

Valerian may be propagated from seeds or root divisions. Seeds have limited viability. When viable, they germinate in about 20 days. Roots may be divided in spring or fall. Thin plants to 12-inch spacing. Valerian grows in many soils, but does best in rich, moist, well-drained loam under full sun or partial shade. Once established, plants self-sow and spread by root runners. Older plants become weedy and overcrowded and lose vitality. Thin them when harvesting their roots.

Valerian has an effect on cats similar to catnip. Intoxicated felines have been known to destroy plants; use chicken-wire fencing if necessary.

Harvest roots in the fall of their second year. Split thick roots to speed drying. Valerian's characteristic unpleasant odor develops as the roots dry.

VERVAIN

Joy of a Healer

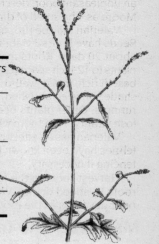

Family: Verbenaceae; other members include teak, lantana

Genus and species: *Verbena officinalis* (European); *V. hastata* (American)

Also known as: Simpler's joy, blue vervain, verbena, herb-of-the-cross, enchanter's herb, Indian hyssop

Parts used: Leaves, flowers, roots

During the Middle Ages, healing herbs were often called simples, and herbalists simplers. Vervain was prescribed so frequently for so many conditions, it became known as simpler's joy. The name has some basis in fact. Vervain appears to act like a mild aspirin, helping to relieve minor pains and inflammations.

Herb-of-the-Cross

In Egyptian mythology, vervain grew from the tears of Isis, goddess of fertility, as she grieved for her murdered brother-husband, Osiris. A thousand years later, vervain entered Christian mythology as the herb pressed into Christ's wounds to stanch his bleeding, hence its name herb-of-the-cross.

Hippocrates recommended vervain for fever and plague. The court physician to Roman Emperor Theodosius the Great prescribed it for tumors of the throat (probably goiters). His fanciful prescription advised cutting vervain root into two pieces, tying one around the patient's throat and hanging the other over a fire. As the heat and smoke shriveled the hanging root, the tumor was supposed to shrink.

The Romans spread vervain throughout Europe, where it became especially popular among the Druids of pre-Christian England, who used it in magic spells, hence its name enchanter's herb.

German abbess/herbalist Hildegard of Bingen prescribed a decoction of vervain and vermouth for "toxic blood [infections], toothache, [and] discharges from the brain to the teeth."

Our word vervain comes from the Celtic *ferfaen*—from *fer*, to drive away, and *faen*, a stone—a reference to its traditional use in treating kidney stones.

Medieval Acne Treatment

During the Middle Ages, vervain became a popular acne remedy. Those with pimples stood outside at night holding a handful of the herb wrapped in a cloth. When a shooting star passed, they rubbed the cloth over their pimples and the blemishes were supposed to disappear.

From acne, vervain evolved into a treatment for other skin problems. Seventeenth-century herbalist Nicholas Culpeper wrote: "The leaves bruised, or the juice mixed with vinegar, does wonderfully cleanse the skin, and take away morphew [dandruff]." Culpeper also recommended vervain to treat jaundice, gout, cough, wheezing, bleeding gums, shortness of breath, fever, plague, gravel (kidney stones), dropsy (congestive heart failure), and "used with hog grease, it helps with swellings and pains of the secret parts [genitals]."

Remedy for War Wounds

Colonists introduced European vervain into North America, and it quickly went wild. They also found the Indians using native American vervain, also known as Indian hyssop, to treat fever and gastrointestinal complaints and to clear cloudy urine.

During the Revolutionary War, military physicians used vervain extensively to relieve pain, loosen bronchial mucus, and induce vomiting. More than a century later, the Eclectics recommended it for fever, colds, cough, intestinal worms, menstrual irregularity, bruises, and as a tonic "during convalescence from acute diseases."

Contemporary herbalists recommend vervain as a tranquilizer, expectorant, menstruation promoter, and treatment for headache, fever, depression, seizures, wounds, dental cavities, and gum disease.

HEALING with Vervain

When in doubt, physicians often say, "Take two aspirin and call me in the morning." An herbalist might say the same thing, substituting vervain for aspirin. No wonder they called this herb simpler's joy.

Pain and Inflammation Relief. Chemically, vervain is quite different from aspirin, but German and Japanese studies suggest it has similar effects, combining mild pain relief with some ability to reduce inflammation. These findings support its traditional use in treating headache, toothache, and wounds.

Laxative. One study suggests the herb also has a mild laxative effect.

Dead-End File. Vervain has never been shown to treat dandruff, induce vomiting, promote menstruation, remove a kidney stone, or do anything except provide mild pain relief.

Rx for Vervain

For a very bitter infusion to help treat headache, mild arthritis, and other minor pains, use 2 teaspoons of dried herb per cup of boiling water. Steep 10 to 15 minutes. Drink up to 3 cups a day. Mask vervain's bitterness with sugar, honey, and lemon, or mix it with an herbal beverage tea.

In a tincture, use $1/2$ to 1 teaspoon up to three times a day.

Medicinal doses of these herbs should not be given to children under age 2. For older children and people over 65, start with a low-strength preparation and increase strength if necessary.

The Safety Factor

European animal studies show vervain depresses heart rate, constricts the bronchial passages, and stimulates the intestine and uterus. Because it may depress heart rate, anyone with congestive heart failure or a history of heart disease should not use it. The possibility of bronchial constriction might cause problems for asthmatics and those with other respiratory conditions. Intestinal stimulation might aggravate chronic gastrointestinal conditions, for example, colitis. And pregnant women should steer clear of vervain because of its possible stimulating effect on the uterus—except possibly at term and under the supervision of a physician to help induce labor.

Other Cautions

Although both vervain species have similar effects, the Food and Drug Administration includes V. *officinalis* among herbs generally regarded as safe but considers V. *hastata* an herb of "undefined safety." For otherwise healthy nonpregnant, non-nursing adults who do not have a history of heart disease or asthma, both vervains are considered relatively safe in amounts typically recommended.

Vervain should be used in medicinal amounts only in consultation with your doctor. If vervain causes minor discomforts, such as stomach or intestinal distress, use less or stop using it. Let your doctor know if you experience unpleasant effects or if the symptoms for which the herb is being used do not improve significantly in two weeks.

Pain-Free Harvest

Vervain is a 3-foot perennial with thin, erect, stiff stems. Its opposite leaves are oblong and toothed near the ground and lance-shaped and deeply lobed higher up. The plant develops slender flower spikes that bear small blue or lilac flowers from early summer through midautumn. The herb's bluish flowers gave it the name blue vervain.

Vervain grows easily from seeds planted in spring after frost danger has passed. Although it's a perennial, this herb is rather short-lived; however, it self-sows. Vervain prefers rich, moist loam under full sun.

Harvest the leaves and flower tops as the plants flower.

WHITE WILLOW

Potent Against Pain

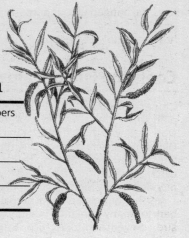

Family: Salicaceae; other members include poplar

Genus and species: *Salix alba*

Also known as: Salicin willow

Parts used: Bark

Look at a white willow and what do you see? Most people see only a stately shade tree. But herbalists also see the potent pain reliever, aspirin. In fact, aspirin was originally created from a chemical in white willow bark, salicin, named for the herb's genus, *Salix*.

From Joy to Weeping

White willow grew on the banks of the Nile, and the ancient Egyptians considered it a symbol of joy. The Hebrews adopted the beautiful tree, and in Leviticus (23:40) God commanded them to celebrate the autumn harvest festival by setting up temporary shelters covered with willow boughs: "Ye shall take . . . boughs of willow . . . and rejoice seven days."

But the willow became a symbol of sorrow after the destruction of the first Temple in Jerusalem, which began the Jews' Babylonian exile. Consider the willow's transformation in Psalm 137: "By the rivers of Babylon, where we sat down, and there we wept, when we remembered Zion, upon the willows, we hanged up our harps, for they that led us there captive asked of us . . . song. . . ." Since that time, the graceful tree has been known as weeping willow.

Cools the Fire of Pain and Desire

Chinese physicians have used white willow bark to relieve pain since 500 B.C., but it took five centuries for that use to work its way to Europe. First-century Greek physician Dioscorides was the first Westerner to recommend willow bark for pain and inflammation, and his prescription did not catch on. A century later, the Roman doctor Galen recommended it only for the vague purpose of "drying up humors."

As the centuries passed, herbalists prescribed white willow bark for many ailments, including suppression of sexual desire. Seventeenth-century English herbalist Nicholas Culpeper noted: "The leaves, bark, and seed are used to stanch bleeding . . . stay vomiting . . . provoke urine . . . take away warts . . . and clear the face and skin from spots and discolourings. . . . The leaves bruised and boiled in wine stays the heat of lust in man or woman, and quite extinguishes it if it be long used." At this time, white willow was not commonly used to treat pain, but Culpeper touted the work of one Mr. Stone, who demonstrated its "great efficacy . . . in intermittent fever [malaria]." Culpeper concluded white willow bark "is likely to become an object worthy of . . . attention."

Culpeper's words proved prophetic. By the 18th century, white willow bark was widely used to treat all sorts of fevers, and its pain-relieving action also returned to vogue. Early colonists introduced the tree into North America and found many Indian tribes using the bark of native willows to treat pain, chills, and fever.

From Salicin to Aspirin

Around 1828, French and German chemists extracted white willow bark's active chemical, salicin. Ten years later, an

Italian chemist purified the aspirin precursor, salicylic acid. Although this potent pain reliever was first discovered in white willow, chemists made the first aspirin from another herb that contains this same chemical—meadowsweet. Salicin was discovered in meadowsweet in 1839. During the mid-19th century, researchers showed both salicin and salicylic acid reduce fever and relieve pain and inflammation. Unfortunately, they also have unpleasant—and potentially hazardous—side effects: nausea, diarrhea, bleeding, stomach ulceration, ringing in the ears (tinnitus), and at high doses, respiratory paralysis and death.

Chemists created acetylsalicylic acid—aspirin—from salicylic acid obtained from meadowsweet (see page 363). The idea was to preserve the benefits of salicylic acid while minimizing its side effects.

Aspirin eventually became the household drug of choice for a broad range of everyday ailments.

Contemporary herbalists recommend white willow bark for headache, fever, arthritis, other pain, and inflammations.

HEALING with White Willow

Contrary to Culpeper, white willow bark won't cure malaria, but it is indeed herbal "aspirin." It contains more salicylates than meadowsweet, making it a more potent natural healer.

Fever, Pain, Inflammation. Try white willow any time you think you need aspirin. Aspirin is a more concentrated source of the active chemicals in the herb (salicylates), so don't expect the herb to be as effective.

Women's Health. Like aspirin, white willow contains enough salicylate to suppress the action of chemicals called prostaglandins, which are involved in menstrual cramps.

Pregnant women should not use white willow, however. In animal studies, aspirin is associated with an increased risk of birth defects. The herb is not as powerful, but it's better to be safe than sorry.

Intriguing Possibility. One laboratory study suggested

white willow may reduce blood sugar (glucose), but the herb's effect on human diabetes, if any, remains unclear.

R_x for White Willow

For a pain-, fever-, and inflammation-relieving infusion, soak 1 teaspoon of powdered bark per cup of cold water for 8 hours. Strain. Drink up to 3 cups a day. White willow tastes bitter and astringent. Add honey and lemon, or mix it with an herbal beverage tea.

White willow should not be given to children under age 2 or to those under 16 with a cold, flu, or chicken pox. For other children and people over 65, start with low-strength preparations and increase strength if necessary.

The Safety Factor

Aspirin upsets some people's stomachs, but most herbalists say white willow bark rarely causes this problem. If stomach upset, nausea, or tinnitus develop, reduce your dose or stop using the herb.

Those with chronic gastrointestinal conditions, such as ulcers and gastritis, should not use this herb.

When children under 16 with colds, flu, or chicken pox take aspirin, they are at risk for Reye's syndrome—a potentially fatal condition involving the brain, liver, and kidneys. White willow has never been linked to Reye's syndrome, but because of it's aspirin-like action, do not give it to children with colds, flu, or chicken pox.

Other Cautions

For otherwise healthy nonpregnant, nonnursing adults who do not have ulcers or gastritis and are not taking other salicylate medications, white willow bark is considered relatively safe in amounts typically recommended.

White willow should be used in medicinal amounts only in consultation with your doctor. If white willow causes minor discomforts, such as stomach upset or ringing in the ears, use less or stop using it. Let your doctor know if you experience unpleasant effects or if the symptoms for which the herb is being used do not improve significantly in two weeks.

A Harvest of Willow

Throughout history, many of the 500 willow species have been used in herbal healing, but for the last 200 years only white willow has been commonly used. It reaches 75 feet and has rough, grayish brown bark, and long, thin leaves on flexible branches, which give the tree a graceful beauty.

White willows grow in almost any moist garden soil under full sun. Buy saplings at nurseries or propagate them from first-year branches several feet in length rooted in water or from foot-long hardwood cuttings taken in spring or fall and rooted the same way. Do not transplant willows. Willows grow quickly and must be pruned regularly.

Harvest the bark from older branches during pruning and dry.

WILD CHERRY

Tasty Cough Syrup

Family: Rosaceae; other members include rose, plum, almond, apricot

Genus and species: *Prunus serotina, P. virginiana*

Also known as: Choke cherry, rum cherry, wild black cherry, Virginia prune bark

Parts used: Inner bark, root bark

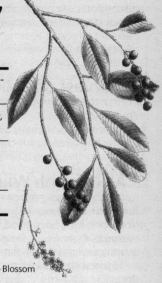

Blossom

Children's cough remedies are often cherry flavored. That flavor is no accident. Since 1820, the bark of the native American wild cherry tree has been listed in the U.S. *Pharmacopoeia* as a phlegm-loosener (expectorant) and mild sedative. But this herb is not just kids' stuff. It also contains a chemical similar to cyanide that might be deadly in very large amounts.

Popular Healer

Early colonists found many Indian tribes using wild cherry bark tea as a tranquilizer, sedative, and treatment for colds, coughs, diarrhea, labor pains, and other ailments. They adopted the Indian uses for the herb and also used it to treat bronchitis, pneumonia, and whooping cough.

During the 19th century, wild cherry bark ranked among

541

the nation's most popular botanical medicines, both by itself and as an ingredient in an enormous number of patent medicines.

Wild cherry bark was a favorite of America's 19th-century Eclectic physicians, who considered it an excellent tranquilizer and mild sedative and a remedy for the dry, hacking cough associated with colds and flu. The Eclectics also recommended the herb as a tonic during convalescence from lengthy illnesses.

Contemporary herbalists recommend wild cherry for colds, cough, asthma, and bronchitis.

HEALING with Wild Cherry

Wild cherry continues to be listed in the U.S. *Pharmacopoeia* as an expectorant and mild sedative.

Cough. Only one scientific source—the Food and Drug Administration (FDA)—disputes wild cherry's value. The FDA concluded wild cherry bark "is of little if any remedial value [except] as a flavoring agent." The FDA recognizes only one expectorant as safe and effective—guaifenesen. Ironically, many lung authorities consider guaifenesen *ineffective*. Try wild cherry and see if it works for you.

Tranquilizer, Sedative. In recommended doses, one chemical in this herb, hydrocyanic acid, appears to act as a mild tranquilizer and sedative. However, hydrocyanic acid is related to cyanide, and unusually large amounts are poisonous. Stick to recommended amounts.

R$_x$ for Wild Cherry

For an infusion that may help treat cough, stress, anxiety, or insomnia, use 1 teaspoon of powdered bark per cup of boiling water. Steep 10 minutes. Drink up to 3 cups a day. Wild cherry has a pleasant aroma but a bitter, astringent taste; adding honey, sugar, and lemon or mixing it with an herbal beverage blend will improve flavor.

In a tincture, take $1/4$ to $1/2$ teaspoon up to three times a day.

Wild cherry should not be given to children under age 2. For older children and people over 65, start with a low-strength preparation and increase strength if necessary.

The Safety Factor

Alert: Wild cherry leaves, bark, and fruit pits all contain hydrocyanic acid, which in large amounts is a cyanide-like poison. Grazing animals have been poisoned by eating large quantities of leaves, which are more toxic than the medicinal bark.

Symptoms of toxicity include spasms, twitching, and difficulty breathing and speaking. If these occur, stop using the herb and seek medical attention immediately.

The medical literature contains no reports of wild cherry bark causing problems at recommended doses. But it has been implicated in birth defects among the offspring of laboratory animals that ingested the herb while pregnant. Pregnant women should not use wild cherry bark.

Other Cautions

Wild cherry bark is included in the FDA's list of herbs generally regarded as safe. For otherwise healthy nonpregnant, nonnursing adults, wild cherry bark is considered relatively safe in amounts typically recommended.

Wild cherry should be used in medicinal amounts only in consultation with your doctor. If wild cherry bark causes minor discomforts, such as stomach upset or diarrhea, use less or stop using it. Let your doctor know if you experience unpleasant effects or if the symptoms for which the herb is being used do not improve significantly in two weeks.

A Giant of a Healer

Wild cherry is one of our largest trees, often reaching 90 feet. It grows in the area bounded by Nova Scotia, Florida, Texas, and Nebraska. The trunk is covered with rough black bark, which breaks off in plates. The root bark must be peeled. Both barks are considered medicinal, and although they look different, they are both known as wild cherry bark.

Wild cherry's oval, serrated leaves are a brilliant green. The tree produces small white flowers in late spring, followed by blackish purple fruits the size of large peas.

Wild cherry grows best in fertile soil under full sun. Authorities recommend planting saplings purchased at nurseries.

Herbalists recommend the young, thin branch bark rather than the older, thicker trunk bark. Collect it in autumn by pruning some branches and stripping them. The bark deteriorates after about a year in storage, so collect it annually.

WITCH HAZEL

The Herb Even Doctors Use

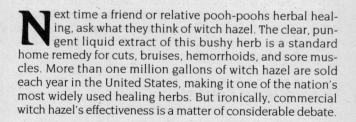

Family: Hamamelidaceae; witch hazel is only member

Genus and species: *Hamamelis virginiana*

Also known as: Winterbloom, snapping hazelnut, hamamelis

Parts used: Leaves, bark

Next time a friend or relative pooh-poohs herbal healing, ask what they think of witch hazel. The clear, pungent liquid extract of this bushy herb is a standard home remedy for cuts, bruises, hemorrhoids, and sore muscles. More than one million gallons of witch hazel are sold each year in the United States, making it one of the nation's most widely used healing herbs. But ironically, commercial witch hazel's effectiveness is a matter of considerable debate.

Nothing to Do with Witches

The "hazel" in this herb's name comes from its similarity to the common hazelnut. As for the "witch," some say early colonists used the shrub to make brooms, witches' favorite form of transportation. Others trace it to witch hazel's winter flowering and the loud "pop" when it disperses its seeds, supposedly evidence of occult influence. Still others claim the shrub's forked branches were used by dousers looking for water, and that dousing was once associated with witchcraft.

The fact is, this herb's name has nothing to do with witchcraft. In medieval Middle English, *witch* had another meaning. It was spelled *wych* or *wyche*, and meant pliant or flexible. Witch hazel's branches are, indeed, flexible—so springy, in fact, the Indians used them to make bows.

Soothes Those Sores

Witch hazel was highly valued in Indian medicine. Many tribes rubbed a decoction on cuts, bruises, insect bites, aching joints, sore muscles, and sore backs. They also drank witch hazel tea to stop internal bleeding, prevent miscarriage, and treat colds, fevers, sore throat, and menstrual pain.

The colonists adopted witch hazel's Indian uses, but the herb remained a folk remedy until the 1840s, when an Oneida medicine man introduced the plant to one Theron T. Pond of Utica, New York. Pond learned of the plant's astringent properties and ability to treat burns, boils, wounds, and hemorrhoids. In 1848, he began marketing witch hazel extract as Pond's Golden Treasure. Later, the name was changed to Pond's Extract, which became a big hit, and witch hazel water has been with us ever since.

Controversy Brews

Early witch hazel water was simply a strained decoction of the shrub's leaves and twigs that contained tannins, which made the extract highly astringent. But by the late 19th century, manufacturers switched to steam distillation, a simpler process but one that left the resulting water with little if any tannin. That's when the controversy erupted.

The Eclectic text, *King's American Dispensatory*, asserted: "The decoction is very useful in hemorrhage, diarrhea, dysentery, swellings, inflammations, tumors, hemorrhoids, epistaxis [nosebleed], and uterine hemorrhage following delivery. . . . [However] since the introduction of the distilled extract [witch hazel] has been largely abandoned. . . . The fluid extract has little to recommend it."

Nonetheless, witch hazel was listed as an astringent and anti-inflammatory in the U.S. *Pharmacopoeia* from 1862 through 1916, and in the *National Formulary*, the pharmacists' reference, from 1916 to 1955. The *National Formulary* finally dropped it because in 1947, the 24th edition of *The Dispensatory of the United States* stated witch hazel: "is so nearly destitute of medicinal virtues, it scarcely deserves official recognition. . . . [Its continued use serves only to fill] the need in American families for an embrocation [liniment] which appeals to the psychic influence of faith."

Yet today, witch hazel can be found on the shelves of every pharmacy.

Contemporary herbalists sidestep the controversy by recommending only the decoction of witch hazel bark, which contains astringent tannins. They are unanimous in their praise of this herb's cooling, astringent action when used externally for cuts, burns, scalds, bruises, inflammations, and hemorrhoids. They recommend it as a gargle for sore throat and sores in the mouth, and internally to treat diarrhea.

HEALING with Witch Hazel

Wouldn't it be ironic if this widely used herbal remedy turned out to be worthless? Fortunately that does not appear to be the case.

Astringent. Witch hazel leaves, twigs, and bark contain fairly high concentrations of tannins, and a Belgian animal study showed it constricts blood vessels, supporting its long-time use as an astringent.

Commercial witch hazel water may not contain tannins, but it does contain other chemicals with reported antiseptic, anesthetic, astringent, and anti-inflammatory action. Witch hazel water is an ingredient in Tucks, Preparation H Cleansing Pads, and several German hemorrhoid preparations.

R_x for Witch Hazel

For an astringent decoction, boil 1 teaspoon of powdered leaves or twigs per cup of water for 10 minutes. Strain and cool. Apply directly or mix into an ointment.

For a bitter, astringent gargle, use 1 teaspoon of bark per cup of boiling water. Steep 10 minutes and strain.

Witch hazel may be used externally on anyone, but dilute it for use on children under age 2.

The Safety Factor

The medical literature contains no reports of harm from using witch hazel externally or as a gargle.

For otherwise healthy nonpregnant, nonnursing adults, witch hazel is considered safe in amounts typically recommended.

If witch hazel causes minor discomforts, such as skin irritation, dilute it or stop using it. Let your doctor know if you experience unpleasant effects or if the symptoms for which the herb is being used do not improve significantly in two weeks.

Colorful Winter Bloomer

Witch hazel's Latin name refers to Virginia, but the shrub grows all over the eastern United States. Most commercial witch hazel is grown in the Carolinas and Tennessee.

Witch hazel is a perennial that drops its leaves each autumn. Its single root sends up several twisting stems that fork into many flexible, hairy branches. Witch hazel blooms long after most other flowers have disappeared, depending on location, from September to December, hence the name winterbloom.

The shrub's spidery yellow flowers appear at the same time its previous year's fruits mature. Its woody seed pods burst open with an audible pop and propel their two hard black seeds up to 25 feet. The seeds are edible and have been compared to hazelnuts, hence the name snapping hazelnut.

As a late-bloomer, witch hazel makes a colorful addition to any garden. Witch hazel grows from seeds or twig cuttings. Seeds should be refrigerated at around 40°F for several months before planting to encourage germination. Cuttings generally produce roots in about ten weeks. Witch hazel grows best in moist, rich, sandy, or peaty soil under partial shade but tolerates poorer soil and full sun.

Harvest the leaves and twigs anytime and dry.

YARROW

The Herbal Bandage

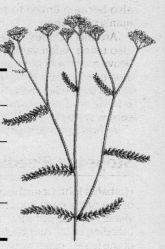

Family: Compositae; other members include daisy, dandelion, marigold

Genus and species: *Achillea mille-folium*

Also known as: Thousand weed, milfoil, soldier's woundwort, herbe militaire, nose bleed, bloodwort, bad man's plaything

Parts used: Leaves, stems, flower tops

Legend has it that during the Trojan War, Achilles stopped the bleeding of his fellow soldiers' wounds by applying yarrow's fernlike leaves. Scientists have discovered the mythological hero may have been right. Yarrow contains substances that may help stop bleeding and have pain-relieving and anti-inflammatory properties potentially helpful in wound treatment. It also appears to have potential as a digestive aid, menstrual remedy, and mild sedative.

Soldier's Woundwort

Achilles defined yarrow's use in herbal healing for more than 2,500 years. Dioscorides, a physician attached to Roman legions, recommended rubbing the crushed plant on wounds. The herb's many popular names—herbe militaire, nose bleed, soldier's woundwort, and bloodwort—attest to its use as a blood stopper during the Middle Ages. (*Wort* is Old English for *plant*.) Perhaps from an association with brawling, yarrow also became linked to ruffians and earned the name, "bad man's plaything."

Around Achilles' time, ancient Chinese physicians were also using Asian yarrow to treat inflammations, bleeding, heavy menstrual flow, and dog and snake bites. The Chinese also used yarrow in the ritual of the I *Ching*, the oracle consulted to predict the future. Coins are typically used today, but the traditional way to cast the I *Ching* involved dried yarrow stems.

India's Ayurvedic physicians used yarrow to treat fevers.

Stops the Bleeding

Herbalist John Gerard recommended yarrow for "swellings . . . of the privie parts." In the 17th century, John Parkinson advised, "If it be put into the nose, assuredly it will stop the bleeding of it." And Nicholas Culpeper wrote: "an ointment of the leaves cures wounds . . . restrains violent bleedings . . . is good for inflammations and ulcers . . . and is excellent for the piles [hemorrhoids]."

Colonists introduced yarrow into North America, and the Indians adopted it enthusiastically as an external treatment for wounds and burns, and internally to treat colds, sore throat, arthritis, toothache, insomnia, and indigestion.

The 19th-century Eclectics considered yarrow a "tonic upon the venous system," but downplayed its age-old role in wound treatment. Their text, *King's American Dispensatory*, recommended it for bloody urine (hematuria), incontinence, hemorrhoids, menstrual cramps, diarrhea, dysentery, and "hemorrhage where the bleeding is small in amount."

Contemporary herbalist Steven Foster recommends yarrow as "an herbal Band-Aid." Other herbalists prescribe yarrow for fevers, urinary tract infections, and as a digestive aid.

Healing with Yarrow

If Achilles had had some yarrow on hand when his vulnerable heel was wounded, he might have survived the Trojan War.

Wound Treatment. Yarrow contains many chemicals that support its traditional use in wound treatment. Two—achilletin and achilleine—spur blood coagulation. Several—azulene, camphor, chamazulene, eugenol, menthol, quercetin, rutin, and salicylic acid—have anti-inflammatory and pain-relieving action. Several others—tannins, terpeniol, and cineol—are antiseptic.

Digestive Aid. Yarrow contains a chemical also present in chamomile and chamazulene, that helps relax the smooth muscle tissue of the digestive tract, making it an antispasmodic. Scientists do not consider yarrow's digestive action as potent as chamomile's, however.

Women's Health. Antispasmodics relax not only the digestive tract but other smooth muscles, such as the uterus, as well, lending some credence to yarrow's use in treating menstrual cramps.

Tranquilizer, Sedative. Yarrow also contains a small amount of a hypnotic chemical, thujone, the effects of which have been compared to marijuana. The thujone in yarrow may account for its traditional use as a sedative. In large amounts, thujone is poisonous, but recommended amounts of yarrow do not contain enough to cause harm.

Intriguing Possibility. Two animal studies show yarrow protects the liver from toxic chemical damage. And a scientifically conducted trial in India showed yarrow helps treat hepatitis. If you have liver disease, ask your physician about using yarrow in addition to standard therapies.

Rx for Yarrow

For wound treatment, press fresh leaves and flower tops into cuts and scrapes on the way to washing and bandaging them.

For a possible tranquilizing infusion to help aid digestion or help treat menstrual cramps, use 1 to 2 teaspoons of dried herb per cup of boiling water. Steep 10 to 15 minutes. Drink up to 3 cups a day. Yarrow tastes tangy and bitter with some astringency. To improve flavor, add honey, sugar, or lemon, or mix it with an herbal beverage blend.

To help promote healing, apply it externally to clean wounds and inflammations.

In a tincture, use $1/2$ to 1 teaspoon up to three times a day.

Medicinal yarrow preparations should not be given to children under age 2. For older children and people over 65, start with low-strength preparations and increase strength if necessary.

The Safety Factor

High doses of yarrow may turn urine dark brown. Do not become alarmed.

The medical literature contains no reports of harm from yarrow; however, those allergic to ragweed might develop a rash.

Thujone-free extracts of yarrow are approved by the Food and Drug Administration for use in beverages. For otherwise healthy nonpregnant, nonnursing adults, yarrow is considered safe in amounts typically recommended.

Yarrow should be used in medicinal amounts only in consultation with your doctor. If yarrow causes minor discomforts, such as a rash or diarrhea, use less or stop using it. Let your doctor know if you experience unpleasant effects or if the symptoms for which the herb is being used do not improve significantly in two weeks.

Fuzzy Plant Is Easy to Grow

Yarrow is an attractive 3-foot perennial covered with delicate hairs. Its feathery leaves are divided into what seem like thousands of tiny leaflets, hence its names, thousand weed and milfoil, a corruption of the French term for 1,000 leaves, *mille feuille*. Yarrow's numerous, tiny, white flowers develop in dense clusters on flat-topped, umbrella-like stalks in summer.

Yarrow grows easily from seeds or root divisions planted in spring or fall. Sow seeds just under the surface of fine soil and keep them moist until they germinate, usually within two weeks. Thin seedlings to 12-inch spacing. Yarrow adapts to many soil types but needs good drainage and does best in moderately rich soil under full sun. Divide plants every few years to keep them growing vigorously.

Harvest yarrow when the plants are in bloom. Hang them to dry.

Chapter 6

Prevention and Treatment: A Fast-Action Guide to Using the Healing Herbs

Which herb do you reach for if you have a cold? A headache? Is there a digestive aid safe enough to give to infants for colic? What about a soothing herbal beverage to help you unwind after a frazzling day at work?

There are more than 100 separate uses for the healing herbs discussed in this book. Those uses have been arranged here in three easy-to-use tables: "Conditions," "Healing Actions," and "Other Uses."

In "Conditions," you'll find a list of all the herbs that can be used to treat and prevent specific symptoms and diseases. Some herbs can be used as natural alternatives to certain medicines—for example, antibiotics or sedatives. They're all listed under "Healing Actions." "Other Uses" highlights a few more unusual uses for the healing herbs—for instance, as insect repellents.

Some Precautions

Before using any herb medicinally, read all about it in chapter 5. The tables in this chapter list only the most potentially hazardous reactions. Before you can use any herb safely, you need to thoroughly familiarize yourself with its effects.

If you have any chronic condition—such as angina, asthma, arthritis, cancer, diabetes, heart disease, or high blood pressure—use healing herbs in conjunction with your regular medical treatment and only in consultation with your physician. Any herb may cause allergic reactions in sensitive individuals. Herb oils are much more concentrated than herbs themselves, and ingesting even small amounts can be hazardous.

A Special Note for Women

With few exceptions, pregnant and nursing women should not ingest medicinal amounts of any healing herb because of possible harm to the fetus or infant.

Most herbal digestive aids are antispasmodics, meaning that they relax the smooth muscle lining of the intestinal tract. The uterus is also a smooth muscle, and it would be reasonable to expect antispasmodic herbs to calm this organ, as well. However, most digestion-enhancing herbs have traditionally been used to stimulate the uterus, that is, to promote menstruation. Using them could conceivably create a risk of miscarriage. This apparent contradiction appears to be dose-related. Ginger, for example, has been shown to be a safe treatment for morning sickness in recommended amounts, though in extremely large amounts (about 20 times the stomach-settling dose), it may induce uterine contractions.

Most digestion-enhancing herbs are also used in cooking. Pregnant women and those attempting to conceive may use culinary amounts. But until the question of uterine effects has been more thoroughly investigated, prudence suggests that pregnant women steer clear of medicinal amounts. This is true even though, for most of these herbs, uterine stimulation has not been experimentally verified. Pregnant women shouldn't use any herb medicinally without the approval and supervision of their obstetricians.

Conditions

Condition	Herbs	Special Precautions
Acne	Basil oil	
Acquired immune deficiency syndrome (AIDS)	Garlic St.-John's-wort	*St.-John's-wort* acts like an MAO inhibitor, a class of drugs that interacts with a number of foods and other drugs. (See page 468.)
Anxiety	Balm Bay Catnip Celery Chamomile Motherwort Passionflower Skullcap Wild cherry Yarrow	*Balm* can interfere with a thyroid-stimulating hormone. If you have a thyroid problem, consult your physician before using it. Long-term use of *celery* can deplete potassium stores.
Arthritis	Angelica Black haw Boneset Chamomile Chaparral Echinacea Fenugreek Gentian Ginger Horsetail Juniper Licorice Meadowsweet	*Angelica* may cause a rash in those exposed to sun. *Fenugreek* has some estrogenic action. Women who have been advised not to take the Pill or who have a history of breast cancer should consult their physician before using it.

(continued)

Conditions (*continued*)

Condition	Herbs	Special Precautions
Arthritis (*continued*)	St.-John's-wort Turmeric Vervain White willow	Long-term use of *horsetail* and *juniper* depletes potassium stores. Long-term use of large amounts of *licorice* may cause water retention, elevated blood pressure, headache, and hormone imbalance (pseudoaldosteronism). *St.-John's-wort* acts like an MAO inhibitor, a class of drugs that interacts with a number of foods and other drugs. (See page 468.) *Vervain* can depress the heart rate and constrict bronchial passages. If you have heart disease or asthma, consult your physician before using it.
Asthma	Angelica Anise Cocoa	*Angelica* may cause a rash in those exposed to sun.

Condition	Herbs	Special Precautions
	Coffee Coltsfoot Ginkgo Kola Tea	*Anise* has some estrogenic action. Women who have been advised not to take the Pill or who have a history of breast cancer should consult their physician before using it. Long-term use of large amounts of *coltsfoot* may cause hepatic veno-occlusive disease, a serious disorder that impairs liver function. *Cocoa, coffee, kola,* and *tea* contain caffeine, which can cause insomnia and possible addiction.
Athlete's foot	Garlic	
Bad breath	Alfalfa Chaparral Parsley	Long-term use of *parsley* can deplete potassium stores.
Bleeding	Blackberry Shepherd's purse Witch hazel	*Shepherd's purse* can cause powerful uterine contractions.

(continued)

Conditions (*continued*)

Condition	Herbs	Special Precautions
Bleeding (*continued*)	Yarrow	
Bronchitis (See also Cough)	Barberry Echinacea Garlic Goldenseal	
Burns (See also Pain)	(for external use on minor burns) Aloe Chamomile Comfrey Echinacea Gotu kola Marsh mallow Passionflower St.-John's-wort Yarrow	Flush burns with cold water before applying herbal remedies. Serious burns require medical attention.
Cancer prevention	Alfalfa Apple Chaparral Garlic Ginseng	
Cancer treatment	Chaparral Mistletoe	*Mistletoe* can slow the heart rate and affect pressure. If you have heart disease, consult your physician before using it.

Condition	Herbs	Special Precautions
Cholera	Barberry Goldenseal	
Cholesterol, high	Alfalfa Apple Fenugreek Garlic Ginger Ginseng Psyllium Red pepper Saffron Skullcap Tea Turmeric	*Fenugreek* has some estrogenic action. Women who have been advised not to take the Pill or who have a history of breast cancer should consult their physician before using it. *Tea* contains caffeine, which can cause insomnia and possible addiction.
Cirrhosis	Ginseng Licorice	Long-term use of large amounts of *licorice* may cause water retention, elevated blood pressure, headache, and hormone imbalance (pseudoaldosteronism).
Cold sores (See Herpes)		
Colds and flu (See also Cough)	Boneset Echinacea Ginger Hyssop	*Savory* is especially good for children because it's so mild.

(*continued*)

Conditions (*continued*)

Condition	Herbs	Special Precautions
Colds and flu (*continued*)	Marsh mallow Rose Savory	
Colic	Coriander Dill Savory Slippery elm	
Congestive heart failure (See also Diuretic in "Healing Actions" table)	Hawthorn	
Conjunctivitis	Barberry	
Constipation	Apple Buckthorn Cascara sagrada Parsley Psyllium Rhubarb Senna Vervain	*Buckthorn, rhubarb, cascara sagrada*, and *senna* may cause severe intestinal cramps. Long-term use of *parsley* can deplete potassium stores. *Vervain* can depress the heart rate and constrict bronchial passages. If you have heart disease or asthma, consult your physician before using it.

Condition	Herbs	Special Precautions
Cough	Angelica Anise Cocoa Coffee Coltsfoot Ephedra Eucalyptus Fenugreek Horehound Hyssop Kola Licorice Marsh mallow Maté Mullein Oregano Pennyroyal Savory Slippery elm Tea Thyme Wild cherry	*Angelica* may cause a rash in those exposed to sun. *Anise* and *fenugreek* have some estrogenic action. Women who have been advised not to take the Pill or who have a history of breast cancer should consult their physician before using either. Long-term use of large amounts of *coltsfoot* may cause hepatic veno-occlusive disease, a serious disorder that impairs liver function. *Ephedra* can elevate blood pressure. It should not be used by people with high blood pressure. Long-term use of large amounts of *licorice* may cause water retention, elevated blood pressure, headache, and

(continued)

Conditions (*continued*)

Condition	Herbs	Special Precautions
Cough (*continued*)		hormone imbalance (pseudoaldosteronism). *Cocoa, coffee, kola, maté,* and *tea* contain caffeine, which can cause insomnia and possible addiction.
Depression	St.-John's-wort	*St.-John's-wort* acts like an MAO inhibitor, a class of drugs that interacts with a number of foods and other drugs. (See page 468.)
Diabetes	Apple Celery Fenugreek Garlic Ginseng Sage	Long-term use of *celery* can deplete potassium stores. *Fenugreek* has some estrogenic action. Women who have been advised not to take the Pill or who have a history of breast cancer should consult their physician before using it.
Diarrhea	Apple Barberry Bayberry	*Bayberry* can change the body's potassium/sodium balance.

Condition	Herbs	Special Precautions
	Blackberry Dill Goldenseal Meadowsweet Mullein Psyllium Raspberry Rhubarb Tea Uva ursi	If you have high blood pressure, heart disease, or kidney disease, consult your physician before using it. Large doses of *rhubarb* have a laxative effect. *Tea* contains caffeine, which can cause insomnia and possible addiction. Long-term use of *uva ursi* can deplete potassium stores.
Dizziness	Ginger Ginkgo	
Ear infection	Echinacea	
Emphysema	Coltsfoot Thyme	Long-term use of large amounts of *coltsfoot* may cause hepatic veno-occlusive disease, a serious disorder that impairs liver function.
Fever	Bayberry Black haw	*Bayberry* can alter the body's potassium/

(*continued*)

Conditions (*continued*)

Condition	Herbs	Special Precautions
Fever (*continued*)	Meadowsweet Parsley White willow	sodium balance. If you have high blood pressure, heart disease, or kidney disease, consult your physician before using it. Long-term use of *parsley* can deplete potassium stores.
Food-poisoning prevention	Rosemary Sage Thyme	
Food-poisoning treatment	Angelica Apple Barberry Bayberry Burdock Catnip Chamomile Cinnamon Clove Dill Echinacea Garlic Ginseng Goldenseal Meadowsweet Mints Mullein	*Angelica* may cause rash in those exposed to sun. *Bayberry* can alter the body's potassium /sodium balance. If you have high blood pressure, heart disease, or kidney disease, consult your physician before using it. *St.-John's-wort* acts like an MAO inhibitor, a class of drugs that interacts with a number of foods and other drugs. (See page 468.)

Condition	Herbs	Special Precautions
Gas	Dill	
Giardiasis	Barberry Elecampane Goldenseal	
Gout (See also Pain)	Nettle	
Gum disease prevention	Chaparral Myrrh	
Hay fever	Nettle Parsley	Long-term use of *nettle* and *parsley* can deplete potassium stores.
Headache (See also Pain)	Feverfew (for migraine) Red pepper (for cluster type)	
Hearing loss in the elderly (cochlear deafness)	Ginkgo	
Heart disease treatment (See also High blood pressure and Cholesterol, high in this table, and Diuretic in "Healing Actions" table)	Ginkgo Hawthorn Passionflower	

(*continued*)

Conditions (*continued*)

Condition	Herbs	Special Precautions
Hemorrhoids	(for external use) Blackberry Mullein Psyllium Shepherd's purse Witch hazel	
Hepatitis	Licorice	Long-term use of large amounts of *licorice* may cause water retention, elevated blood pressure, headache, and hormone imbalance (pseudoaldosteronism).
Herpes—cold sores and genital (See also Pain)	(for external use) Balm Comfrey Hyssop Licorice Marjoram Mint oils Uva ursi (for internal use) Echinacea Ginseng	

Condition	Herbs	Special Precautions
High blood pressure (See also Diuretic in "Healing Actions" table)	Barberry Black Cohosh Feverfew Garlic Ginger Mistletoe Motherwort Saffron Valerian	*Black cohosh* can depress the heart rate. If you have congestive heart failure, consult your physician before using it. *Mistletoe* can slow the heart rate and affect blood pressure. If you have heart disease, consult your physician before using it. *Valerian* is a sedative and can cause drowsiness.
Hives	Parsley	Long-term use of *parsley* can deplete potassium stores.
Impotence (caused by poor blood flow)	Ginkgo	
Insomnia	Balm Celery Hop Motherwort Passionflower Skullcap Valerian Wild cherry	*Balm* interferes with a thyroid-stimulating hormone. If you have a thyroid problem, consult your physician before using it.

(continued)

Conditions (*continued*)

Condition	Herbs	Special Precautions
Insomnia (*continued*)	Yarrow	Long-term use of *celery* can deplete potassium stores.
Intermittent claudication (leg pain)	Ginkgo	
Jet lag	Cocoa Coffee Ephedra Ginseng Kola Maté Tea	*Ephedra* can elevate blood pressure. People with high blood pressure should not use it. *Cocoa, coffee, kola, maté,* and *tea* contain caffeine, which can cause insomnia and possible addiction.
Lead poisoning	Apple Garlic	
Leprosy (Hansen's disease)	Garlic Gotu kola	
Liver disease prevention	Ginseng Licorice Turmeric	Long-term use of large amounts of *licorice* may cause water retention, elevated blood pressure, headache, and hormone imbalance (pseudoaldosteronism).

Condition	Herbs	Special Precautions
Macular degeneration (a condition that leads to blindness)	Ginkgo	
Menopausal discomforts	Anise Black cohosh Fennel Fenugreek Red clover	*Anise, black cohosh, fennel, fenugreek,* and *red clover* all have some estrogenic action. Women who have been advised not to take the Pill or who have a history of breast cancer should consult their physician before using these herbs. Women with heart disease should consult their physician before using *black cohosh*; it can depress the heart rate.
Menstrual discomforts (See also Pain)	Anise Black cohosh Black haw Fennel Fenugreek Feverfew Red clover Yarrow	*Anise, black cohosh, fennel, fenugreek,* and *red clover* all have some estrogenic action. Women who have been advised not to take the Pill or who have a history of breast cancer should consult their physician before using any of these herbs.

(continued)

Conditions (*continued*)

Condition	Herbs	Special Precautions
Menstrual discomforts (*continued*)		Women with heart disease should consult their physician before using *black cohosh*; it can depress the heart rate.
Menstruation, delayed	Celery Fenugreek Motherwort Parsley Rhubarb Saffron Shepherd's purse	*Shepherd's purse* can cause powerful uterine contractions. *Fenugreek* has some estrogenic action. Women who have been advised not to take the Pill or who have a history of breast cancer should consult their physician before using it. *Mistletoe* can slow the heart rate and affect blood pressure. If you have heart disease, consult your physician before using it. *Rhubarb* can cause severe intestinal cramps. Long-term use of *celery* or *parsley* can deplete potassium stores.

Condition	Herbs	Special Precautions
Menstruation, heavy	Goldenseal Shepherd's purse	*Shepherd's purse* can cause powerful uterine contractions.
Migraine (See Headache)		
Miscarriage prevention	Raspberry	Use herbs for this purpose only during the final five weeks of pregnancy.
Morning sickness	Ginger Mints Raspberry	Pregnant women should use medicinal amounts of herbs only in consultation with their doctor.
Motion sickness prevention	Ginger	
Mouth sores (See also Pain, in this table, and Anti-virals and Immune system stimulant in "Healing Actions" table)	Blackberry	
Nausea	Ginger	
Pain (See also Anesthetic in "Healing Actions" table)	Black haw Meadowsweet Passionflower	*Vervain* can depress the heart rate and constrict bronchial passages. If you have

(*continued*)

Conditions (*continued*)

Condition	Herbs	Special Precautions
Pain (*continued*)	Red pepper Vervain White willow	heart disease or asthma, consult your physician before using it.
Pinkeye (See Conjunctivitis)		
Poison ivy	Aloe	
Postpartum hemorrhage	Goldenseal Shepherd's purse	*Shepherd's purse* can cause powerful uterine contractions.
Premenstrual syndrome (See also Diuretic in "Healing Actions" table)	Buchu Celery Dandelion Horsetail Juniper Nettle Parsley Sarsaparilla Uva ursi	All herbs with diuretic action can deplete potassium stores. Do not use diuretics for weight loss. Long-term use of *uva ursi* can deplete potassium stores.
Prostate cancer	Anise Black cohosh Fennel Red clover	*Black cohosh* slows the heart rate. If you have heart disease, consult your physician before using it.
Psoriasis	Echinacea Gotu kola	

Condition	Herbs	Special Precautions
Scalds (See Burns)		
Sore throat	Fenugreek Licorice Marsh mallow Mullein Sage Slippery elm	*Fenugreek* has some estrogenic action. Women who have been advised not to take the Pill or who have a history of breast cancer should consult their physician before using it. Long-term use of large amounts of *licorice* may cause water retention, elevated blood pressure, headache, and hormone imbalance (pseudoaldosteronism).
Stress	Balm Bay Catnip Celery Chamomile Ginseng Motherwort Passionflower Skullcap Wild cherry Yarrow	*Balm* can interfere with a thyroid-stimulating hormone. If you have a thyroid problem, consult your physician before using it. Long-term use of *celery* can deplete potassium stores.

(continued)

Conditions (*continued*)

Condition	Herbs	Special Precautions
Stroke prevention (See also High blood pressure, and Cholesterol, high, in this table, and Diuretic in "Healing Actions" table)	Ginkgo	
Stroke treatment	Ginkgo	
Sunburn (See Burns)		
Tinnitus (ringing in the ears)	Ginkgo	
Toothache (See also Pain)	(for external use) Allspice oil Clove oil	Use only a drop or two of *allspice oil* or *clove oil*. Ingestion of even small amounts can cause poisoning.
Tooth-decay prevention	Chaparral Mints Tea	
Ulcer prevention	Chamomile Papaya	
Ulcer treatment	Chamomile Licorice	Long-term use of large amounts of *licorice* may cause water retention, elevated blood pressure, headache, and

Condition	Herbs	Special Precautions
		hormone imbalance (pseudoaldosteronism).
Urethritis	Uva ursi	Long-term use of *uva ursi* can deplete potassium stores.
Urinary incontinence	Cranberry	
Urinary tract infection prevention	Cinnamon Cranberry	
Urinary tract infection treatment	Barberry Cinnamon Dill Garlic Goldenseal Uva ursi	Long-term use of *uva ursi* can deplete potassium stores.
Varicose veins	Gotu kola	
Vertigo (See Dizziness)		
Whooping cough (pertussis)	Echinacea	
Wound healing (See also Pain)	(for external use) Aloe Blackberry Comfrey Echinacea	

(*continued*)

Conditions (*continued*)

Condition	Herbs	Special Precautions
Wound healing (*continued*)	Eucalyptus Garlic Gotu kola Marsh mallow Mints Passionflower St.-John's-wort Shepherd's purse Slippery elm Turmeric Uva ursi Witch hazel Yarrow	
Yeast infection (Candidiasis)	Barberry Chamomile Cinnamon Dandelion Echinacea Garlic Goldenseal	Long-term use of *dandelion* can deplete potassium stores.

Healing Actions

Uses	Herbs	Special Precautions
Anesthetic	(for external use) Allspice oil Balm Cinnamon oil Clove oil Mint oils Tarragon oil	
Antibiotic (for *bacterial* infections such as strep throat)	Apple Barberry Bayberry Boneset Burdock Catnip Chamomile Cinnamon Clove Dill Echinacea Garlic Ginseng Goldenseal Licorice Meadowsweet Mints Myrrh St.-John's-wort	*Bayberry* can alter the body's potassium/sodium balance. If you have high blood pressure, heart disease, or kidney disease, consult your physician before using it. Long-term use of large amounts of *licorice* may cause water retention, elevated blood pressure, headache, and hormone imbalance (pseudoaldosteronism). St.-John's-wort acts like an MAO inhibitor, a class of drugs that interacts with a number of foods and other drugs. (See page 468.)

(*continued*)

Healing Actions (*continued*)

Uses	Herbs	Special Precautions
Antibiotic (for *fungal* infections such as yeast infections)	Aloe Barberry Burdock Chamomile Cinnamon Clove Dandelion Echinacea Garlic Goldenseal Licorice St.-John's-wort	Long-term use of *dandelion* may deplete potassium stores. *St.-John's-wort* acts like an MAO inhibitor, a class of drugs that interacts with a number of foods and other drugs. (See page 468.)
Antibiotic (for *parasitic* infections such as intestinal worms)	Basil oil Clove Elecampane Garlic	
Antibiotic (for *protozoan* infections such as giardia)	Barberry Bayberry Echinacea Elecampane Garlic Goldenseal Turmeric	*Bayberry* can change the body's potassium/sodium balance. If you have high blood pressure, heart disease, or kidney disease, consult your physician before using it.
Antidepressant	St.-John's-wort	*St.-John's-wort* acts like an MAO inhibitor, a class of drugs that interacts with a number of foods and other drugs. (See page 468.)

Uses	Herbs	Special Precautions
Anti-inflammatory	Angelica Black haw Boneset Chamomile Chaparral Echinacea Fenugreek Gentian Ginger Horsetail Juniper Licorice Meadowsweet St.-John's-wort Turmeric Vervain	*Angelica* may cause a rash in those exposed to sun. *Fenugreek* has some estrogenic action. Women who have been advised not to take the Pill or who have a history of breast cancer should consult their physician before using it. Long-term use of *vervain*, *horsetail*, or *juniper* may deplete potassium stores. Long-term use of large amounts of *licorice* may cause water retention, elevated blood pressure, headache, and hormone imbalance (pseudoaldosteronism). *St.-John's-wort* acts like an MAO inhibitor, a class of drugs that interacts with a number of foods and other drugs. (See page 468.)

(*continued*)

Healing Actions (continued)

Uses	Herbs	Special Precautions
Anti-inflammatory (continued)		*Vervain* may depress the heart rate and constrict bronchial passages. If you have heart disease or asthma, consult your physician before using it.
Antiperspirant	Sage	
Antiseptic (first aid for minor burns, cuts, and wounds)	(for external use) Aloe Apple leaves Balm Bay Blackberry Catnip Chamomile Chaparral Cinnamon Clove Coriander Echinacea Eucalyptus Garlic Hop Kelp Licorice Mints Myrrh Passionflower Rosemary	

Uses	Herbs	Special Precautions
	Sage St.-John's-wort Tarragon Thyme Turmeric Yarrow	
Antiviral	Balm Boneset Chamomile Cinnamon Echinacea Ginger Ginseng St.-John's-wort	*Balm* may interfere with a thyroid-stimulating hormone. If you have a thyroid problem, consult your physician before using it. *St.-John's-wort* acts like an MAO inhibitor, a class of drugs that interacts with a number of foods and other drugs. (See page 468.)
Decongestant	Angelica Anise Cocoa Coffee Ephedra Eucalyptus Kola Mints Pennyroyal Rosemary Tea	*Angelica* may cause a rash in those exposed to sun. *Anise* has some estrogenic action. Women who have been advised not to take the Pill or who have a history of breast cancer should consult their physician before using it.

(*continued*)

Healing Actions (*continued*)

Uses	Herbs	Special Precautions
Decongestant (*continued*)		*Ephedra* may elevate blood pressure. People with high blood pressure should not use it.
		Cocoa, coffee, kola, and *tea* contain caffeine, which can cause insomnia and possible addiction.
Digestive aid	Allspice Angelica Anise Balm Caraway Catnip Chamomile Cinnamon Clove Cocoa Comfrey Coriander Dandelion Dill Fennel Feverfew Gentian Ginger Goldenseal Hop Marjoram	*Angelica* may cause a rash in those exposed to sun. *Anise* and *fenugreek* have some estrogenic action. Women who have been advised not to take the Pill or who have a history of breast cancer should consult their physician before using it. *Balm* may interfere with a thyroid-stimulating hormone. If you have a thyroid problem, consult your physician before using it.

Uses	Herbs	Special Precautions
	Marsh mallow Mints Oregano Papaya Passionflower Pennyroyal Red pepper Rosemary Sage Savory Slippery elm Thyme Turmeric Yarrow	*Cocoa* contains caffeine, which can cause insomnia and possible addiction. Long-term use of *comfrey* may cause hepatic veno-occlusive disease, a serious disorder that can impair liver function. Long-term use of *dandelion* may deplete potassium stores.
Diuretic (for water retention, high blood pressure)	Buchu Celery Dandelion Horsetail Juniper Nettle Parsley Sarsaparilla Uva ursi	All herbs with diuretic action can deplete potassium stores. Do not use diuretics for weight loss.
Immune system stimulant	Barberry Basil Boneset Chamomile Echinacea Ginger Ginseng Goldenseal	Long-term use of large amounts of *licorice* may cause water retention, elevated blood pressure, headache, and hormone imbalance (pseudoaldosteronism).

(*continued*)

Healing Actions (*continued*)

Uses	Herbs	Special Precautions
Immune system stimulant (*continued*)	Gotu kola Licorice Marsh mallow Mistletoe St.-John's-wort	*Mistletoe* can slow the heart rate and affect blood pressure. If you have heart disease, consult your physician before using it. *St.-John's-wort* acts like an MAO inhibitor, a class of drugs that interacts with a number of foods and other drugs. (See page 468.)
Labor stimulant (See also Menstruation, delayed, in "Conditions" table)	Shepherd's purse	Using herbs to induce labor requires medical supervision.
Laxative	Apple Buckthorn Cascara sagrada Psyllium Rhubarb Senna Vervain	*Buckthorn, rhubarb*, and *senna* may cause severe intestinal cramps. Intestinal cramps are also possible with *cascara sagrada*. *Vervain* may depress the heart rate and constrict bronchial passages. If you have heart disease or asthma, consult your physician before using it.

Uses	Herbs	Special Precautions
Sedative	Balm Celery Hop Motherwort Passionflower Skullcap Valerian Wild cherry Yarrow	*Balm* may interfere with a thyroid-stimulating hormone. If you have a thyroid problem, consult your physician before using it. Long-term use of *celery* may deplete potassium stores.
Stimulant	Cocoa Coffee Ephedra Ginseng Kola Maté Tea	*Ephedra* may elevate blood pressure. People with high blood pressure should not use it. *Cocoa, coffee, kola, maté,* and *tea* contain caffeine, which can cause insomnia and possible addiction.
Tranquilizer	Balm Bay Catnip Celery Chamomile Motherwort Passionflower Skullcap Wild cherry Yarrow	*Balm* may interfere with a thyroid-stimulating hormone. If you have a thyroid problem, consult your physician before using it. Long-term use of *celery* may deplete potassium stores.

(continued)

Healing Actions (*continued*)

Uses	Herbs	Special Precautions
Weight-loss aid	Coffee Ephedra	*Coffee* contains caffeine, which can cause insomnia and possible addiction. *Ephedra* may elevate blood pressure. People with high blood pressure should not use it.

Other Uses

Condition	Herbs	Special Precautions
Heavy metal, toxic, protection from	Apple Garlic Kelp	
Insect repellent (cockroaches)	Bay Eucalyptus	
Insect repellent (flies, fleas, gnats, mosquitoes)	Pennyroyal oil	*Pennyroyal oil* is poisonous. Do not ingest.
Memory improvement	Ginkgo Ginseng	
Nutrient absorption improvement	Ginseng	

Other Uses (*continued*)

Uses	Herbs	Special Precautions
Radiation, protection from	Kelp Tea	*Tea* contains caffeine, which can cause insomnia and possible addiction.
Radiation therapy	Echinacea Ginseng Mistletoe Tea	*Mistletoe* can slow the heart rate and affect blood pressure. If you have heart disease, consult your physician before using it. *Tea* contains caffeine, which can cause insomnia and possible addiction.
Reaction time improvement	Ginkgo	
Smoking cessation	Ephedra	*Ephedra* may elevate blood pressure. People with high blood pressure should not use it.

REFERENCES

Journals and Periodicals

American scientists have pretty much left the field of healing herbs wide open for scientists from other countries. There's *some* research going on in the United States, but most healing herb research takes place in Germany, Eastern Europe, and Asia and is published in foreign-language journals.

As a result, studies that are several years old often represent the very latest information available in the English language. These older studies are still valid and valuable.

The references here list articles from the English-language scientific literature.

These references follow standard scientific format. For journals they list author, year of publication, journal title, volume:number (in a few cases):page number. For magazines they list author, year of publication, magazine title, date:page number.

The journals cited can be found at most university and medical school libraries. Recent journals are typically displayed in easily accessible reading rooms. Most older journals are usually stored nearby. Journal libraries are not difficult to use once you understand their organization. Ask a librarian to orient you.

Those with microcomputers, modems, and the necessary software may retrieve articles using MEDLINE, the National Library of Medicine's computerized database, or the Natural Products Alert (NAPRALERT) database at the University of Illinois College of Pharmacy in Chicago.

Those who live near Cincinnati may use the Lloyd Library, which houses one of the world's largest collections of botanical literature.

Alfalfa

Free, B. L. and L. D. Satterlee. 1975. *Journal of Food Science* 40:88.

Gestetner, B. et al. 1971. *Journal of Science, Food, and Agriculture* 22:168.

Keeler, R. F. 1975. *Lloydia* 38:56.

Manilow, M. R. et al. 1977. *American Journal of Clinical Nutrition* 30:2061.

————. 1977. *Steroids* 29:105.

————. 1978. *Atherosclerosis* 30:27.

————. 1981. *Food and Cosmetic Toxicology* 19:444.

————. 1981. *Journal of Clinical Investigations* 67:156.

————. 1981. *Lancet* I:615.

————. 1984. *Science* 216:415.

Polk, I. 1982. *Journal of the American Medical Association* 247:1493.

Roberts, J. L. and J. A. Hayashi. 1983. *New England Journal of Medicine* 308:1361.

Smith-Barbaro, P. et al. 1981. *Journal of the National Cancer Institute* 67:495.

Wattenberg, L. 1975. *Cancer Research* 35:3326.

Worthington-Roberts, B. and M. A. Breskin. 1983. *American Pharmacy* 23:421.

Allspice

Veek, M. E. and G. F. Russell. 1973. *Journal of Food Science* 38:1028.

Aloe

Collins, C. E. and C. Collins. 1935. *American Journal of Roentgenology and Radiation Therapy* 33:396.

Ghannam, N. et al. 1986. *Hormone Research* 24:288.

Haggers, J. P. et al. 1979. *American Journal of Medical Technology* 41:293.

Kupchan, G. and S. Karmin. 1976. *Journal of Natural Products* 39:223.

Morrow, D. M. et al. 1980. *Archives of Dermatology* 116:1064.

Rodriguez-Bigas, M. et al. 1988. *Plastic and Reconstructive Surgery* 81:386.

Winters, W. D. et al. 1981. *Economic Botany* 35:89.

Angelica

Ioannou, Y. M. et al. 1982. *Cancer Research* 42:119.

Ivie, G. W. et al. 1981. *Science* 213:909.

Opdyke, D. L. J. 1975. *Food and Cosmetic Toxicology* 13 (Suppl.):
713.

Anise

Albert-Puelo, M. 1980. *Journal of Ethnopharmacology* 2:337.

Duke, J. A. 1988. *HerbalGram* 15:11.

Embong, M. B. et al. 1977. *Canadian Journal of Plant Science*
57:681.

Gerhbein, L. L. 1977. *Food and Cosmetic Toxicology* 15:173.

Okley, H. M. and M. F. Grundon. 1971. *Journal of the Chemical
Society* 19:1157.

Opdyke, D. L. J. 1975. *Food and Cosmetic Toxicology* 13
(Suppl.):715.

Apple

Delbarre, F. et al. 1977. *American Journal of Clinical Nutrition*
30:463.

El-Nakeeb, M. A. and R. T. Yousef. 1970. *Planta Medica* 18:201.

Fisher, H. et al. 1964. *Science* 146:1063.

————. 1966. *Journal of Atherosclerosis Research* 6:292.

Ginter, E. et al. 1982. *International Journal of Vitamin and Nutrition
Research* 21:51.

Jenkins, D. J. A. et al. 1977. *Annals of Internal Medicine* 86:22.

Leveille, G. A. and H. E. Sauberlich. 1966. *Journal of Clinical
Nutrition* 88:209.

Mathe, D. et al. 1977. *Journal of Nutrition* 107:466.

Miranda, P. M. and D. L. Horowitz. 1978. *Annals of Internal
Medicine* 88:482.

Smith-Barbaro, P. et al. 1981. *Journal of the National Cancer
Institute* 67:495.

Balm

Aufmkolk, M. et al. 1984. *Endocrinology* 115:527.

————. 1984. *Hormone Metabolism Research* 16:183.

Forster, H. B. et al. 1980. *Planta Medica* 40:309.

Herrmann, E. C. and L. S. Kucera. 1967. *Proceedings of the Society of Experimental Biology and Medicine* 124:869.

Kucera, L. S. et al. 1965. *Annals of the New York Academy of Sciences* 130:481.

Kucera, L. S. and E. C. Herrmann. 1967. *Proceedings of the Society of Experimental Biology and Medicine* 124:865.

Barberry and Oregon Grape

Choudhry, V. P. et al. 1972. *Indian Pediatrics* 9:143.

Cordell, G. A. and N. R. Farnsworth. 1970. *Lloydia* 40:1.

Desai, A. B. et al. 1971. *Indian Pediatrics* 8:462.

Gupte, S. 1975. *American Journal of Diseases of Children* 129:886.

Hahn, F. E. and J. Ciak. 1976. *Antibiotics* 3:577.

Kumazawa, Y. et al. 1984. *International Journal of Immunopharmacology* 6:587.

Sabir, M. and N. Bhide. 1971. *Indian Journal of Physiology and Pharmacology* 15:111.

Sack, R. B, and J. L. Froehlich. 1982. *Infection and Immunology* 35:471.

Sharma, R. et al. 1970. *Indian Pediatrics* 7:496.

Subbaiah, T. V. and A. H. 1967. Amin. *Nature* 215:527.

Sun, D. et al. 1988. *Antimicrobial Agents and Chemotherapy* 32:1370.

Basil

Balambal, R. et al. 1985. *Journal of the Association of Physicians* (India) 33:507.

Drinkwater, N. R. et al. 1976. *Journal of the National Cancer Institute* 57:1323.

Godhwani, B. et al. 1988. *Journal of Ethnopharmacology* 24:193.

Jain, M. L. and S. R. Jain. 1972. *Planta Medica* 22:66.

Miller, E. C. et al. 1983. *Cancer Research* 43:1124.

Bay

Garmon, L. 1982. *Science News* Sept. 12.

MacGregor, J. T. et al. 1974. *Journal of Agricultural and Food Chemistry* 22:777.

Bayberry

Kapadia, G. J. et al. 1976. *Journal of the National Cancer Institute* 57:207.

Paul, B. D. et al. 1974. *Journal of Pharmaceutical Sciences* 63:958.

Yoshizawa, S. et al. 1987. *Phytotherapy Research* 1:44.

Blackberry

Alonso, R. et al. 1980. *Planta Medica* Suppl.: 102–106.

Fong, H. H. S. et al. 1972. *Journal of Pharmaceutical Sciences* 61:1818.

Black Cohosh

Benoit, P. S. et al. 1976. *Lloydia* 39:160.

Costello, C. H. and E. V. Lynn. 1950. *Journal of the American Pharmaceutical Association* 39:177.

Farnsworth, N. R. and A. B. Seligman. 1971. *Tile and Till* 57:52.

Genazzani, E. and L. Sorrentin. 1962. *Nature* 194:544.

Jarry, H. et al. 1985. *Planta Medica* 55:316.

Jarry, H. and G. Harnischfeger. 1985. *Planta Medica* 55:46.

Black Haw

Jarboe, C. H. et al. 1966. *Nature* 212:837.

———. 1967. *Journal of Medicinal Chemistry* 10:488.

Blue Cohosh

Benoit. P. S. et al. 1976. *Lloydia* 39:160.

Chandrasekhar, K. and G. H. R. Sarma. 1974. *Journal of Reproduction and Fertility* 38:236.

DiCarlo, F. I. et al. 1964. *Journal of the Reticuloendothelial Society* 1:24.

Ferguson, H. C. and L. D. Edwards. 1954. *Journal of the American Pharmaceutical Association* 43:16.

McShefferty, J. and J. B. Stenlake. 1956. *Journal of the Chemical Society* 449:2314.

Boneset

Benoit, P. S. et al. 1976. *Lloydia* 39:160.

Lee, K. H. et al. 1977. *Phytochemistry* 16:1068.

Rodriguez, E. et al. 1976. *Phytochemistry* 15:1573.
Tsuda, A. et al. 1963. *Canadian Journal of Chemistry* 8:1919.
Vollmar, A. et al. 1986. *Phytochemistry* 25:377.
Wagner, H. 1972. *Phytochemistry* 11:1504.

Buchu
Kaiser, R. et al. 1975. *Journal of Agricultural and Food Chemistry* 23:943.

Buckthorn
Belkin, M. et al. 1952. *Journal of the National Cancer Institute* 13:742.
Breimer, D. D. and A. J. Baars. 1976. *Pharmacology* 14 (Suppl.):30–47.
Kupchan, S. M. and A. Krim. 1976. *Lloydia* 39:223.
Van Os, F. H. L. 1976. *Pharmacology* 4 (Suppl.):18.

Burdock
Bryson, P. D. et al. 1978. *Journal of the American Medical Association* 239:2157.
Dombradi, G. 1970. *Chemotherapy* 15:250.
Morita, K. et al. 1984. *Mutation Research* 129:1:25.
Tsujita, J. et al. 1979. *Nutrition Reports International* 20:635.

Caraway
Harries, N. et al. 1978. *Journal of Clinical Pharmacy* 2:171.
Opdyke, D. L. J. 1973. *Food and Cosmetic Toxicology* 11:1051.

Cascara Sagrada
Breimer, D. D. and A. J. Baars. 1976. *Pharmacology* 14 (Suppl.):30.
Evans, F. J. et al. 1975. *Journal of Pharmacy and Pharmacology* 27:91.
Fairbairn, J. W. et al. 1977. *Journal of Pharmaceutical Sciences* 66:1300.
Fairbairn, J. W. and S. Simic. 1964. *Journal of Pharmacy and Pharmacology* 16:450.
Van Os, F. H. L. 1976. *Pharmacology* 14 (Suppl.):18.

Catnip

Harvey, J. et al. 1978. Lloydia 41:367.

Jackson, B. and A. Reed. 1969. Journal of the American Medical Association 207:1349.

Poundstone, J. 1969. Journal of the American Medical Association 208:360.

Tucker, A. and S. Tucker. 1988. Economic Botany 42:214.

Celery Seed

Adams, R. M. 1969. Occupational Contact Dermatitis, 190. Philadelphia: Lippincott.

Ames, B. 1983. Science 221:1256.

Anon. 1989. University of California, Berkeley, Wellness Letter 6:3:8.

Best, C. H. and D. A. Scott. 1923 Journal of Metabolic Research 3:177.

Bermingham, D. J. et al. 1961. Archives of Dermatology 83:73.

Bjeldanes, L. F. and I. Kim. 1978. Journal of Food Science 43:143.

Bjeldanes, L. F. and I. Kim. 1977. Journal of Organic Chemistry 42:233.

Farnsworth, N. R. and A. B. Seligman. 1971. Tile and Till 57:52.

Jain, S. R. and M. R. Jain. 1973. Planta Medica 24:127.

Kiangsu Institute of Modern Medicine. 1977. Encyclopedia of Chinese Drugs, vol. 2:1122. Shanghai, People's Republic of China: Shanghai Scientific and Technical Publications.

Sharaf, A. A. et al. 1963. Planta Medica 2:159.

Chamomile

Achterrath-Tuckerman, U. et al. 1980. Planta Medica 39:38.

Aggag, M. E. and R. T. Yousef. 1972. Planta Medica 22:140.

Benner, M. H. and H. J. Lee. 1973. Journal of Allergy and Clinical Immunology 52:307.

Farnsworth, N. R. and B. M. Morgan. 1972. Journal of the American Medical Association 221:410.

Forrester, H. B. et al. 1980. Planta Medica 40:309.

Grochulski, A. and B. Borkowski. 1972. Planta Medica 21:289.

Habersang, S. et al. 1979. Planta Medica 37:115.

Hausen, B. M. et al. 1984. Planta Medica 50:229.

Isaac, O. 1979. Planta Medica 35:118.

Jakovlev, V. et al. 1979. *Planta Medica* 35:2:3.

———. 1983. *Planta Medica* 49:67.

Loggia, R. D. et al. 1982. *Pharmaceutical Research Communications* 14:153.

Szelenyi, I. et al. 1979. *Planta Medica* 35:218.

Wagner, H. 1985. In: *Economic and Medicinal Plant Research* (vol. I) United Kingdon: Academic Press.

Chaparral

Boxer, S., Ed. 1987. *Discover* 8:13.

Burk, D. and M. Woods. 1963. *Radiation Research Supplement* 3:212.

Chang, J. et al. 1984. *Inflammation* 8:143.

Lisanti, V. F. and B. Eichel. 1963. *Journal of Dental Research* 42:1030.

Mirjano, K. and G. Chiou. 1984. *Ophthalmic Research* 16:256.

Nakadate, T. et al. 1985. *Japanese Journal of Pharmacology* 38:161.

Pardini, R. S. et al. 1970. *Biochemical Pharmacology* 19:2699.

Smart, C. R. et al. 1969. *Cancer Chemotherapy Reports* (Part I) 53:147.

———. 1970. *Rocky Mountain Medical Journal* Nov.:39.

Cinnamon

Halbert, E. and D. G. Wheeden. 1966. *Nature* 212:1603.

Opdyke, D. L. J. 1975. *Food and Cosmetic Toxicology* 13 (Suppl.):545.

———. 1975. *Food and Cosmetic Toxicology* 13 (Suppl.):749.

Clove

Abraham, S. K. and P. C. Kesavan. 1978. *Indian Journal of Experimental Biology* 16:518.

Hackett, P. H. et al. 1985. *Journal of the American Medical Association* 253:3551.

Opdyke, D. L. J. 1975. *Food and Cosmetic Toxicology* 13 (Suppl.):545.

———. 1975. *Food and Cosmetic Toxicology* 13 (Suppl.):749.

Rasheed, A. et al. 1984. *New England Journal of Medicine* 310:50.

Takechi, M. and Y. Tanaka. 1981. *Planta Medica* 42:1:69.

Cocoa

Anon. 1989. *University of California, Berkeley, Wellness Letter* 5:5:1.

Coffee

Anon. 1982. *American Journal of Public Health* 72:610.

Anon. 1989. *Family Practice News* Feb. 15:28.

Anon. 1980. *FDA Drug Bulletin* 10:3:19.

Anon. 1977. *Medical Letter* Aug. 12:19:6.

Check, W. 1979. *Journal of the American Medical Association* 241:1221.

Ferguson, T. 1980. *Medical Self-Care* 11:8.

Graedon, J. and T. Graedon. 1989. *Medical Self-Care* 50:22.

Greden, J. 1974. *American Journal of Psychiatry* 131:1089.

Rosenberg, L. et al. 1989. *American Journal of Epidemiology* 128:570.

Stamford, B. 1989. *The Physician and Sportsmedicine* 17:193.

Coltsfoot

Bergner, P. 1989. *Medical Herbalism* 1:1:1.

Delaveau, P. et al. 1980. *Planta Medica* 40:49.

Hirono, I. et al. 1979. *Journal of the National Cancer Institute* 63:469.

Hwang, S. B. et al. 1987. *European Journal of Pharmacology* 141:269.

Kraus, C. et al. 1985. *Planta Medica* 51:89.

Roulet, M. et al. 1988. *Journal of Pediatrics* 112:433.

Comfrey

Ames, B. et al. 1987. *Science* 236:271.

Bergner, P. 1989. *Medical Herbalism* 1:1.

Furuya, T. and K. Araki. 1968. *Chemical and Pharmaceutical Bulletin* 16:2515.

Gracza, L. et al. 1985. *Archives of Pharmacy* 312:1090.

Heinerman, J. 1985. *Herb Report* 2:1.

Henry Doubleday Society. 1979. *British Medical Journal* 6163:596.

Hirono, I. et al. 1978. *Journal of the National Cancer Institute* 61:865.

————. 1979. *Journal of the National Cancer Institute* 63:469.

Huxtable, R. J. et al. 1986. *New England Journal of Medicine* 315:1095.

Macalister, C. J. 1912. *British Medical Journal* 1:10.

Mascolo, N. et al. 1987. *Phytotherapy Research* 1:1:28.
Ridker, P. M. et al. 1985. *Gastroenterology* 88:1050.
Roitman, J. N. 1981. *Lancet* 1:944.
Steuart, G. 1987. *Herb, Spice, and Medicinal Plant Digest* 5:4:9.
Taylor, A. and N. C. Taylor. 1963. *Proceedings of the Society for Experimental Biology and Medicine* 114:772.
Weston, C. F. M. et al. 1987. *British Medical Journal* 295:183.

Coriander
Farnsworth, N. R. and A. B. Seligman. 1971. *Tile and Till* 57:52.
Mascolo, N. et al. 1987. *Phytotherapy Research* 1:28.

Cranberry
Blatherwick, N. R. and M. L. Long. 1923. *Journal of Biological Chemistry* 57:815.
Dugan, C. and P. S. Cardaciotto. 1966. *Journal of Psychiatric Nursing* 8:467.
Kahn, H. D. 1967. *Journal of the American Dietetic Association* 51:251.
Konowalchuk, J. and J. I. Speirs. 1978. *Applied Environmental Microbiology* 35:1219.
Moen, D. V. 1962. *Wisconsin Medical Journal* 61:282.
Soloway, M. and R. A. Smith. 1988. *Journal of the American Medical Association* 260:1465.
Zinsser, H. H. et al. 1968. *New York State Journal of Medicine* 68:3001.

Dandelion
Farnsworth, N. R. and A. B. Seligman. 1971. *Tile and Till* 57:52.
Mascolo, N. et al. 1987. *Phytotherapy Research* 1:1:28.
Racz-Kotilla, E. et al. 1974. *Planta Medica* 26:212.
Wat, C. K. et al. 1979. *Journal of Natural Products* 42:103.

Echinacea
Bergner, P. 1989. *Townsend Letter for Doctors* July:353.
Stimpel, M. et al. 1984. *Infection and Immunology* 46:845.
Voaden, D. J. and M. Jacobson. 1972. *Journal of Medicinal Chemistry* 15:619.
Wacker, A. and W. Hilbig. 1978. *Planta Medica* 33:89.

Elecampane

Vichkanova, S. A. 1977. *Chemical Abstracts* 87:162117.

Ephedra

Anon. 1989. *Lawrence Review of Natural Products* June.

Bailey, C. J. et al. 1986. *General Pharmacology* 17:243.

Dulloo, A. G. and D. S. Miller. 1986. *American Journal of Clinical Nutrition* 43:388.

Kasahara, Y. et al. 1985. *Planta Medica* 54:325.

Low, R. B. et al. 1984. *Addictive Behaviors* 9:335.

Eucalyptus

Garmon, L. 1982. *Science News* Sept.12.

Maruzella, J. C. and P. A. Henry. 1958. *Journal of the American Pharmaceutical Association* 47:294.

Fennel

Albert-Puleo, M. 1980. *Journal of Ethnopharmacology* 2:337.

Forster, H. B. et al. 1980. *Planta Medica* 40:4:309.

Gershbein, L. L. 1977. *Food and Cosmetic Toxicology* 15:173.

Harries, N. et al. 1978. *Journal of Clinical Pharmacology* 2:171.

Marcus, C. and E. P. Lichtenstein. 1979. *Journal of Agricultural and Food Chemistry* 27:1217.

Sekizawa, J. and T. Shibamoto. 1982. *Mutation Research* 101:127.

Fenugreek

Arbo, M. S. and Al-Kafawi, A. A. 1969. *Planta Medica* 17:14.

Bever, B. O. and G. R. Zahnd. 1979. *Quarterly Journal of Crude Drug Research* 17:139.

Ribes, G. et al. 1984. *Annals of Nutrition and Metabolism* 28:37.

Sauvaire, Y. and J. C. Baccon. 1978. *Lloydia* 41:588.

Singhal, P. C. et al. 1982. *Current Science* 51:136.

Valette, G. et al. 1984. *Atherosclerosis* 50:105.

Feverfew

Awang, D. V. C. 1989. *Canadian Pharmaceutical Journal* 122:266.

Berry, J. I. 1984. *Pharmacy Journal* 232:611.

Groenwagen, W. A. et al. 1986. *Lancet* I:44.

Heptinstall, S. et al. 1985. *Lancet* I:1071.

Johnson, E. S. et al. 1985. *British Medical Journal* 291:569.

Murphy, J. J. et al. 1988. *Lancet* II:189.

Romo, J. et al. 1970. *Phytochemistry* 9:1615.

Garlic (and Onions, Leeks, Chives, and Shallots)

Amonkar, S. V. and A. Banerji. 1971. *Science* 174:1343.

Anon. 1980. *Chinese Medical Journal* 93:123.

Barona, F. E. and M. R. Tansey. 1977. *Mycologia* 69:793.

Barrie, S. A. et al. 1987. *Orthomolecular Medicine* 2:1:15.

Belman, S. 1983. *Carcinogenesis* 4:8:1063.

Bordia, A. K. 1973. *Lancet* II:1491.

———. 1978. *Atherosclerosis* (1978) 30:355.

———. 1981. *American Journal of Clinical Nutrition* 34:2100.

Bordia, A. K. and H. C. Bansal. 1973. *Lancet* II:1491.

Bordia, A. K. et al. 1977. *Atherosclerosis* 26:379.

———. 1977. *Atherosclerosis* 28:155.

Boullin, D. J. 1981. *Lancet* I:776.

Caporaso, R. et al. 1983. *Antimicrobial Agents and Chemotherapy* 23:700.

Ernst, E. et al. 1985. *British Medical Journal* 291:139.

Jain, R. C. 1977. *American Journal of Clinical Nutrition* 30:1380.

Jain, R. C. and D. B. Konar. 1976. *Artery* 2:6:531.

Jain, R. C. and C. R. Vyas. 1975. *American Journal of Clinical Nutrition* 28:684.

Jain, R. C. et al. 1973. *Lancet* II:1491.

Kendler, B. S. 1987. *Preventive Medicine* 16:5:670.

Lau, B. H. S. et al. 1987. *Nutrition Research* 7:139.

Lybarger, J. A. et al. 1982. *Journal of Allergy and Clinical Immunology* 69:448.

Makheja, A. N. et al. 1979. *Lancet* I:781.

Marsh, C. L. et al. 1987. *Journal of Urology* 137:2:359.

Nagai, K. 1973. *Japanese Journal of the Association of Infectious Diseases* 47:111.

Sparins, V. L. et al. 1986. *Nutrition and Cancer* 8:3:211.

Tansey, M. R. and J. A. Appleton. 1975. *Mycologia* 67:2:409.

You, W. C. et al. 1989. *Journal of the National Cancer Institute* 81:162.

Gentian

Glatzel, H. 1969. *Hippokrates* 40:23:916.

Glatzel, H. and K. Hackenberg. 1967. *Planta Medica* 15:3:223.

Ginger

Babbar, O. P. 1982. *Indian Journal of Experimental Biology* 20:572.

Backon, J. 1986. *Medical Hypotheses* 20:271.

Bergner, P. 1989. *Townsend Letter for Doctors* March:115.

Cai, L. P. 1984. *Journal of New Chinese Medicine* 2:22.

Dorso, C. R. et al. 1980. *New England Journal of Medicine* 303:756.

Gujral, S. et al. 1978. *Nutrition Reports International* 17:183.

Hikino, H. 1985. *Economic Medicinal Plant Research* 1:53.

Mattes, H. W. D. 1980. *Phytochemistry* 19:2643.

Suekawa, M. et al. 1984. *Journal of Pharmacobio-Dynamics* 7:836.

Mowrey, D. B. and D. E. Clayson. 1982. *Lancet* I:655.

Shoji, N. et al. 1982. *Journal of Pharmaceutical Sciences* 71:10:1174.

Thompson, E. H. et al. 1973. *Journal of Food Science* 38:652.

Ginkgo

Bauer, U. 1988. In: *Rokan (Gingko Biloba): Recent Results in Pharmacology and Clinic*, E. W. Funfgeld, ed., 212. Berlin: Springer-Verlag.

Braquet, P. 1987. *Drugs of the Future* 12:7:643.

Cahn, J. 1984. In: *Proceedings of the International Symposium on the Effects of Gingko Biloba on Organic Cerebral Impairment*, 43. London: John Libbey.

Chatterjee, S. S. 1984. In: *Proceedings of the International Symposium on the Effects of Gingko Biloba on Organic Cerebral Impairment*, 5. London: John Libbey.

Dubreuil, C. 1988. In: *Rokan (Gingko Biloba)*, 237.

Guillon, J. M. 1988. In: *Rokan (Gingko Biloba)*, 153.

Haguenauer, J. P. et al. 1988. In: *Rokan (Gingko Biloba)*, 260.

Lebuisson, D. A. et al. 1988. In: *Rokan (Gingko Biloba)*, 231.

Lefort, J. et al. 1984. *British Journal of Pharmacology* 82:565.

Meyer, B. 1988. In: *Rokan (Gingko Biloba)*, 245.

Pidoux, B. et al. 1983. *Journal of Cerebral Blood Flow and Metabolism* 3(Suppl):S556.

Sikora, R. et al. 1989. *Journal of Urology* 141:188A.

Taillandier, J. et al. 1988. In: *Rokan (Gingko Biloba)*, 291.

Vorberg, G. 1985. *Clinical Trials Journal* 22:149.

Weitbrecht, W. V. and W. Jansen. 1984. *Proceedings of the International Symposium on the Effects of Gingko Biloba on Organic Cerebral Impairment*, 91. London: John Libbey.

Wilford, J. N. 1988. *New York Times* March 1:C3.

Ginseng

Baldwin, C. A. et al. 1986. *Pharmacy Journal* 237:583.

Baranov, A. I. 1982. *Journal of Ethnopharmacology* 6:339.

Barna, P. 1985. *Lancet* II:548.

Ben-Hur, E. and S. Fulder. 1981. *American Journal of Chinese Medicine* 9:48.

Brekhman, I. I. and I. V. Dardymov. 1969. *Annual Review of Pharmacology* 9:419.

———. 1969. *Lloydia* 32:46.

Farnsworth, N. R. et al. 1985. *Economic and Medicinal Plant Research* 1:156.

Fulder, S. 1977. *New Scientist* 1:138.

Golikov, A. P. and N. Ikonnikov. 1962. In: *Proceedings of the Symposium on Eleutherococcus and Ginseng*, ed. I. I. Brekhman, 51. Vladivostok, U.S.S.R.: The Academy of Sciences.

Hallstrom, C. and S. Fulder. 1982. *Comparative Medicine of the East and West* 6:277.

Han, B. H. et al. 1979. *Korean Biochemical Journal* 12:1:33.

Hong, S. P. et al. 1976. *Korean Journal of Pharmacognosy* 7:111.

Hyuchenok, R. Y. 1972. *Medicines of the Far East*, U.S.S.R. Academy of Sciences, 83.

Khatnashvili, T. M. 1964. In: *Materials for the Conference on Problems of Medical Therapy at the Oncology Clinic*, 163. Leningrad, U.S.S.R.

Kim, C. et al. 1970. *Lloydia* 33:43.

———. 1976. *American Journal of Clinical Medicine* 4:163.

Kim, E. et al. 1971. *Korean Journal of Pharmacognosy* 2:23.

Liberti, L. E. and A. Der Marderosian. 1978. *Journal of Pharmaceutical Sciences* 67:1487.

Matsuda, H. et al. 1986. *Chemical and Pharmaceutical Bulletin* 34:1153.

———. 1986. *Chemical and Pharmaceutical Bulletin* 34:2100.

Michinori, K. et al. 1981. *Journal of Natural Products* 44:405.

Oshima Y. and K. Sato. 1987. *Journal of Natural Products* 50:188.

Otsuka, H. et al. 1977. *Planta Medica* 32:9.

Petkov, V. D. and A. H. Mosharrof. 1987. *American Journal of Chinese Medicine* 15:19.

Popov, I. M. and W. J. Goldwag. 1973. *American Journal of Chinese Medicine* 1:267.

Salto H. and Y. U. Lee. 1978. *Proceedings of the Third International Ginseng Symposium* 3:109.

Schultz, F. H. et al. 1980. *Federation Proceedings* 39:554.

———. 1981. *Proceedings of the Third National Ginseng Conference,* Asheville, North Carolina 3:45.

———. 1987. *Proceedings of the First National Herb Growing and Marketing Conference,* Purdue University 1:186.

Siegel, R. K. 1979. *Journal of the American Medical Association* 241:1614.

Singh, V. K. et al. 1983. *Planta Medica* 47:234.

———. 1984. *Planta Medica* 50:462.

Tong, L. S. et al. 1980. *American Journal of Chemical Medicine* 8:3:254.

Yamamoto, M. et al. 1974. *Proceedings of the First International Ginseng Symposium.*

———. 1983. *American Journal of Chinese Medicine* 11:88.

———. 1983. *American Journal of Chinese Medicine* 11:96.

Yokozawa, T. et al. 1975. *Chemical and Pharmaceutical Bulletin* 23:3095.

Zhang, J. S. et al. 1987. *Radiation Research* 112:156.

Zuin, M. et al. 1987. *Journal of International Medical Research* 15:276.

Goldenseal

Choudhry, V. P. et al. 1972. *Indian Pediatrics* 9:143.

Cushman, M. et al. 1979. *Journal of Medical Chemistry* 22:3:331.

Desai, A. B. et al. 1971. *Indian Pediatrics* 8:462.

Farnsworth, N. R. and A. B. Seligman. 1971. *Tile and Till* 57:52.

Fitzpatrick, F. K. 1954. *Antibiotics and Chemotherapy* 4:5:528.

Genest, K. and D. W. Hughes. 1969. *Canadian Journal of Pharmaceutical Sciences* 4:41.

Gupta, S. 1975. *American Journal of Diseases of Children* 129:886.

Hahn, F. E. and J. Ciak. 1976. *Antibiotics* 3:577.

Hartwell, J. L. 1971. *Lloydia* 34:103.

Kumazawa, Y. et al. 1984. *International Journal of Immunopharmacology* 6:587.

Lahiri, S. C. and N. K. Dutta. 1967. *Journal of the Indian Medical Association* 48:1:1.

Nishino, H. et al. 1986. *Oncology* 43:131.

Sabir, M. and Bhide, N. 1971. *Indian Journal of Physiology and Pharmacology* 15:111.

Sack, R. B. and J. L. Froehlich. 1982. *Infection and Immunology* 35:471.

Sharda, D. C. 1970. *Journal of Indian Medical Association* 54:1:22.

Sharma, R. et al. 1970. *Indian Pediatrics* 7:496.

Subbaiah, T. V. and A. H. Amin. 1967. *Nature* 215:527.

Sun, D. et al. 1988. *Antimicrobial Agents and Chemotherapy* 32:1370.

Gotu Kola

Bossé, J. P. et al. 1979. *Annuals of Plastic Surgery* 3:1:13.

Dutta, T. and U. P. Basu. 1968. *Indian Journal of Experimental Biology* 6:181.

Fam, A. 1973. *International Surgery* 58:451.

Morisset, R. et al. 1987. *Phytotherapy Research* 1:3.

Natarajan, S. and P. P. Paily. 1973. *Indian Journal of Dermatology* 18:82.

Pointel, J. P. et al. 1987. *Angiology* 38:46.

Ramaswamy, A. S. et al. 1970. *Journal of Research in Indian Medicine* 4:160.

Tenni, R. et al. 1988. *Italian Journal of Biochemistry* 37:69.

Hawthorn

Ammon, H. P. T. and M. Handel. 1981. *Planta Medica* 43:318.

Beretz, A. et al. 1980. *Planta Medica* 39:241.

Iwamoto, M. et al. 1981. *Planta Medica* 42:1.

Petkov, V. 1979. *American Journal of Chinese Medicine* 7:197.

Thompson, E. B. et al. 1974. *Journal of Pharmaceutical Sciences* 63:1936.

Wagner, H. and J. Grevel. 1982. *Planta Medica* 45:98.

Wegrowski, J. et al. 1984. *Biochemical Pharmacology* 33:3491.

Hop

Fenselau, C. and P. Talalay. 1973. *Food and Cosmetic Toxicology* 11:597.

Schmalreck, A. F. et al. 1975. *Canadian Journal of Microbiology* 21:205.

Wolfart, R. et al. 1983. *Planta Medica* 48:120.

Horehound

Krejci, I. and R. Zadina. 1959. *Planta Medica* 7:1.

Horsetail

Phillipson, J. D. and C. Melville. 1960. *Journal of Pharmacy and Pharmacology* 12:506.

Hyssop

Herrmann, E. C. and L. S. Kucera. 1967. *Proceedings of the Society for Experimental Biology and Medicine* 124:874.

Opdyke, D. L. J. 1978. *Food and Cosmetic Toxicology* 16(Suppl. 1):783.

Juniper

Bousquet, J. et al. 1984. *Clinical Allergy* 14:249.

Janku, J. et al. 1957. *Experientia* 13:255.

Mascolo, N. et al. 1987. *Phytotherapy Research* 1:1:28.

Opdyke, D. L. J. 1976. *Food and Cosmetic Toxicology* 14:307.

Kelp

Biard, J. F. et al. 1980. *Planta Medica* Suppl.:136.

Funayama, S. and H. Hikino. 1981. *Planta Medica* 41:29.

Iritani N. and J. Nogi. 1972. *Atherosclerosis* 15:87.

Mautner, H. G. et al. 1953. *Journal of the American Pharmaceutical Association* 42:5:294.

Searl, P. B. et al. 1981. *Proceedings of the Western Pharmacology Society* 24:63.

Skoryna, S. C. et al. 1966. *Proceedings of the Fifth International Seaweed Symposium*, 396. Elmsford, N.Y.: Pergamon Press.

———. 1964. *Canadian Medical Association Journal* 91:285.

Sutton A. et al. 1971. *International Journal of Radiation Biology* 19:79.

Tanaka, Y. et al. 1968. *Canadian Medical Association Journal* 99:169.
————. 1968. *Canadian Medical Association Journal* 98:1179.

Kola

Yarbrough, C. C. 1974. *Journal of the American Medical Association* 230:701.

Licorice

Abe, N. et al. 1982. *Microbiology and Immunology* 26:535.
————. 1987. *European Journal of Cancer and Oncology* 23:10:1549.
Anderson, S. et al. 1971. *Scandinavian Journal of Gastroenterology* 6:683.
Bardhan, K. D. et al. 1978. *Gut* 19:779.
Blachley, J. D. and J. P. Knochel. 1980. *New England Journal of Medicine* 302:784.
Borst, J. G. et al. 1953. *Lancet* 264:657.
Chamberlain, T. J. 1970. *Journal of the American Medical Association* 213:1343.
Chandler, R. F. 1985. *Canadian Pharmaceutical Journal* 118:420.
Cliff, J. M. and M. Thompson. 1970. *Gut* 11:167.
Conn, J. W. et al. 1968. *Journal of the American Medical Association* 205:492.
Doll, R. et al. 1962. *Lancet* II:793.
Epstein, M. T. et al. 1977. *British Medical Journal* 19:488.
Fujisawa. K. et al. 1980. *Asian Medical Journal* 23:745.
Gibson, M. R. 1978. *Lloydia* 41:348.
Glick, L. 1982. *Lancet* II:817.
Guslandi, M. et al. 1980. *Clinical Therapy* 3:40.
Guslandi, M. 1981. *Lancet* I:387.
Kassir, Z. A. 1985. *Irish Medical Journal* 78:153.
LaBroody, S. J. et al. 1979. *British Medical Journal* 6174:1308.
Lai, F. et al. 1980. *New England Journal of Medicine* 303:463.
Lewis, J. R. 1974. *Journal of the American Medical Association* 229:460.
Martin, D. F. and J. P. Miller. 1981. *Lancet* I:609.
Mitscher, L. A. et al. 1980. *Journal of Natural Products* 43:259.
Nagy, G. S. 1978. *Gastroenterology* 74:7.
Pompei, R. et al. 1979. *Nature* 281:689.
————. 1980. *Experentia* 36:304.

Segal, R. et al. 1985. *Journal of Pharmaceutical Sciences* 74:1:79.
Sharaf, A. and N. Goma. 1965. *Journal of Endocrinology* 31:289.
Suzuki, H. et al. 1984. *Asian Medical Journal* 26:423.
Tanaka, S. et al. 1987. *Planta Medica* 53:1:5.
Tangri, K. K. et al. 1965. *Biochemical Pharmacology* 14:8:1277.
Trupie, A. G. G. et al. 1969. *Gut* 10:299.
Wilson, J. A. C. 1972. *British Journal of Clinical Practice* 26:563.

Marjoram
Herrmann, E. C. and L. S. Kucera. 1967. *Proceedings of the Society for Experimental Biology and Medicine* 124:874.
Van Den Broucke, C. O. and J. A. Lemli. 1980. *Planta Medica* 38:317.

Marsh Mallow
Tomoda, M. et al. 1980. *Chemical and Pharmaceutical Bulletin* 28:824.
————. 1987. *Planta Medica* 53:8.

Maté
Vassalo, A. et al. 1985. *Journal of the National Cancer Institute* 75:1005.

Meadowsweet
Fang, V. et al. 1968. *Journal of Pharmaceutical Sciences* 57:2111.

Mints (Peppermint, Spearmint, etc.)
Harries, N. et al. 1978. *Journal of Clinical Pharmacy* 2:171.
Herrmann, E. C. and L. S. Kucera. 1967. *Proceedings of the Society for Experimental Biology and Medicine* 124:874.
Marauzella, J. C. and N. A. Sicurella. 1960. *Journal of the American Pharmaceutical Association* 49:11:692.
Sanyal, A. and K. C. Varma. 1969. *Indian Journal of Microbiology* 9:1:23.

Mistletoe
Bloksma, N. et al. 1979. *Immunobiology* 156:309.
Bloksma, N. et al. 1982. *Planta Medica* 46:221.

Franz, H. et al. 1981. *Biochemistry Journal* 195:481.
Hall, H. A. et al. 1986. *Annals of Emergency Medicine* 15:1320.
Kwaja, T. A. et al. 1980. *Experientia* 36:599.
Luther, P. et al. 1980. *International Journal of Biochemistry* 11:429.
Mack, R. B. 1984. *North Carolina Medical Journal* 45:791.
Petkov, V. 1979. *American Journal of Chinese Medicine* 7:197.
Rentea, R. et al. 1981. *Laboratory Investigations* 44:43.
Vester, F. and J. Niehaus. 1965. *Experientia* 21:197.

Motherwort
Xia, Y. X. 1983. *Journal of Traditional Chinese Medicine* 3:3:185.

Mullein
Benoit, P. S. et al. 1976. *Lloydia* 39:160.
Fitzpatrick, F. K. 1954. *Antibiotics and Chemotherapy* 4:528.
Tyler, V. E. 1986. *Proceedings of the First National Herb Growing and Marketing Conference*, Purdue University 1:52.

Myrrh
Arora, R. B. et al. 1972. *Indian Journal of Medical Research* 60:929.
Delaveau, P. et al. 1980. *Planta Medica* 40:49.
Malhotra, S. C. and M. M. S. Ahuja. 1971. *Indian Journal of Medical Research* 59:1621.
Mester, L. et al. 1979. *Planta Medica* 37:367.

Nettle
Duke, J. 1984. *HerbalGram* 1:4:10.
Mittman, P. 1988. National College of Naturopathic Medicine.

Oregano
Simon, J. 1986. *Proceedings of the First National Herb Growing and Marketing Conference*, Purdue University 1:24.

Papaya
Chen, C. et al. 1981. *American Journal of Chinese Medicine* 9:205.
Singh, S. and S. Devi. 1978. *Indian Journal of Medical Research* 67:499.

Parsley

Busse, W. W. et al. 1984. *Journal of Allergy and Clinical Immunology* 73:801.

Middleton, E. and G. Drzewiecki. 1984. *Biochemical Pharmacology* 33:333.

Petkov, V. 1979. *American Journal of Chinese Medicine* 7:197.

Wickelgren, I. 1989. *Science News* July 136:5.

Passionflower

Aoyagi, N. et al. 1974. *Chemical and Pharmaceutical Bulletin* 22:1008.

Birner, J. and J. M. Nicholls. 1973. *Antimicrobial Agents and Chemotherapy* 3:105.

Lutmoski, J. et al. 1975. *Planta Medica* 27:112.

Nicholls, J. M. et al. 1973. *Antimicrobial Agents and Chemotherapy* 3:110.

Speroni, E. and A. Minghetti. 1988. *Planta Medica* 54:488.

Pennyroyal

Allen, W. T. 1987. *Lancet* II:1022.

Buechel, D. W. et al. 1983. *Journal of the American Osteopathic Association* 82:793.

Early, E. F. 1961. *Lancet* II:580.

Sullivan, B. et al. 1979. *Journal of the American Medical Association* 242:2873.

Psyllium

Anon. 1989. *Tufts University Diet and Nutrition Letter* 7:9:1.

Agha, F. P. et al. 1984. *American Journal of Gastroenterology* 79:319.

Anderson, J. W. et al. 1988. *Archives of Internal Medicine* 148:292.

Arthurs, Y. and J. F. Fielding. 1983. *Irish Journal of Medicine* 76:253.

Bell, L. P. et al. 1989. *Journal of the American Medical Association* 261:1195.

Connaughton, J. and C. F. McCarthy. 1982. *Irish Journal of Medicine* 75:93.

Duckett, S. 1980. *New England Journal of Medicine* 303:583.

Ershoff, B. H. 1976. *Journal of Food Science* 41:949.

Moesgaard, F. et al. 1982. *Diseases of the Colon and Rectum* 25:454.
Shub, H. A. et al. 1978. *Diseases of the Colon and Rectum* 21:582.
Suhonen, R. et al. 1983. *Allergy* 38:363.
Tomoda, M. et al. 1987. *Planta Medica* 53:1:8.

Raspberry

Bamford, D. S. et al. 1970. *British Journal of Pharmacology* 40:161.
Burn, J. H. and E. R. Withell. 1941. *Lancet* II:6149:1.
Fong, H. H. S. et al. 1972 *Journal of Pharmaceutical Sciences* 61:1818.

Red Clover

Dewick, P. 1977. *Phytochemistry* 16:93.
Duke, J. 1989. *HerbalGram* 18/19:13.
Hartwell, J. 1970. *Lloydia* 3:97.

Red Pepper

Anon. 1989. *Environmental Nutrition* Sept. 8.
Bernstein, J. et al. 1987. *Journal of the American Academy of Dermatology* 17:93.
Graham, D. Y. et al. 1988. *Journal of the American Medical Association* 260:3473.
Hawk, R. J. and L. E. Millikan. 1988. *International Journal of Dermatology* 27:336.
Locock, R. A. 1985. *Canadian Pharmaceutical Journal* 118:516.
Rquebert, J. 1978. *Annales Pharmaceutiques Francaises* 36:361.
Sambaiah, K. and N. Satyanarayana. 1980. *Indian Journal of Experimental Biology* 18:898.
Visudhiphan, S. et al. 1982. *American Journal of Clinical Nutrition* 35:1452.
Wang, J. P. et al. 1984. *Thrombosis Research* 36:497.
Watson, C. P. N. et al. 1988. *Pain* 33:333.

Rhubarb

Burkitt, R. W. 1921. *Lancet* Sept. 3.
Chirikdjian, J. J. et al. 1983. *Planta Medica* 48:34.
Dong-hai, J. et al. 1980. *Pharmacology* 20 (Suppl.):128.
Fairbairn, J. W. 1976. *Pharmacology* 14 (Suppl.):48.

Rose

Anderson, T. W. et al. 1972. *Canadian Medical Association Journal* 107:503.

———. 1975. *Canadian Medical Association Journal* 112:823.

Coulehan, J. L. et al. 1974. *New England Journal of Medicine* 290:6.

———. 1976. *New England Journal of Medicine* 295:973.

Hume, R. and E. Weyers. 1973. *Scottish Medical Journal* 18:3.

Pitt., H. A. and A. M. Costrini. 1979. *Journal of the American Medical Association* 241:908.

Rosemary

Chang, S. S. 1977. *Journal of Food Science* 42:1102.

Mascolo, N. et al. 1987. *Phytotherapy Research* 1:1:28.

Opdyke, D. L. J. 1974. *Food and Cosmetic Toxicology* 12 (Suppl.):977.

Rao, B. G. V. N. and S. S. Nigam. 1970. *Indian Journal of Medical Research* 58:627.

Saffron

Chisolm, G. M. et al. 1972. *Atherosclerosis* 14:327.

Gainer, J. L. and G. M. Chisolm. 1974. *Atherosclerosis* 19:135.

Grisola, S. 1974. *Lancet* 7871:41.

Jones, J. R. 1975. *Experientia* 31:548.

Sage

Chang, S. S. 1977. *Journal of Food Science* 42:1102.

Opdyke, D. L. J. 1976. *Food and Cosmetic Toxicology* 14(Suppl.):857.

St.-John's-Wort

Busse, W. W. et al. 1984. *Journal of Allergy and Clinical Immunology* 73:801.

Hobbs, C. 1989. *HerbalGram* 18/19:24.

James, J. S. 1989. *AIDS Treatment News* Feb. 24.

———. 1989. *AIDS Treatment News* June 2.

———. 1989. *AIDS Treatment News* Nov. 17.

Meruelo, D. et al. 1988. *Proceedings of the National Academy of Sciences* 85:5230.

Suzuki, O. et al. 1984. *Planta Medica* 50:272.

Sarsaparilla
Fitzpatrick, F. K. 1954. *Antibiotics and Chemotherapy* 4:5:528.
Hobbs, C. 1988. *HerbalGram* 17:10.
Thurmon, F. M. 1942. *New England Journal of Medicine* 227:128.

Savory
Duke, J. 1987. *HerbalGram* 14:6.
Opdyke, D. L. J. 1976. *Food and Cosmetic Toxicology* 14(Suppl.):859.

Senna
Anon. 1978. *Morbidity and Mortality Weekly Report* 27:248.
Prior, J. and I. White. 1978. *Lancet* II:947.

Shepherd's Purse
Kuroda, K. and T. Kaku. 1969. *Life Sciences* 8:3:151.
Kuroda, K. and K. Takagi. 1968. *Nature* 220:5168:707.
————. 1969. *Archives of International Pharmacodynamics* 178:2:382.

Skullcap
Kimura, Y. 1981. *Chemical and Pharmaceutical Bulletin* 20:2308.
————. 1982. *Chemical and Pharmaceutical Bulletin* 20:219.

Tarragon
Deans, B. S. and K. P. Svoboda. 1988. *Journal of Horticultural Science* 63:503.
Robbins, R. C. 1967. *Journal of Atherosclerosis Research* 7:3.
Van Duuren, B. L. et al. 1971. *Journal of the National Cancer Institute* 46:1039.

Tea
Anon. 1989. *University of California, Berkeley, Wellness Letter* 5:4:1.
Anon. 1988. *HerbalGram* 15:5.
Anon. 1984. *HerbalGram* Spring:3.
Kaiser, H. E. 1967. *Cancer* 20:614.
Kapadia, G. J. 1976. *Journal of the National Cancer Institute* 57:207.
Muramatsu, K. et al. 1986. *Journal of Nutrition Science and Vitaminology* 32:613.
Yoshizawa, S. et al. 1987. *Phytotherapy Research* 1:44.

Thyme

Sourgens, H. et al. 1982. *Planta Medica* 45:78.

Van den Broucke, C. O. and J. A. Lemli. 1980. *Planta Medica* 38:317.

Turmeric

Arora, R. et al. 1971. *Indian Journal of Medical Research* 60:138.

Basu, A. B. 1971. *Indian Journal of Pharmacy* 33:131.

Chandra, D. and S. S. Gupta. 1972. *Indian Journal of Medical Research* 60:138.

Dhar, M. L. et al. 1968. *Indian Journal of Experimental Biology* 6:232.

Garg, S. K. 1974. *Planta Medica* 26:225.

Ghatak, N. and N. Basu. 1972. *Indian Journal of Experimental Biology* 10:235.

Kiso, Y. et al. 1983. *Planta Medica* 49:185.

Kuttan, R. et al. 1985. *Cancer Letters* 29:197.

Lutmoski, J. et al. 1974. *Planta Medica* 26:9.

Srivastava R. et al. 1985. *Thrombosis Research* 40:413.

Uva Ursi

Frohne, D. 1970. *Planta Medica* 18:1.

Valerian

Bounthanh, C. et al. 1981. *Planta Medica* 41:21.

Hendricks, H. et al. 1981. *Planta Medica* 42:62.

Leathwood, P. et al. 1982. *Pharmacology, Biochemistry, and Behavior* 17:65.

Leathwood, P. and F. Chaufford. 1985. *Planta Medica* 54:144.

Riedel, E. et al. 1982. *Planta Medica* 46:219.

Vervain

Inouye, H. et al. 1974. *Planta Medica* 25:285.

White Willow

Anon. 1988. *American Family Physician* 38:197.

Sallis, R. E. 1989. *American Family Physician* 39:209.

Yarrow

Albert-Puelo, M. 1978. *Economic Botany* 32:71.

Busse, W. W. et al. 1984. *Journal of Allergy and Clinical Immunology* 73:801.

Duke, J. 1987. *HerbalGram* 12:7.

Middleton, E. and G. Drzewiecki. 1984. *Biochemical Pharmacology* 33:3333.

Sama, S. K. et al. 1976. *Indian Journal of Medical Research* 64:738.

Books

Boyle, Wade. *Herb Doctors: Pioneers in 19th-Century American Botanical Medicine*. East Palestine, Ohio: Buckeye Naturopathic Press, 1988.

Brinker, Francis J. *The Toxicology of Botanical Medicines*. 2nd ed. Portland, Ore.: Eclectic Medical Institute, 1987.

Conrow, Robert and Arlene Hecksel. *Herbal Pathfinders: Voices of the Herb Renaissance*. Santa Barbara, Calif.: Woodbridge Press, 1983.

Coulter, Harris L. *Divided Legacy*. Berkeley, Calif.: Homeopathic Educational Services, 1982.

Culpeper, Nicholas. *Culpeper's Complete Herbal and English Physician*. 1826 ed. Avon, England: Pitman Press, 1981.

Cumston, Charles Greene. *An Introduction to the History of Medicine*. New York: Dorset Press, 1987.

De Waal, M. *Medicinal Herbs in the Bible*. York Beach, Maine: Samuel Weiser, 1984.

Der Marderosian, Ara and Lawrence Liberti. *Natural Product Medicine*. Philadelphia: George F. Stickley, 1988.

Dobelis, Inge N., ed. *Magic and Medicine of Plants*. Pleasantville, N.Y.: Reader's Digest, 1986.

Duke, James A. *Handbook of Medicinal Herbs*. Boca Raton, Fla.: CRC Press, 1985.

Ehrenreich, Barbara and Deirdre English. *Witches, Midwives, and Nurses: A History of Women Healers*. Detroit: Black and Red, 1973.

Felter, Harvey Wickes and John Uri Lloyd. *King's American Dispensatory*. 18th ed., 1898. Portland, Ore.: Eclectic Medical Publications, 1983.

Foster, Steven. *Echinacea Exalted!* Brixley, Mo.: Ozark Beneficial Plant Project, 1985.

————. *Herbal Bounty.* Salt Lake City: Peregrine Smith Books, 1984.

Foster, Steven and James A. Duke. *A Field Guide to Medicinal Plants: Eastern and Central North America* (Peterson Field Guide #40). Boston: Houghton Mifflin, 1990.

Fulder, Stephen. *Ginseng: Magical Herb of the East.* Northamptonshire, England: Thorsons Publishing, 1988.

Funfgeld, E. W., ed. *Rokan Ginkgo Biloba: Recent Results in Pharmacology and Clinic.* Berlin and New York: Springer-Verlag, 1988.

Gilman, Alfred G., Louis S. Goodman, Theodore W. Rall, and Ferid Murad, eds., 7th ed. *Goodman and Gilman's The Pharmacological Basis of Therapeutics.* New York: Macmillan, 1985.

Grieve, Maud. *A Modern Herbal.* New York: Dover, 1971.

Griffith, H. Winter. *The Complete Guide to Vitamins, Minerals, Supplements, and Herbs.* Tucson: Fisher Books, 1988.

Hallowell, Michael. *Herbal Healing: A Practical Introduction.* Bath, England: Ashgrove Press, 1985.

Harris, Ben Charles. *Comfrey: What You Need to Know.* New Canaan, Conn.: Keats Publishing, 1982.

Harris, Lloyd J. *The Book of Garlic.* Berkeley, Calif.: Aris Books, 1979.

Herbrandson, Dee. *Shaker Herbs and Their Medicinal Uses.* New Gloucester, Maine: Shaker Heritage Society, Sabbathday Lake, 1985.

Heyn, Birgit. *Ayurvedic Medicine.* Northamptonshire, England: Thorsons Publishing, 1987.

Hoffman, David. *The Holistic Herbal.* Dorset, England: Element Books, 1983.

Hou, Joseph P. *Ginseng: The Myth and the Truth.* North Hollywood, Calif.: Wilshire Book Co., 1978.

Kloss, Jethro. *Back to Eden.* Loma Linda, Calif.: Back to Eden Books, 1988.

Kowalchik, Claire and William H. Hylton, eds. *Rodale's Illustrated Encyclopedia of Herbs.* Emmaus, Pa.: Rodale Press, 1987.

Kreig, Margaret B. *Green Medicine: The Search for Plants That Heal.* Chicago: Rand McNally, 1964.

Lad, Vasant and David Frawley. *The Yoga of Herbs.* Santa Fe, N.M.: Lotus Press, 1986.

Law, Donald. *The Concise Herbal Encyclopedia.* New York: St. Martin's Press, 1973.

Leung, Albert Y. *Encyclopedia of Common Natural Ingredients Used in Food, Drugs, and Cosmetics.* New York: John Wiley & Sons, 1980.

Lewis, Walter and Memory P. F. Elvin-Lewis. *Medical Botany.* New York: John Wiley & Sons, 1974.

Lust, John. *The Herb Book.* New York: Bantam, 1974.

Marti-Ibaez, Felix. *The Epic of Medicine.* New York: Bramhall House, 1962.

McIntyre, Michael. *Herbal Medicine for Everyone.* London: Penguin, 1988.

Millspaugh, Charles F. *American Medicinal Plants.* 1892 ed. New York: Dover, 1974.

Morse, Flo. *The Story of the Shakers.* Woodstock, Vt.: Countryman Press, 1986.

Mowrey, Daniel B. *The Scientific Validation of Herbal Medicine.* Lehi, Utah: Cormorant Books, 1986.

————. *Next Generation Herbal Medicine.* Lehi, Utah: Cormorant Books, 1988.

Murray, Michael. *The 21st Century Herbal.* Bellevue, Wash.: Vita-Line, 1987.

Reid, Daniel P. *Chinese Herbal Medicine.* Boston: Shambhala, 1987.

Schechter, Steven. *Fighting Radiation with Foods, Herbs, and Vitamins.* Brookline, Mass.: East West Health Books, 1988.

Simon, James E. and Lois Grant, eds. *Proceedings of the First National Herb Growing and Marketing Conference.* West Lafayette, Ind.: Purdue University Cooperative Extension Service, 1987.

————. *Proceedings of the Second National Herb Growing and Marketing Conference.* West Lafayette, Ind.: Purdue University Cooperative Extension Service, 1987.

Simon, James E., Arlene Kestner, and Maureen A. Buehrle. *Proceedings of the Fourth National Herb Growing and Marketing Conference*. Silver Spring, Pa.: International Herb Growers and Marketers Association, 1989.

Spoerke, David. *Herbal Medications*. Santa Barbara, Calif.: Woodbridge Press, 1980.

Starr, Paul. *The Social Transformation of American Medicine*. New York: Basic Books, 1982.

Stuart, Malcolm, ed. *The Encyclopedia of Herbs and Herbalism*. New York: Grosset & Dunlap, 1979.

Strehlow, Wighard and Gottfried Hertzka. *Hildegard of Bingen's Medicine*. Santa Fe, N.M.: Bear and Co., 1988.

Tannahill, Reay. *Food in History*. New York: Stein & Day, 1973.

Tierra, Michael. *The Way of Herbs*. New York: Pocket Books, 1983.

Tyler, Varro E. *The New Honest Herbal*. Philadelphia: George F. Stickley, 1987.

Tyler, Varro E., Lynn R. Brady, and James E. Robbers. *Pharmacognosy* 9th ed. Philadelphia: Lea and Febiger, 1988.

Weed, Susun S. *Wise Woman Herbal for the Childbearing Years*. Woodstock, N.Y.: Ash Tree Publishing, 1985.

Weil, Andrew. *Natural Health, Natural Medicine*. Boston: Houghton Mifflin, 1990.

Weiner, Michael A. *Earth Medicine, Earth Food*. New York: Macmillan, 1980.

————. *Weiner's Herbal*. New York: Stein & Day, 1980.

————. *The People's Herbal*. New York: Perigee/Putnam, 1984.

Weiss, Rudolph Fritz. *Herbal Medicine*. Beaconsfield England: Beaconsfield Publishers, 1988.

Weiss, Gaea and Shandor Weiss. *Growing and Using the Healing Herbs*. Emmaus, Pa.: Rodale Press, 1985.

Wheelwright, Edith Grey. *Medicinal Plants and Their History*. New York: Dover, 1974.

Willard, Terry. *Textbook of Modern Herbology*. Calgary, Alberta: Progressive Publishing, 1988.

Wren, R. C. *Potter's New Cyclopaedia of Botanical Drugs and Preparations*. Essex, England: C. W. Daniel, 1988.

Index

Create Your Own Medical Library with
☑ BANTAM MEDICAL REFERENCE BOOKS

THE BANTAM MEDICAL DICTIONARY
by the editors of Market House Books

Offering the latest authoritative definitions in simple language, this exhaustive reference covers anatomy, physiology, all the major medical and surgical specialties from cardiology to tropical medicine. It also discusses fields such as biochemistry, nutrition, pharmacology, psychology, psychiatry, and dentistry.

❏ 28498-3 $6.99/$8.99 in Canada

THE PILL BOOK
7th edition

More than 25 newly approved drugs and 140 new brand names in this completely revised edition

Profiles of the 1,500 most commonly prescribed drugs in the United States: generic and brand names, dosages, side effects, adverse reactions, and warnings. Includes 32 pages of actual-size color photographs of prescription pills, as well as information on drugs with food, sex, pregnancy, alcohol, children, and the elderly.

❏ 57452-3 $6.99/$8.99 in Canada

Ask for these books at your local bookstore or use this page to order.

Please send me the books I have checked above. I am enclosing $____ (add $2.50 to cover postage and handling). Send check or money order, no cash or C.O.D.'s, please.

Name _____

Address _____

City/State/Zip _____

Send order to: Bantam Books, Dept. HN 13, 2451 S. Wolf Rd., Des Plaines, IL 60018
Allow four to six weeks for delivery.

Prices and availability subject to change without notice.

HN 13 11/96

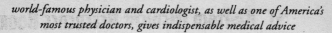

From the Editors of *Prevention* Magazine Health Books

THE DOCTORS BOOK OF HOME REMEDIES

This complete, practical guide contains more than 2,300 accessible healing tips for the most common medical complaints, including bladder infections, depression, emphysema, headaches, PMS, toothaches, and much more.

___29156-4 $6.99/$8.99 in Canada

THE DOCTORS BOOK OF HOME REMEDIES II

The sequel to the bestselling *The Doctors Book of Home Remedies*, with more than 1,200 all-new doctor-tested tips anyone can use to heal everyday health problems.

___56984-8 $6.99/$8.99

THE DOCTORS BOOK OF HOME REMEDIES FOR CHILDREN

For the first time, here is complete, time-tested home remedy advice for child health care, from infancy through age 12.

___56985-6 $6.99/$8.99

HIGH-SPEED HEALING
The Fastest, Safest, and Most Effective Shortcuts to Lasting Relief

In addition to quick relief for everything from allergies to vertigo, arthritis to wrinkles, you'll find hundreds of effective treatment tips for the most common medical complaints as well as more serious concerns, complete with worksheets, visualization exercises, and immunity-boosting strategies.

___56476-5 $6.99/$7.99
